MW00685429

A Strategy for Assessing and Managing Occupational Exposures

Second Edition

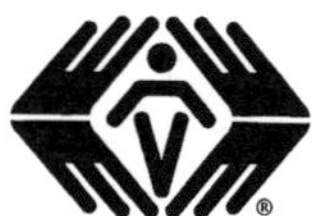

American Industrial Hygiene Association
Exposure Assessment Strategies Committee

John R. Mulhausen, Ph.D., CIH, and
Joseph Damiano, MS, CIH, CSP

This book was developed by experts with background, training, and experience in exposure assessment and management, working with information and conditions existing at the time of publication. The American Industrial Hygiene Association (AIHA), as publisher, and the authors have been diligent in ensuring that the material and methods addressed in this book reflect prevailing occupational health and safety and industrial hygiene practices. It is possible, however, that certain procedures discussed will require modification because of changing federal, state, and local regulations, or heretofore unknown developments in research.

AIHA and the authors disclaim any liability, loss, or risk resulting directly or indirectly from use of the practices and/or theories discussed in this book. Moreover, it is the reader's responsibility to stay informed of any changing federal, state, or local regulations that might affect the material contained herein, and the policies adopted specifically in the reader's workplace.

Specific mention of manufacturers and products in this book does not represent an endorsement by AIHA.

Copyright 1998 by the American Industrial Hygiene Association. All rights reserved. No part of this publication may be reproduced in any form or by any other means — graphic, electronic, or mechanical, including photocopying, taping, or information storage or retrieval systems — without prior written consent of the publisher.

ISBN 0-932627-86-2

AIHA Press
American Industrial Hygiene Association
2700 Prosperity Avenue, Suite 250
Fairfax, VA 22031

Tel.: (703) 849-8888
Fax: (703) 207-3561
http://www.aiha.org
e-mail: infonet@aiha.org

Stock No. 327-EA-98

Table of Contents

Figures and Tables Used in this Book

Figures Used in this Book

Tables Used in this Book

Contributors

Authors

Joseph Damiano, MS, CIH, CSP
Aluminum Company of America

John R. Mulhausen, Ph.D., CIH
3M Company

Contributing Authors

Christopher J. Cole, MS, CIH, CSP
Advanced Lighting Technologies, Inc.

M. Cathy Fehrenbacher, MS, CIH
U.S. Environmental Protection Agency

James W. Gordon, CIH
Celanese

Neil C. Hawkins, Sc.D., CIH
Dow Chemical Company

Paul Hewett, Ph.D., CIH
National Institute for Occupational Safety and Health

Michael A. Jayjock, Ph.D., CIH
Rohm & Haas Toxicology Laboratory

Jeffrey R. Miller, MSPH, CIH, CSP
Radian International LLC

Mark Nicas, Ph.D., CIH
University of California–Berkeley

Samuel K. Norwood, Ph.D., CIH
Dow Chemical Company

James C. Rock, Ph.D., CIH, PE
Texas A&M University

John E. Wright, CIH
Harsco Corporation

Foreword and Acknowledgments

When the first edition of *A Strategy for Occupational Exposure Assessment* was published in 1991, members of the AIHA Exposure Assessment Strategies Committee were already discussing a second edition. Because of our desire to treat this book as a "living document," we knew a second edition was inevitable. Some concepts in the first edition obviously needed to be refined, new discoveries and theories needed to be addressed, and it should be the goal of any practicing industrial hygienist to strive for continuous improvement.

In 1991, little did we know that we were embarking on what can best be called an "adventure in industrial hygiene." Development of this second edition forced us to look carefully at the topography of industrial hygiene practice. The landscape, we found, was intriguing yet imperfect. The art and science of exposure assessment was rapidly progressing beyond the discussions presented in the first edition. Exciting new ideas were being considered as work continued on improving exposure assessment approaches to make them more successful and practical.

In generating this second edition, we used the first edition as a springboard: the best of the ideas from that book are included. We started by working to capture the essence of professional judgment — still the cornerstone of a practical exposure assessment strategy — and then, building on this capability, propose what we believe is a best practice for assessing and managing occupational exposures to chemical, physical, and biological agents.

Our Audience and Our Customers

The primary audience for the second edition is the industrial hygiene professional. We encourage all industrial hygienists to read this text, though it should be most useful for those professionals with at least three years experience.

This text was written with our principal customer in mind: the worker exposed to chemical, physical, or biological agents. The text was also written to support the efforts of our colleagues who are equally interested and supportive of worker health protection. They include: industrial management, labor leaders, governmental authorities, occupational physicians, occupational health nurses, safety engineers, toxicologists, and epidemiologists.

A Consensus Document

This second edition is not a literature review. It does not provide a comprehensive, nor balanced, review of the literature on occupational exposure assessment; rather, it is a consensus document describing how the members of the AIHA Exposure Assessment Strategies Committee believe occupational exposures should be assessed and managed by industrial hygienists. As a consensus document, all members and corresponding members of the EASC voted in 1997 to accept and support the document as presented. No doubt, however, if you were to interview these members individually, you would find differences of opinion on specific elements. In generating the second edition, we strived for consensus; it was not our intent to build a homogeneous view of occupational exposure assessment.

Because the committee would like this to be a "living document," we are interested in users' experiences as the ideas and tools offered in this book are applied. We are particularly interested in validation efforts, enhancements to the process, and practical tools for implementing the strategy in the workplace. Those of you who are interested in learning more and who want to actively contribute are encouraged to become involved in the AIHA Exposure Assessment Strategies Committee. Your contributions and efforts will be the impetus for a third edition.

Acknowledgments

The second edition was drafted and redrafted several times. There were countless discussions, debates, meetings, and telephone conference calls. It would have been more fun if we had been paid to do this, but we enjoyed the adventure nevertheless. We took pleasure in the response from numerous members of the industrial hygiene community who had vigorously supported and applied the exposure assessment strategy proposed in the first edition. They were among those who offered constructive thoughts on how to improve the strategy.

These ideas were put forth in a variety of forums. Some of you published papers on exposure assessment, and we were monitoring the literature. Some of you attended the professional development courses sponsored by the Exposure Assessment Strategies Committee, and we listened to your questions. Some of you presented platform papers or participated in roundtable discussions on exposure assessment at past AIHCEs, and we were in the audience listening. Thank you for your enthusiasm, and please accept our apologies if we have failed to acknowledge your contributions.

Unfortunately, it is impossible to acknowledge all of the ideas, events, and colleagues who influenced this second edition. We are, of course, greatly indebted to the contributing authors. All members of the EASC provided technical review of the second edition. The contributing authors served as both critics and writers.

Our greatest acknowledgment, of course, must be extended to the editors and authors of the first edition, principally Neil Hawkins, Sam Norwood, and Jim Rock. The editors and members of the EASC who authored the first edition were truly pioneers. They proposed a new strategy for occupational exposure assessment that for the first time bridged the methodologies reported by statisticians and the experienced professional judgment practices of the industrial hygienist.

Joseph Damiano
John R. Mulhausen

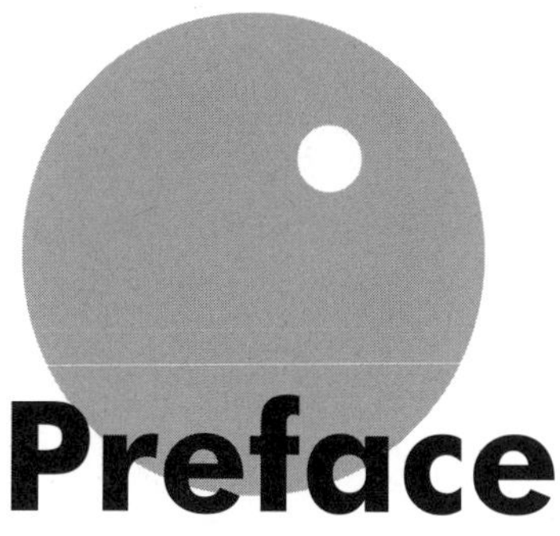

Preface

The AIHA Exposure Assessment Strategies Committee has made an effort in this book to enhance the exposure assessment paradigm proposed in the first edition of *A Strategy for Occupational Exposure Assessment.* The strategy for assessing and managing occupational exposures is a framework for practicing industrial hygienists everywhere. Each element is essential. Every tool and every guidance offered in this book has been developed to help industrial hygienists effectively allocate resources for ensuring worker health protection.

It is not realistic to expect any practitioner or organization to adopt the comprehensive approach outlined in this book in its entirety in one step. The gap, we expect, will be large. Most organizations, for example, have focused on assessing workplace exposures to environmental agents with assigned occupational exposure limits (OELs); however, the scope of the comprehensive approach is the assessment of all environmental agents, regardless whether a formal OEL exists. Moreover, this strategy is applied to *all* workers on *all* days, not just to those workers and days believed to have the highest exposures.

Clearly the comprehensive approach we put forth requires a commitment. It should be viewed as best practice and a worthwhile long-term goal for your organization. No program will do everything needed immediately. Approach the process in tiers, always using the system to apply your resources to the most important risks. Strive for continuous improvement. There is much flexibility in this strategy, and industrial hygienists are encouraged to tailor the strategy to suit the circumstances in their workplace and the needs of their workers.

Although the strategy offered in this book is consistent with the first edition, many differences are apparent. We prefer to call these differences enhancements.

Certainly the most obvious change is the change in title. The committee feels strongly that there is an interdependence between exposure assessment and exposure management. Exposure assessment is judging an exposure, and judgments are made in the context of available exposure information and the potential health effects caused by the specific environmental agent. Moreover, there is a dynamic relationship between exposure assessment and the application of health hazard control practices. To adequately explain exposure assessment, we must present the full process; in our view, that full process provides for effective management of occupational exposures. In a sense, the strategy for assessing and managing occupational exposures is industrial hygiene.

Among the other new features are:

- Attention is given to the consistency between the comprehensive exposure assessment approach recommended in this text and risk assessment/risk management methodologies.
- The term "homogeneous exposure group" is no longer used. The designation of groups of workers with like exposures is a practical tool for stratifying the work force to facilitate exposure assessments. It is not necessary for the exposures for employees in these groups to be exactly alike. Since statistical rigor is frequently unnecessary in classifying workers for exposure assessment, we decided to maintain the same basic concept and change HEG to similar exposure group (SEG).
- The OEL, whether formally established or loosely defined, is identified as an essential tool for judging any and all workplace exposures.
- The qualitative exposure assessment and the quantitative exposure assessment are not separate and consecutive steps in the exposure assessment process. Rather, exposure assessments are made in view of all available data, both qualitative and quantitative.
- Exposure monitoring is not essential to exposure assessment. Many occupational exposures can be assessed without monitoring data.
- Uncertainty in the exposure profile, health effects information, and the OEL must be weighed in judging exposures and in determining management strategies.
- There is clearer recognition of the cyclic, continuous improvement nature of a practical exposure assessment and management strategy. Successive iterations through the characterization, assessment, prioritization, and follow-up efforts of the strategy result in increasing understanding and control of exposures.
- Although traditional industrial hygiene practice emphasizes personal monitoring to measure exposure to air contaminants and noise, modeling techniques are becoming more widely accepted and may be required for prospectively assessing an exposure that has not yet begun.
- There is increased recognition of the importance of dermal exposures.
- There are "critical" similar exposure groups in which the misclassification of workers in various SEGs might cause some workers to be inadvertently exposed to an excessive health risk. The industrial hygienist can use analysis of variance techniques to evaluate the homogeneity of the critical SEG and then reclassify workers in view of sampling data.
- We recognize that it is good practice to begin collecting exposure data or use modeling techniques to quantify exposures when exposure estimates exceed 10% of the OEL.
- Occupational exposure histories can be maintained through six relational databases:
  - Workplace data;
  - Environmental agent data;
  - Worker data;

- SEG data;
  - Monitoring data; and
  - Exposure assessment data.
- Finally, a spreadsheet software tool is provided to help the reader get started with the use of statistical tools. These tools help industrial hygienists form a better understanding of the exposure profile and aid in the exposure assessment judgment.

Joseph Damiano
John R. Mulhausen

1
Introduction

Why Is Exposure Assessment Important?

Industrial hygiene is defined as the science and art of anticipating, recognizing, evaluating, and controlling health hazards in the workplace. Clearly the identification, characterization, and assessment of exposures is implied in this traditional definition, so why spend all this effort to write a book about what industrial hygienists have been doing for years?

The answer lies in an examination of the growing number of real and perceived risks and changing social requirements that industrial hygiene programs must be prepared to manage, and in the approaches that will be effective in understanding and managing those risks. Industrial hygiene programs today must be prepared to manage a broader range of risks than in the past. The standards to which those programs are held accountable have increased. Whereas in the past programs could be less rigorous, they must now be thorough, systematic, well-documented, and efficient.

Growing Variety of Present and Future Risks

The workplace today is becoming more complex. The variety of risks associated with workplace exposure to chemical, physical, and biological agents is increasing. Although the first priority of the industrial hygienist is to protect the health of workers, health risk is not the only risk he or she is asked to manage. Others would be regulatory risks, legal risks, and risks related to the anxiety inherently associated with many people's response to exposures.

Industrial hygienists must consider that organizations today are accountable to many more — and more varied — stakeholders than in the past. These new stakeholders include employees, owners, customers, labor unions, regulators, stockholders, the press, and the communities in which the organization operates. Industrial hygienists are relied on to satisfy the workplace exposure concerns of these stakeholders.

When evaluating risk to employees and the organization, industrial hygienists must remember that their programs will be held accountable not only for today's state of the art but tomorrow's as well. It is not sufficient to limit the question to: "Are employee exposures below established exposure limits?" Instead, industrial hygienists must ensure that exposures are characterized well enough — and controlled well enough — to keep present risks within acceptable limits and to put the organization in the position to manage future risks. Among the questions that must be considered are:

- How might this exposure affect employee health?
- How "good" is the exposure limit?
- What other risks are presented by this exposure?

Compliance with current limits is not sufficient. Most chemicals have no occupational exposure limits, and the information used to set existing limits is often incomplete. Also, existing limits are not always designed to protect the most sensitive workers. These limits might even be out of date.

Each day, new toxicological and epidemiological information is gathered. This means new exposure limits will be generated for environmental agents that formerly had none, and that many of the limits currently in place will change. Experience has shown that most exposure limits are lowered when they are changed, and there is no reason to believe that trend will not continue.

Unfortunately, when new limits are set or old limits are changed, there may be a population of workers who have been exposed to an environmental agent for some time at levels above the new limit. Industrial hygienists today must focus on how to position their programs so they are best able to manage changes and minimize any future risks. Having a historical database for all exposures should allow identification of employees who were exposed above the lowered exposure limit and enable the extent of their past overexposures to be estimated. An appropriate strategy could then be developed for medical management of the health of those employees.

Efficient and Effective Programs

At the same time industrial hygienists are being asked to manage a growing variety of risks, the efficacy, efficiency, and cost-effectiveness of their programs are being scrutinized more carefully. Economic factors demand that each organizational unit demonstrate its worth and its ability to operate waste-free — industrial hygiene programs are no exception. The ability to understand, prioritize, and manage exposures and risks efficiently requires a more systematic, better-documented approach to industrial hygiene than has typically been practiced in the past.

Industrial Hygiene Program Management

The better the industrial hygienist understands exposures, the better he or she is able to direct and prioritize the industrial hygiene program. This is true whether the goal of the exposure assessment process is regulatory compliance, a comprehensive description of all exposures, or a diagnostic evaluation of health hazard controls. The system for exposure assessment must be integrated with other systems for defining, prioritizing, and managing worker health protection. Assessment results are used to determine the needs and priority for health hazard controls, build exposure histories, and demonstrate regulatory compliance.

Exposure assessment is at the heart of industrial hygiene programs as it supports all of the functional elements (see Figure 1.1). A well-rationalized program relies on a thorough understanding of

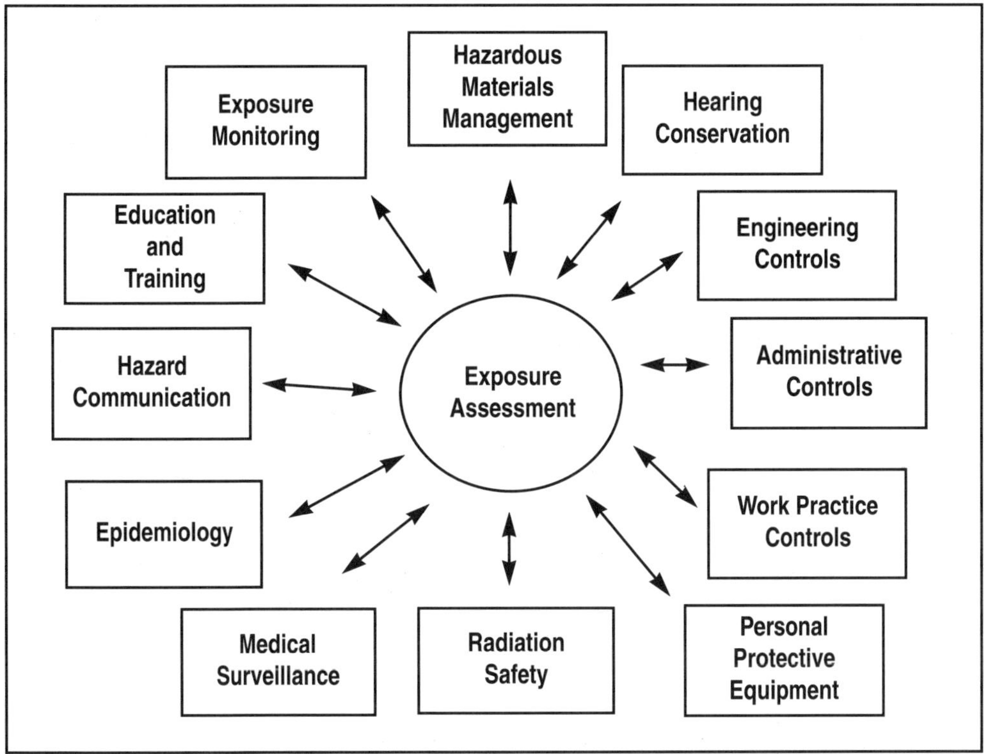

Figure 1.1 — Exposure assessment's central role in industrial hygiene program management.

what is known — and not known — about exposures. For example, to understand where best to spend precious resources on a monitoring program, industrial hygienists must understand potential exposures that need better characterization or careful routine tracking. A thorough characterization of exposures allows the industrial hygienist to focus worker training programs, better target medical surveillance programs, and define specific requirements for personal protective equipment (PPE).

Better Prioritization of Control Efforts and Expenditures

The better our understanding of exposures and the risks they pose, the more assurance we have that we are controlling the most important (highest risk) exposures first. Control efforts (whether engineering, work practice, or PPE programs) are usually costly to implement and maintain. It is therefore critical that those efforts be appropriately prioritized, deployed, and managed.

A thorough understanding of exposures allows prioritization of control efforts to use limited funds wisely. The right combination of control efforts — including short-term, long-term, temporary, and permanent controls — can be implemented based on the prioritized exposure assessments. Plans can be made for improving controls and moving from short-term solutions such as personal protective equipment to long-term solutions such as local exhaust ventilation. Management will be assured that money is being spent first on the controls needed most and not wasted on unnecessary control efforts.

Better Understanding of Worker Exposures

A full understanding of exposures, combined with work history, allows for better characterization of individual worker exposures and better management of employee medical concerns. The management of issues related to public health in the community in which the organization operates may be enhanced if there is a well-developed understanding of occupational exposures. Exposure histories, along with health effects information, can indicate the risk a person or group of people has of developing an occupational illness or disease. By understanding exposures, medical practitioners can better target clinical examinations, medical surveillance, or other diagnostic techniques to detect health effects early. When combined with individual medical histories, a comprehensive characterization of exposures greatly improves the power of epidemiological studies and

Exposure Assessment vs. Risk Assessment

For the industrial hygienist, exposure assessment and risk assessment are inextricably mixed such that they cannot be reasonably separated. Consider the following relationship between health risk and exposure:

$$\text{Health Risk} = (\text{Exposure})(\text{Toxicity})$$

In the world of industrial hygiene, evaluation of exposure is fully half the assessment of health risk. The other half is evaluation of the health effects per unit exposure, or the toxicity of the agent to which the worker is exposed. Thus, any exposure in an industrial hygiene sense is only meaningful in its relationship to the health effects the exposure might cause.

This book will not go into detail on the evaluation of agent toxicity. It is mentioned here, however, to highlight the important connection and interaction between the *toxicity* and the *exposure* in eventually determining the health risk.

The industrial hygienist's ultimate goal is to provide reasonable assurance of worker health. In this regard, what one does about risk is called risk management. Control of health hazards can be considered a risk management function. Here again, there is interaction with risk assessment in that good risk management is almost always predicated on good risk assessment, which in turn is driven by the quality of the industrial hygienist's exposure assessments.(1-3)

better positions health care providers to answer questions about an individual's exposures and how they might have affected his or her health.

Shifting State of the Art: Compliance Monitoring to Comprehensive Exposure Assessment

In the past several years, characterization of exposures has received the attention of occupational hygiene professionals and regulatory agencies worldwide.(4-7) The state-of-the-art approach has shifted from compliance monitoring, which focuses on the maximum-risk employee to determine whether exposures are above or below established limits, to comprehensive exposure assessment, which emphasizes characterization of all exposures for all workers on all days.

Regulations in many countries now mandate some periodic review of exposures throughout an organization.(8-10) Although current regulations vary widely in scope and enforcement, the trend is clear — and the reasoning behind the trend indisputable: A comprehensive approach to assessing occupational exposures better positions an organization to understand the risks associated with the exposures and better positions the organization to manage those risks.

No longer is a compliance-based approach to industrial hygiene the primary focus of the profession. If industrial hygienists accept a broadened definition of risk and agree that their customers — workers and the organizations that employ them — are looking to them to help manage those risks, they should come to the conclusion that industrial hygiene practice must embrace a comprehensive and systematic approach to the evaluation of exposures and the risks they pose. This approach will include logical systems and strategies for evaluating all exposures, interpreting and assessing the many present and future risks those exposures might pose, and efficiently managing those exposures that present unacceptable risks.

Overview of Exposure Assessment Strategy

An overview of the exposure assessment strategy discussed in this text is shown in Figure 1.2. The strategy is cyclic in nature and is used most effectively in an iterative manner that strives for continuous improvement. Early cycles will begin by collecting available information that is relatively easy to obtain. The results of initial exposure assessments based on that information will be used to prioritize follow-up control and information-gathering efforts. Resources should be focused on those exposures with the highest priority based on the potential health risk they present. As those exposures are better understood and controlled, they will drop in priority and the next cycles through the strategy will focus on the next tier priority exposures.

The major steps in the strategy are:

1. *Start:* Establish the exposure assessment strategy.
2. *Basic Characterization:* Gather information to characterize the workplace, work force, and environmental agents.
3. *Exposure Assessment:* Assess exposures in the workplace in view of the information available on the workplace, work force, and environmental agents. The assessment outcomes include a) groupings of workers having similar exposures; b) definition of an exposure profile for each group of similarly exposed workers; and c) judgments about the acceptability of each exposure profile.
4. *Further Information Gathering:* Implement prioritized exposure monitoring or the collection of more information

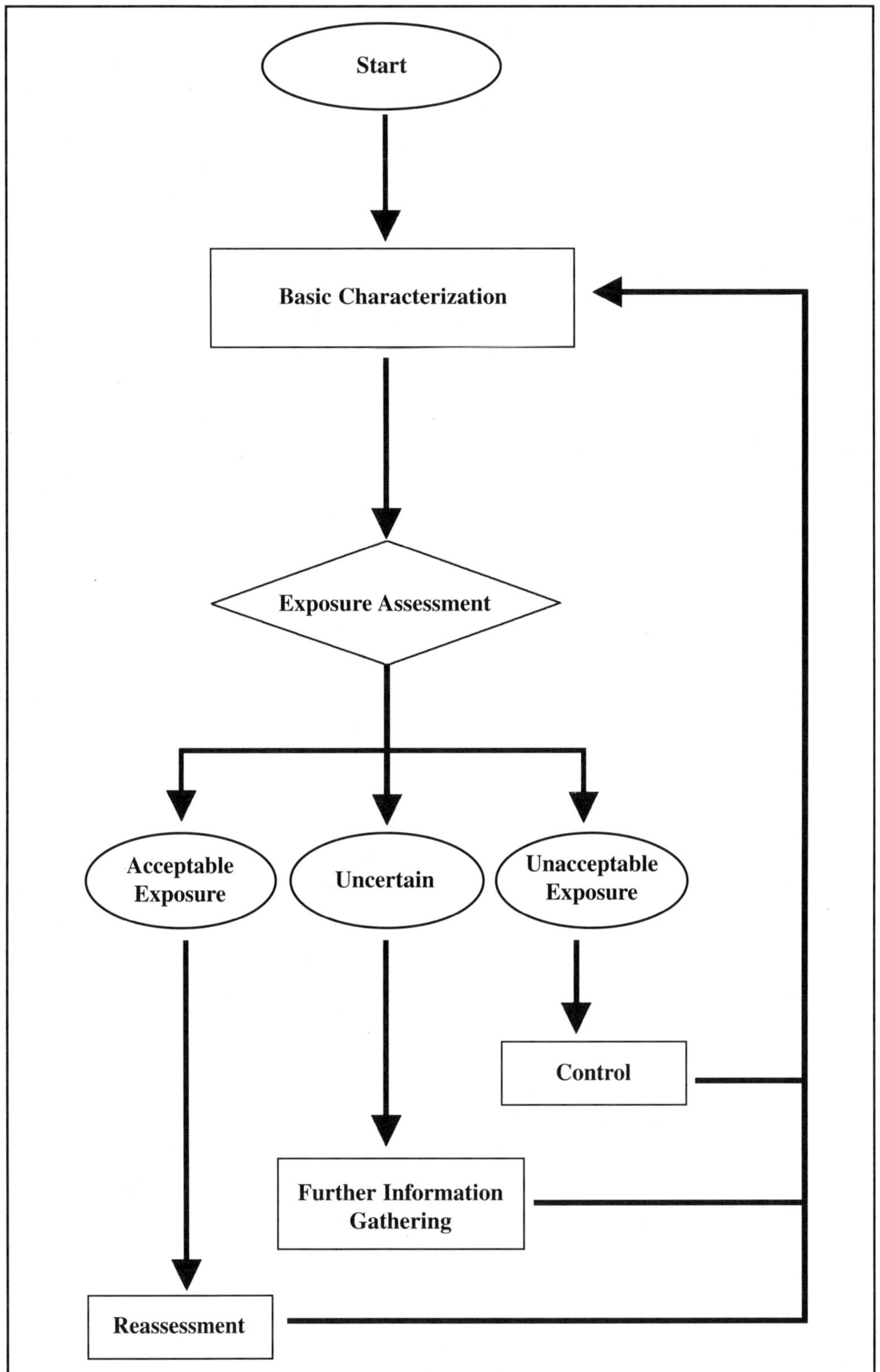

Figure 1.2 — A strategy for assessing and managing occupational exposures.

on health effects so that uncertain exposure judgments can be resolved with higher confidence.

5. *Health Hazard Control:* Implement prioritized control strategies for unacceptable exposures.
6. *Reassessment:* Periodically perform a comprehensive re-evaluation of exposures. Determine whether routine monitoring is required to verify that acceptable exposures remain acceptable.
7. *Communications and Documentation:* Although there is no element in Figure 1.2 for "communications and documentation," the communication of exposure assessment findings and the maintenance of exposure assessment data are assumed throughout as essential features of an effective process.

The following paragraphs describe each of the seven steps:

1. Start: Establish the Exposure Assessment Strategy

In establishing an organization's exposure assessment strategy, the following issues should be carefully addressed:

- Role of the industrial hygienist;
- Exposure assessment goals; and
- Written exposure assessment program.

2. Basic Characterization

Begin the exposure assessment process by collecting and organizing basic information needed to characterize the workplace, work force, and environmental agents. Gather information that will be used to understand the tasks being performed, materials being used, processes being run, and controls in place so that a picture of exposure conditions can be made.

3. Exposure Assessment

Define Similar Exposure Groups

Similar exposure groups (SEGs) are groups of workers having the same general exposure profile for the agent(s) being studied because of the similarity and frequency of the tasks they perform, the materials and processes with which they work, and the similarity of the way they perform the tasks. Data about jobs, processes, tasks, control equipment, and materials that have been gathered and organized in the basic characterization phase is used to divide workers into SEGs. Individual workers may be members of more than one SEG.

Define Exposure Profiles

An exposure profile is an estimate of the exposure intensity and how it varies over time for an SEG. Information used for defining the exposure profile may include qualitative or quantitative data, or both. At the start of the exposure assessment process, few quantitative data may be available, so most early exposure profiles will be based on qualitative information. As the information gathering and assessing cycle progresses, SEGs may be redefined and their exposure profiles modified based on new information.

Make Judgments on Acceptability of the Exposure Profiles for Each SEG

A judgment is made about the exposure, using the exposure profile and information collected on the agent's toxicity. This judgment is used to prioritize control efforts or the collection of more information based on the environmental agent's estimated level of exposure, severity of health effects, and the uncertainty associated with the exposure profile and health effects information. In this system:

- Exposures judged unacceptable are put on a prioritized list for control;
- Exposures not certain enough for a decision are put on a prioritized list for further information gathering; and
- Exposures judged acceptable are documented as such and may be put on a list for periodic routine reassessment to verify that exposures continue to be acceptable.

Unacceptable Exposures — Implementing Health Hazard Controls

Exposure profiles for groups of similarly exposed workers that are judged unacceptable should be put on a list for control. The list should be prioritized such that higher exposures to higher toxicity agents will be corrected first. The prioritization factors may include the uncertainty associated with the judgment, the number of workers exposed and the frequency of exposure.

Uncertain Exposures — Collecting Additional Information

Exposure profiles that are not well-understood, or for which acceptability judgments cannot be made with high confidence, must be further characterized by collecting additional information. The type of information needing to be collected may vary from one SEG to another. The exposure profile for one SEG may be well-understood, but the toxicity data may be scarce. In that case it is important to collect, or in some cases generate, toxicological or epidemiological data.

Another SEG may have little data or prior knowledge available on which to base an estimate of the exposure profile. If so, it is important to generate information to better characterize the exposure profile — either through exposure monitoring, modeling, or biological monitoring.

Acceptable Exposures — No Action or Define a Routine Monitoring Program

Exposures that are judged acceptable may need no further action, other than documentation, until it is time for a reassessment; however, collection of additional information (such as monitoring, toxicological, or epidemiological data) might be needed to 1) validate the judgment of "acceptability" or 2) ensure that the operation does not go out of control.

4. Further Information Gathering

Information gathering efforts should be prioritized. Higher priority should be given to information needs associated with higher exposure estimates, higher toxicity estimates, and higher uncertainty estimates. In some cases, if exposure and toxicity estimates are high enough, consideration should be given to the use of personal protective equipment or another interim control while the information is gathered or generated.

Information needs will vary for each exposure profile and judgment. The types of information that might be needed include:

Exposure Monitoring

If an exposure profile is not well-characterized, personal monitoring of worker exposures might be needed. This may include noise monitoring, air monitoring, dermal exposure monitoring, or other environmental measurements.

Exposure Modeling

Exposure modeling frequently is used to estimate the potential exposures associated with new processes and products. As tools for using mathematical modeling techniques to predict exposures based on workplace and worker parameters become more sophisticated, they should be used more often to estimate exposure profiles. They have the advantage of being less expensive and time-consuming than actual measurement of environmental agents in the workplace.

Biological Monitoring

Biological monitoring might be needed to assess the exposure profile if there are concerns about exposure through skin absorption or inadvertent ingestion. Due to the medical and ethical issues involved, the industrial hygienist should work closely with a physician whenever biological monitoring is considered.

Toxicological Data Generation

If the toxicity of the materials used in the workplace is not well-understood, it is difficult to judge the exposure's acceptability no matter how well the exposure profile is characterized. In those cases, the aid of toxicologists or other experts might be needed to obtain further health effects data on the environmental agents of interest.

Epidemiological Data Generation

Epidemiology programs are useful for identifying new relationships between exposures and illness. They can help determine whether illness outbreaks are related to work exposure. They help assure management and workers that if illnesses or diseases are work-related they will be identified and dealt with appropriately. The results of epidemiological studies add to the available toxicological data for an environmental agent and enable better judgments on the exposure's acceptability or unacceptability. One of the biggest weaknesses in current epidemiology practice is the lack of useful exposure data.

5. Health Hazard Controls

It is critical that industrial hygiene control programs be deployed and adjusted in view of exposure assessment findings. Exposure assessment findings can also be used to prioritize the implementation of health hazard controls. Diagnostic monitoring can be used to identify and measure the specific sources of unacceptable exposures, evaluate the effectiveness of existing controls, and determine whether new or modified controls are effective.

6. Reassessment

It is important for exposure profiles and SEGs to be kept up-to-date. This requires the entire exposure assessment process to be updated on a timely basis or maintained through a comprehensive management-of-change process. This will ensure that exposures continue to be well-understood and that the organization's industrial hygiene programs continue to respond to changing priorities.

7. Communications and Documentation

Exposure assessment findings must be communicated in a timely and effective fashion to all affected workers and others who are involved in worker health protection. The entire exposure assessment process, including follow-up recommendations and closure on the recommendations, must be documented. Lists of SEGs, their exposure profiles, and the judgment on their acceptability should be stored permanently so that individual exposure histories can be generated. Information on baseline and routine monitoring programs, as well as hazard control plans, must be kept — as should evidence that the recommendations were acted on appropriately.

Summary

Industrial hygienists throughout the world have recognized that a systematic and comprehensive approach to exposure assessment is an effective mechanism for managing industrial hygiene programs. A thorough understanding of exposures allows the industrial hygiene program, including control efforts, to be prioritized to protect employees and manage exposure-related risks. It also puts the industrial hygienist in position to better manage the unpredictable changes that will occur both in knowledge of the health effects of environmental agents and in society's tolerance of workplace exposures. Coupled with good work history information, comprehensive exposure assessments will enable better epidemiology and refinement of our understanding of the relationship between occupational exposures and disease.

Development of a comprehensive exposure assessment program is encouraged because a comprehensive program is the best way for organizations to understand and manage the ever-broadening realm of occupational health-related risks. A framework for systematic and comprehensive exposure assessment is portrayed in this book, and though goals for different exposure assessment programs vary widely, all programs should benefit from the guidance set forth in the following chapters and appendices.

References

1. **Jayjock, M.A., and N.C. Hawkins:** A Proposal for Improving the Role of Exposure Modeling in Risk Assessment. *Am. Ind. Hyg. Assoc. J. 54(12):*733-741 (1993).
2. **Hawkins, N.C., M.A. Jayjock, and J. Lynch:** A Rationale Framework for Establishing the Quality of

Human Exposure Assessment. *Am. Ind. Hyg. Assoc. J. 53(1):*34-41 (1992).

3. **Claycamp, H.G.:** Commentary — Industrial Health Risk Assessment: Industrial Hygiene for Technology Transition. *Am. Ind. Hyg. Assoc. J. 57(5):*423-427 (1996).
4. **Hawkins, N.C., S.K. Norwood, and J.C. Rock:** *A Strategy for Occupational Exposure Assessment.* Akron, Ohio: American Industrial Hygiene Association, 1991.
5. **American Industrial Hygiene Association:** White Paper — A Generic Exposure Assessment Standard. *Am. Ind. Hyg. Assoc. J. 55(11):*1009-1012 (1994).
6. **Organization Resources Counselors, Inc.:** *A Proposed Generic Workplace Exposure Assessment Standard.* Washington, D.C.: Organization Resources Counselors, Inc., 1992.
7. **British Occupational Hygiene Society:** *Sampling Strategies for Airborne Contaminants in the Workplace* (Technical Guide No. 11) by I.G. Guest, J.W. Chessie, R.J. Gardner, and C.D. Money. Leeds, United Kingdom: H & H Scientific Consultants Ltd., 1993.
8. **United Kingdom Health and Safety Executive:** *The Control of Substances Hazardous to Health (COSHH) Regulations and Approved Codes of Practice.* London: Her Majesty's Stationery Office Publications Centre, 1988.
9. **Australia National Occupational Health and Safety Commission:** *Control of Workplace Hazardous Substances.* Canberra, Australia: Australian Government Publishing Service, 1993.
10. **Comité Européen de Normalisation:** *Workplace Atmospheres — Guidance for the Assessment of Exposure by Inhalation of Chemical Agents for Comparison with Limit Values and Measurement Strategy* (EN 689). Brussels, Belgium: Comité Européen de Normalisation, February 1995.

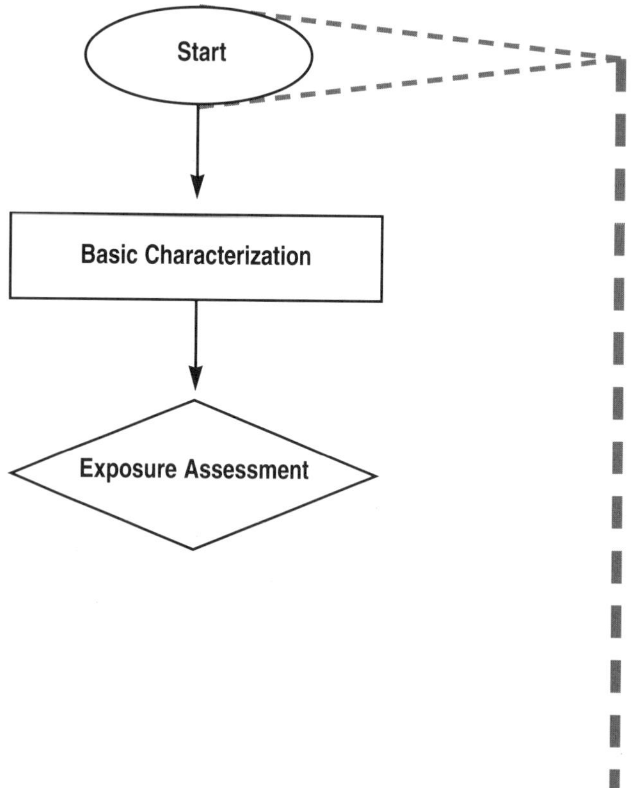

Purpose/Goals

Establish an exposure assessment strategy.

Tools

- *A Strategy for Assessing and Managing Occupational Exposures* and other references
- Involvement of organization's industrial hygienists and other technically knowledgeable professionals

Outcome

- Written exposure assessment program
- Defined goals for the exposure assessment program
- Defined roles for the industrial hygienist and other participants

2

Start: Establishing the Exposure Assessment Strategy

In establishing an organization's exposure assessment strategy, the following issues should be carefully addressed:

- Role of the industrial hygienist;
- Exposure assessment goals; and
- Written exposure assessment program.

Role of the Industrial Hygienist

The exposure assessment must be performed by, or under the supervision of, an industrial hygienist. It is not necessary for the industrial hygienist to perform the entire exposure assessment, but it is critical that he or she direct the overall system and be intimately involved in making professional judgments on the acceptability of exposure profiles. The industrial hygienist's training, skills, and experience qualifies him or her to direct efforts for collecting critical information for basic characterization, supervise designation of SEGs and identify important occupational exposures.

Directing follow-up efforts is another area in which industrial hygienists are well-equipped. They can best determine what monitoring strategies are needed to collect essential data,

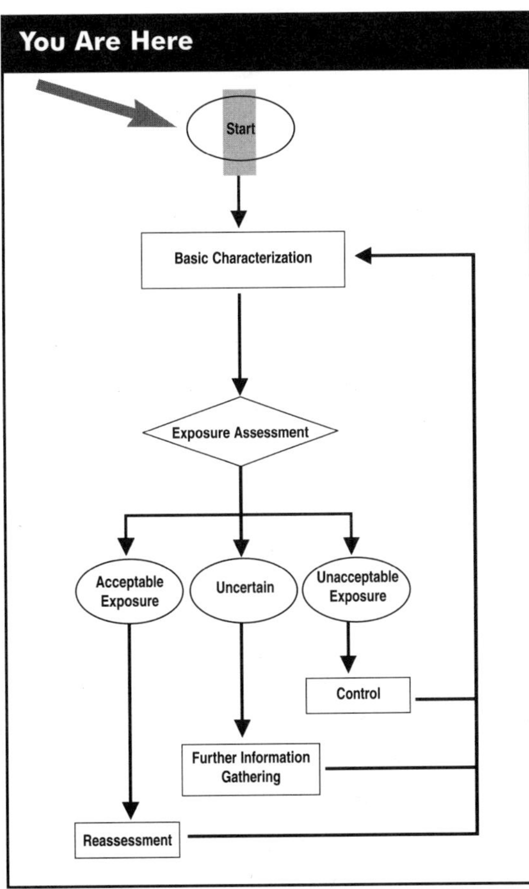

Professional Judgment

Professional judgment is the application and appropriate use of knowledge gained from formal education, observation, experimentation, inference, and analogy. It is fed by the sum and substance of what industrial hygienists know and learn. It allows an industrial hygienist with even a minimum amount of data to estimate the exposure in nearly any scenario. Given an adequate technical background and at least a minimal amount of health effects data, it also allows the industrial hygienist to set a working exposure limit. Comparison of the estimated exposure with the exposure limit and any mitigating circumstances allows for assessment of acceptability and represents the heart of the exposure assessment process.[1,2]

Within this process, the industrial hygienist develops and uses rules and presumptions to arrive at a decision. The extent that these rules and presumptions are rationally known and true is the extent to which the judgments will be valid and appropriately protective. This also means there is a threshold of data every industrial hygienist must have to render a decision. This threshold will vary for different practitioners based on their individual knowledge-base and skill set. All professionals conducting these evaluations, however, must consider and decide as an ethical issue where this threshold occurs for them personally.

The flexibility of this exposure assessment and management strategy not only permits but forces subjective decisions based on professional judgment. Professional judgment is vital to identifying SEGs. It also is essential for making exposure judgments, in planning monitoring campaigns, and in recommending changes needed to reduce exposures to acceptable levels through health hazard controls. Even when monitoring data are abundant, the industrial hygienist must judge whether the data have been appropriately collected and how these data should be properly interpreted.

Throughout this text, comments and examples are provided to illustrate the professional judgment underlying proper application of an occupational exposure assessment strategy. This information is intended to allow new and developing practitioners to study the process and learn from it.

and they should have the best overall sense of effective options for health hazard controls. Industrial hygienists have the expertise to make program modifications and prioritizations that take advantage of the results of the exposure assessment.

The participation of other technically knowledgeable professionals (such as engineers, environmental scientists, toxicologists, safety professionals, physicians, nurses, and epidemiologists) is a proven way to streamline the exposure assessment program and improve the quality of assessments. Interaction of industrial hygienists with colleagues in the occupational health professions will enhance worker protection and augment effec-

Nonroutine Operations

Nonroutine operations are difficult to assess. They are characterized by some of the following features:

- Short lead time;
- Short duration;
- Transient work force;
- Nonrepetitiveness;
- Variable work sites;
- Poorly defined tasks;
- Variable work practices;
- Multiple environmental agents; and
- Limited health effects data on the environmental agents.

Among the nonroutine operations are construction, research and development, environmental remediation, and hazardous waste cleanup. Maintenance and repair is more often routine than nonroutine.

Exposure assessments of nonroutine operations aim most frequently to identify potential health hazards and demonstrate compliance. A distant third-place objective is baseline determination of an SEG's average exposure and variability of exposure. The latter usually occurs only accidentally (i.e., enough data of sufficient type and quality for statistical analyses are collected only because the nonroutine operation was of sufficient duration). Realistically, when a nonroutine operation is complete, there are no more opportunities to collect data.

The fundamental concepts of the exposure assessment and management strategy presented in this book can be applied to any work operation. Clearly, it is a more difficult venture in unplanned and nonroutine operations than those that are planned and routine. For application to nonroutine operations, the strategy must be recognized as a flexible tool. If this strategy were highly prescriptive with few options or opportunities to customize, it would be less useful to the industrial hygiene community as a whole. Instead, a strategy is offered that requires industrial hygienists to exercise professional judgment on how best to apply the tool.

Some specific recommendations for applying the strategy to the nonroutine scenario appear in subsequent chapters. In assessing exposures in nonroutine operations, for example, monitoring frequently is performed to verify that appropriate levels of personal protective equipment have been selected. In managing exposures in nonroutine operations, PPE is often prescribed conservatively to compensate for the high uncertainty in the exposure assessment.

tive implementation of the exposure assessment and management strategy.

Exposure Assessment Goals

Before the process "starts," the exposure assessment goals must be determined. These goals should be clearly articulated and should lead to one of two general exposure assessment strategies: the Comprehensive Strategy or the Compliance Strategy.

Organizations are encouraged to adopt the Comprehensive Strategy. This strategy is directed at assessing all exposures for all workers on all days. In addition to ensuring compliance with existing occupational exposure limits (OELs), this strategy provides an understanding of the day-to-day distribution of exposures. Exposure assessment findings can be used to address present-day health risks and to construct exposure histories. If a historical database is maintained, the exposure assessment data may be used to address future health issues for individual workers or groups of workers. In the latter case, the data may be used to support epidemiological studies.

The goals of a system for comprehensive exposure assessment include:

1. Characterize exposures to all potentially hazardous chemical, physical, and biological agents, including those without formal OELs.
2. Characterize the exposure intensity and temporal (hour-to-hour/day-to-day) variability faced by all workers.
3. Assess the potential risks (e.g., risk of potential harm to employee health, risk of noncompliance with governmental regulations, etc.).
4. Prioritize and control exposures that present unacceptable risks.
5. Identify exposures that need additional information gathering (e.g., baseline monitoring).
6. Document exposures and control efforts, and communicate exposure assessment findings to all affected workers and those involved in worker health protection (e.g., management, labor representatives, medical staff, engineering staff, etc.).
7. Maintain a historical record of exposures for all workers so that future health issues can be addressed and managed relative to actual exposure information.
8. Accomplish the preceding steps with efficient and effective allocation of time and resources.

The Compliance Strategy is directed at assessing compliance with OELs and usually uses worst-case monitoring with a focus on exposures during the time of the survey. This strategy provides little insight into the day-to-day variation in exposure levels and is not amenable to development of exposure histories that accurately reflect exposures and health risk. In many organizations with more limited funding, however, the Compliance Strategy is an appropriate first step.

Because a comprehensive approach to exposure assessment provides a more complete understanding of exposures than the compliance approach, it enables better management of industrial hygiene-related risks. Those risks include not only potential noncompliance with regulations or exposure limits but also potential short-term or long-term damage to employee health; legal liability; and societal and community concerns. It helps provide assurance to an organization's management, customers, and employees (and the communities in which the organization operates) that occupational health risks are understood and that the proper steps are in place to manage the risks.

Written Exposure Assessment Program

A written exposure assessment program is an important reference tool for documenting how an organization will administer occupational exposure assessments. It specifies the strategies, methods, and criteria used in performing the assessments. The written program should address the following:

- Goals of the occupational exposure assessment program;
- Role and responsibilities of the industrial hygienist and other technical support staff;
- Methods for systematized information gathering to form a basic characterization of the workplace, work force, and environmental agents;
- Methods for defining SEGs and the exposure profile for each group;
- Criteria for making a judgment as to whether the exposure profile for an SEG is acceptable, unacceptable, or uncertain;
- Systems for prioritizing and gathering the additional information needed to better characterize uncertain exposures and make a more confident judgment about their acceptability — whether exposure monitoring data or health effects information;
- Exposure thresholds and criteria for conducting monitoring (e.g., baseline monitoring if the exposure estimate is greater than 10% of the OEL);

- A system for ensuring that unacceptable exposures are prioritized and controlled;
- Systems for communicating and documenting exposure assessment findings and health hazard control recommendations; and
- Systems and criteria for periodic reassessment of workplace exposures, including routine monitoring programs to ensure that acceptable exposures remain acceptable.

References

1. **Rock, J.C.:** Can Professional Judgment be Quantified? *Am. Ind. Hyg. Assoc. J. 47(6):*A- 370 (1986).
2. **Roach, S.A.:** A Commentary on the December 1986 Workshop on Strategies for Measuring Exposure. *Am. Ind. Hyg. Assoc. J. 48(12):*A-322–A-332 (1987).

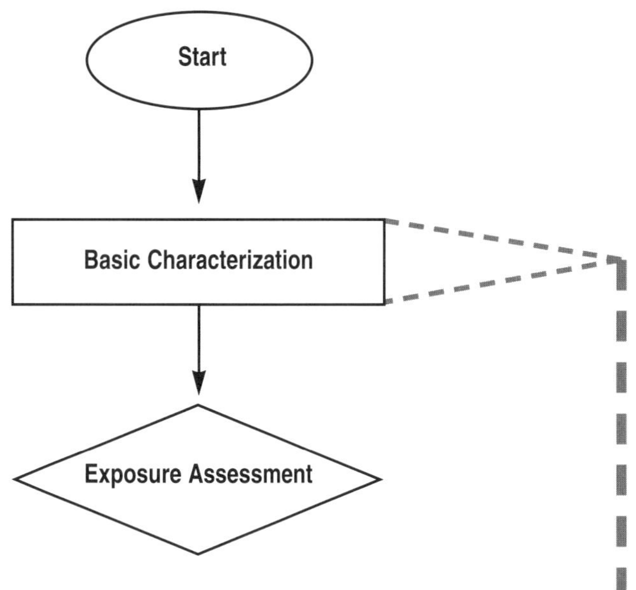

Purpose/Goals

Collect and organize available information on the workplace, work force, agents, historical exposure data, biological monitoring data, etc.

Tools

- Workplace characterization
  Process/operation description
  Chemical, physical, and biological agent inventory
- Work force characterization
  Job title description
  Task analysis
  Number of workers
- Characterization of agents
  Health effects data
  Occupational exposure limits (OELs)
- Characterization of existing controls
- Past assessments/results
- Historical exposure data
- Environmental emission data
- Past biological monitoring data

Outcome

Complete summary of available essential information on workers, tasks, agents, potential exposures, and potential health effects.

3 Basic Characterization and Information Gathering

Thorough characterizations of the workplace, the work force, and the environmental agents are needed before the industrial hygienist can apply various qualitative and quantitative tools for occupational exposure assessments. The basic characterization builds on the traditional "walk-through" survey industrial hygienists have practiced for many years. Information is gathered to support the judgment of occupational exposures, priority setting, and development of health hazard controls.

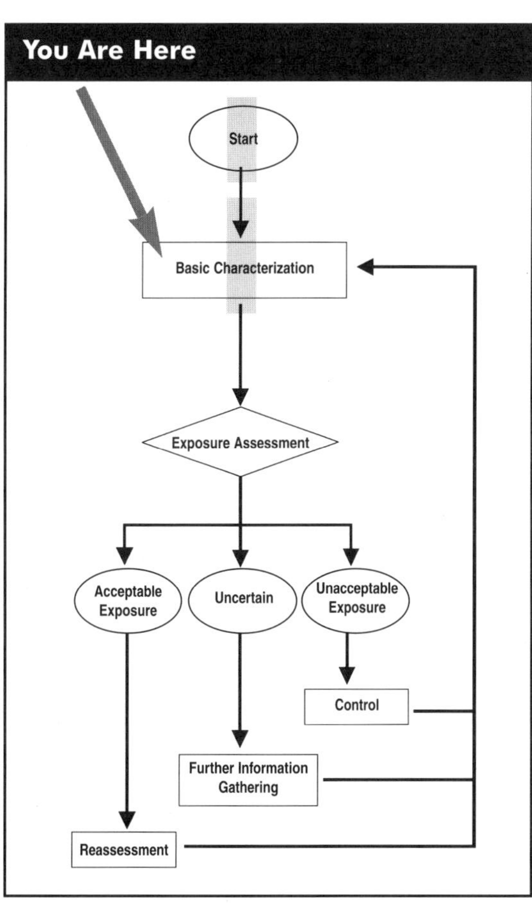

To assess exposures and evaluate health risks, industrial hygienists must have sufficient comprehension of many factors. At a minimum, the following questions must be answered:

- What are the chemical, physical, and biological agents in the work environment?
- What health effects are associated with excessive exposure to the environmental agents?
- What are the occupational exposure limits for each agent?
- How is the work force organized and staffed?
- What are the significant sources of exposure? What processes and operations, and what tasks and work practices,

pose significant potential for worker exposure to the environmental agents?

- What controls are in place, and how are they used?

In performing the basic characterization phase of exposure assessment, the industrial hygienist should seek the assistance and counsel of professional colleagues in related disciplines such as operations management, engineering, occupational safety, environmental protection, toxicology, epidemiology, and occupational medicine. Important information sources and collection methods are listed in Table 3.1.

Table 3.1 — Sources of Information

Collection Method	*Type of Information*
Walkaround survey (i.e., facility tour and observations)	Operations Processes Tasks Personal protective equipment Exposure controls Division of labor Environmental agents Direct-reading instrument measurements
Interviews of workers, managers, and engineers	Tasks Work practices Health issues Processes Exposure controls Maintenance Environmental agents
Interviews of medical and safety staff	Health problems Patterns of problems Work practices Exposure history Environmental agents
Records: Process standards Standard operating procedures Production Personnel Medical Engineering Environmental reports Process flow diagrams	Historic conditions Chemical inventories Usage amounts Tasks Work histories Performance of engineering controls Past environmental monitoring results Past biological monitoring results
Governmental and nongovernmental standards	Current exposure limits Proposed exposure limits
Literature	Epidemiological studies Toxicological studies Emerging issues

Gathering Workplace Information

Preparation of a schematic diagram or a written description of the processes can be used to adequately describe most workplaces. These documents can serve to highlight unit operations and work areas with exposure potential, and they can provide details of the production activities and process chemistry. In some cases, a written description provides a mechanism for defining a work environment that is not in a fixed location (e.g., transportation, utility services, maintenance) or is unusual (e.g., exposures of artists in a workshop).

Process flow diagrams are particularly helpful in characterizing continuous, semicontinuous, and batch operations. For industrial hygienists, the key elements of a process flow diagram are the sources of potential exposure. Sources of potential exposure include equipment and tasks that potentially bring a worker into contact with an environmental agent. For this reason, unit operations and associated equipment should be identified (e.g., reactors, filter presses, pumps, in-line filters, sampling points). Likewise, a material entering or leaving the process should be classified by the transfer method (e.g., pipeline, tank truck, drumming, bagging) since this highlights possible handling problems that could lead to exposure. The disposition of all byproduct streams leaving the process (e.g., noncondensable vapors to vent, waste water to treatment system via trench) should be identified as possible sources of exposure. For processes involving a curing reaction, consider that the hazard may exist until the agent has been fully cured.

The workplace characterization should consider other factors that affect exposure potential, such as ventilation systems, open-top tanks, open sumps, trenches, and use of personal protective equipment.

Maintenance and repair activities should also be characterized. Significant exposures to chemical, physical, and biological agents may be associated with scheduled process unit and equipment overhaul, and for equipment repair and servicing on the production floor and in maintenance shops. Most maintenance exposures are associated with specific tasks that can be identified and characterized.

When gathering information to use in assessing dermal contact, consider sources of contact such as 1) direct handling of the environmental agent (e.g., manual weighing of powders, bench-scale pouring of liquids); 2) handling of materials that can be directly contaminated (e.g., packaging); and 3) secondary contamination (e.g., contact with contaminated surfaces).

Contaminated work surfaces, tools, clothing, and personal protective equipment can be significant sources of dermal exposure. Consider the quality of housekeeping. Look for surfaces and areas outside the immediate process area where contaminants might be transferred inadvertently due to movement, spillage, worker activities, etc. Investigate whether tools, equipment, and other materials leaving the process area might become contaminated and serve as secondary sources of the agent. For example, pencils, door handles, water fountains, telephones, and other equipment may be contaminated and serve as secondary sources of exposure. The same can be said for break rooms, lunch rooms, and office areas. Contaminants can adhere to shoes and be tracked into uncontaminated areas. Surfaces, tools, and equipment in laboratories might become contaminated from production workplace sampling activities. Do not overlook operations of short duration that cannot be performed with gloves.[1-3] OSHA's personal protective equipment standard includes guidance on hazard assessment and PPE selection that can help in gathering workplace information.[4]

Gathering Work Force Information

The goal of the work force characterization is to understand the division of labor and work practices. Detailed knowledge of the routine and nonroutine work assignments, work schedules, and tasks must be acquired. The work force characterization should be based on a variety of resources, including the plant roster, job descriptions, worker interviews, management interviews and, most important, careful observation of work practices and the workplace.

Many organizations have personnel record keeping systems that provide a roster of individuals assigned to specific departments and job classes. The duties and activities of workers in each job class should be reviewed carefully to ensure that each group represents a unique exposure potential. In some cases, job classifications should be subdivided so that significant differences in job activities can be related to specific individuals.

In some organizations, there may not be a personnel job classification scheme, or it may not be available or well-maintained. If the plant's personnel record system cannot be used as a resource, the industrial hygienist will need to identify work groups and link individual workers to the groups. If in grouping workers, the industrial hygienist deviates from the personnel system, accurate records will be needed relating the exposure groups identified by the industrial hygienist to the personnel record keeping system. Incongruence between industrial hygiene and personnel job classification schemes could make investigation of future health issues difficult.

For each of the work groups, a brief outline of work duties and tasks is needed. For groups with only a negligible exposure potential (e.g., clerical, control room operators, etc.) the work duties may be adequately covered by defining the percentage of time spent in the general process areas. However, for most work groups more details are needed about the specific operations, the work activities, and the frequency of those activities.

A work activity description can be prepared in the form of a time distribution, showing each major work area (reactor train, bagging station, analytical lab, etc.) and time spent on each task that has potential for significant exposure to an environmental agent (e.g., process sampling, product bagging, titration analysis). By observation and worker interview, the specific unit operations and tasks that could lead to worker exposure should be identified, as should the frequency and duration of these tasks (e.g., once an hour for 10 minutes, once a shift for 30 minutes, or twice a year for four hours).

The industrial hygienist should collect information on work schedules identifying hours per day, days per week, shift rotation, and perhaps the average number of hours worked per week, month, or year. Moreover, the magnitude and frequency of overtime work should be determined. It is important that several workers be interviewed (on different shifts, if appropriate) to get a clear picture of actual work practices.

Many workplaces rely on contract labor to perform routine and nonroutine work. It is important for contractors to be included in the exposure assessment process. The mechanism and requirements for assessing the exposure of contract labor should be established in the contract. Larger or more sophisticated contractors may have their own exposure assessment capabilities. For other contractors, it might be more effective to rely on the skill and expertise of the client.

The industrial hygienist's observation of work activities must include the potential for skin contact and exposure via dermal absorption. Skin contact is the primary route of exposure for some chemical agents (e.g., methylene dianiline). As OELs are reduced to smaller and smaller values, the importance of the dermal route of exposure in contributing to the total body burden increases dramatically. For benzene, the contribution of skin absorption to the daily dose among tire-manufacturing workers was estimated to have increased from 4% to 30%, with a reduction in inhalation exposures from 10 ppm to 1 ppm. If the OEL

Nonroutine Operations

Expect and accept continuous change in nonroutine operations. Find consistency in a seemingly inconsistent operation. The operation may seem to be different each time it is performed, but there is frequently some underlying consistency. For example, environmental remediation techniques are often specific to certain conditions (e.g., washing of lead-contaminated soil). This operation may be new to your organization, but it has been performed in other places. Find out where, and use this valuable experience to help you assess your nonroutine operation. Then share your knowledge with others.

for benzene were reduced to 0.1 ppm as an 8-hour time-weighted average (TWA), the dermal route of exposure could account for 60% of the total dose.(2) Although data are generally limited on the potential for a substance to be absorbed through the skin, these data should be accessed when available.

Gathering Information on Environmental Agents

Each potentially hazardous chemical, physical, and biological agent in the workplace should be identified. For each agent, information describing its use, physical properties, routes of exposure, potential health effects, and pertinent OELs should be gathered.

A site's inventory of hazardous materials and associated material safety data sheets (MSDSs) can be a good foundation for identifying environmental agents. The MSDS inventory should cover the greatest majority of chemical agents in the workplace, including raw materials, products, byproducts, additives, solvents, refractories, insulations, lubricants, coatings, resins, welding rods, and compressed gases. Various categories of environmental agents are summarized in Table 3.2. The presence of process off-gases, byproducts, waste products, and products of pyrolysis or combustion should be identified to make the inventory of chemical agents complete.

Likewise, the presence of potentially hazardous physical and biological agents (e.g., noise, ionizing radiation, microwave fields, laser radiation, hot environments, pathogenic microorganisms) must be identified.

Each environmental agent should be linked to one or more work groups. Typically, these inventories will break down first by process/department; second by job description; and third, if

Table 3.2 — Categories of Environmental Agents

Category	*Description*
Raw materials	Primary inputs to the process (e.g., reactants, solvents, slurry media, filter aids) that support the main reaction.
Intermediates	Products not to be sold, but to be used as raw materials later in the process.
Products	Desired materials formed by the manufacturing process.
Byproducts	Secondary materials formed by the manufacturing process, usually in small quantities, which are possibly separated from the products as waste streams.
Additives	Supplementary materials (e.g., inhibitors, surfactants, catalysts, pigments) added to the final product to enhance the process or products.
Maintenance and construction materials	Refractories, solvents, insulations, welding fumes, lubricants, adhesives, etc., to which maintenance workers are exposed.
Laboratory chemicals	Materials used for the preparation of samples or performance of wet chemistry and instrumental analyses; usually handled in gram (g) or milliliter (mL) quantities.
Hazardous waste	Generally mixtures of solid and liquid material that are known individually and collectively to be hazardous.
Physical agents	Radioactive materials; noise, vibration, ionizing radiation, nonionizing radiation, heat, etc.
Biological agents	Organisms and biologically active materials produced by living organisms. Examples are spores, casts, endotoxins, etiological agents, etc.

helpful, by task. The inventory should include information on the application or source of each environmental agent.

Quantities and Physical Properties

Industrial hygienists should also understand the approximate quantities and use rates of chemical agents used in the process. Exact amounts are not required, since only a general range (grams, tons, etc.) is needed for assessment of exposure potential. Bulk quantity information is often available from warehouse records or production reports. Also, environmental reporting data can be a source of usage amounts.

Physical property data (e.g., boiling points, vapor pressure, particle size distribution, wavelength of laser radiation) for each agent, under conditions of use, may also be needed to assess exposure potential. The vapor pressure and temperature will assist in determining whether the contaminant will exist as a vapor, aerosol, or both. Also, consider handling conditions that might impact whether a chemical agent can be contacted through the skin. Agents used at high temperatures, for example, might not be available for dermal contact, except under accidental situations.

Health Effects Data and OELs

The health effects data must be sufficient to differentiate acceptable and unacceptable exposure levels. Material safety data sheets are a convenient source of health effects data, but many MSDSs also have inadequate health effects information — all too often because of a lack of toxicological data.

Textbooks that summarize the epidemiological and toxicological literature on various chemical, physical, and biological agents are available.[5-7] This scientific literature should be used as needed to develop a better understanding of the potential health effects of the environmental agents in the workplace.

In this book, the generic term "occupational exposure limit" is used to represent the limit selected or established for the purpose of judging exposure profiles as either acceptable or unacceptable. The OEL can be one or more of the following: 1) regulatory; 2) authoritative; 3) internal; or 4) working.

Regulatory OELs

Regulatory OELs are set and enforced by governmental agencies. In the United States, "permissible exposure limits (PELs)" are promulgated by the Occupational Safety and Health Administration (OSHA).[8] Other workplace OELs are set by the U.S. Mine Safety and Health Administration (MSHA),[9] the U.S. Environmental Protection Agency (primarily for new chemicals), and some state regulatory agencies. In Europe, OELs are established by the European Commission (EC) and its member countries.[10]

Authoritative OELs

Authoritative OELs are those set and recommended by organizations such as the American Conference of Governmental Industrial Hygienists (ACGIH), the American Industrial Hygiene Association (AIHA), or the National Institute for Occupational Safety and Health (NIOSH). ACGIH's values are known as threshold limit values (TLVs®) and biological exposure indices (BEIs®);[11] AIHA's are known as workplace environmental exposure limits (WEELs®);[12] and NIOSH's as recommended exposure limits (RELs).[13]

Internal OELs

Authoritative or regulatory OELs are available for only about 600 of the 70,000 chemicals used in industry. The lack of data has prompted some private organizations to devise internal OELs for substances with no regulatory or authoritative OELs,[(14)] or when the regulatory or authoritative OEL is dated. The organization may initiate testing or may request the substance's manufacturer to perform toxicological studies. Many chemical manufacturers have established OELs for their products.

Working OELs

In the absence of a formal OEL from a regulatory, authoritative, or internal source the industrial hygienist must identify a "working OEL" to differentiate acceptable from unacceptable exposures. A working OEL is an informal limit created in the course of performing an exposure assessment. Working OELs are established in the absence of formal OELs, or they may be established in the presence of a formal OEL when there is significant uncertainty about the adequacy of the formal OEL. A working OEL will be based on whatever data are available — including epidemiological or toxicological information, if any has been generated. It may be based on analogy with another environmental agent for which there is a regulatory, authoritative, or internal OEL. Working OELs are sometimes stated in ranges (e.g., 0.1–1.0 mg/m^3), or they incorporate large safety factors, in order to account for any lack of data.

Because there are no regulatory or authoritative OELs for the majority of chemicals used in industry, it might take significant time (perhaps years in organizations using many different chemicals) to fully develop and apply internal and working OELs in a new exposure assessment program. The effort should be prioritized and managed within the organization. There should be an established procedure for setting and documenting internal OELs and a framework for selecting and applying working OELs. Priority should be given to materials for which significant toxicity is apparent and for which there is significant exposure potential.

Considerations for Using OELs

In assessing health effects data and reviewing existing OELs, the following questions should be examined:

- Why was an existing OEL set at its particular level? What safety factors were used in deriving the OEL? What potentially important health effects were not evaluated? [One essential source for this information is ACGIH's *Docu-*

mentation of Threshold Limit Values and Biological Exposure Indices[6]]

- How adequate are the health effects data that support the OEL? Were the health effects data based on animal or human studies? Were the health effects studies acute or chronic?
- Are the health effects reversible or irreversible? What are the target organs? Do the health effects include reproductive, teratogenic, or carcinogenic effects; immediate death; or disability?
- Does the agent have warning properties (odor or irritation) at levels less than the exposure limit or only at levels greater than the OEL? Does the agent have warning properties at levels less than or greater than concentrations that are immediately dangerous to life or health (IDLH)?
- Should the OEL be adjusted in the presence of a nontraditional work schedule?[14]
- Are there concurrent exposures in the workplace that pose additive or synergistic health risks?
- Are data available on the skin absorption rate? Although data are generally limited on the potential for a substance to be absorbed through the skin, these data should be used when available. If data on skin absorption are not available, it is possible to develop a rough prediction based on surrogate information available on a similar substance. If skin absorption data are unavailable and cannot be estimated, the default of 100% absorption may be acceptable to make an initial exposure assessment.

OEL Averaging Times

At a minimum, each OEL consists of an exposure level and an averaging time. The two are interdependent and must be carefully considered and defined together. The "averaging time" refers to the time span for which an average exposure is estimated. The appropriate averaging time is set by the sponsor of the OEL and, in principle, can extend over any length of time from seconds and minutes, to a single shift, to multiple shifts, to months and years. In practice, three averaging times account for the majority of authoritative and regulatory OELs: eight hours, 15 minutes (for short-term exposure limits [STELs]), and instantaneous (for ceiling limits). The averaging times for internal or working OELs are usually similar.

As the averaging time and exposure level for an OEL are set by the OEL-setting agency or organization as a unit, the two must be used together as they were defined. To be in compli-

Be Careful when Applying 8-Hour OELs over Longer Periods

Unless one is reasonably certain about the toxic effects of any 8-hour exposure, exposures should not be amortized over longer periods. For example, cadmium is a classically chronic toxicant and one might be tempted to calculate and evaluate a worker's exposure over periods longer than a single day. Assuming that cadmium exposure occurs only once a week, the industrial hygienist might be inclined to estimate exposure over the entire week: That is, given a one-day 8-hour time-weighted average exposure of 10 $\mu g/m^3$, the weekly average amortized over five days is 10/5 or 2 $\mu g/m^3$. If there were a reasonable degree of certainty that 10 $\mu g/m^3$ of cadmium inhaled for one day presented no adverse health effect during that exposure, then this approach would be valid. Unfortunately, the toxicological database for cadmium (and many other environmental agents) might not be sufficient to make this determination with any confidence.

ance with OELs, the defined averaging time corresponding to the defined exposure level must be followed.

When setting an internal or working OEL, industrial hygienists have more flexibility for determining appropriate averaging times and exposure levels, but the two must still be defined as a unit. Choosing an appropriate averaging time for an OEL requires knowledge of the environmental agent's uptake, distribution, storage, elimination, and toxic action. If the toxic agent acts very quickly, then very short averaging times are appropriate (ceiling or STEL OELs). If the toxic material acts slowly — through some combination of accumulation of the toxic agent or metabolites, or accumulation of bodily damage — then longer averaging times may be appropriate.

The agent's biological half-life, which may vary from minutes to years, influences its ability to accumulate and exert harmful effects. If the half-life is relatively short, as is the case with many solvents, exposures are best assessed and controlled on a shift-by-shift basis (e.g., 8-hour TWA). Longer biological half-lives may warrant longer integration periods (e.g., a week or month). Some materials associated with chronic toxicity will have a biological half-life of a year or more. When biological dampening occurs as a result of slow uptake or clearance (repair), the accumulated body burdens in critical organs and tissues are not significantly affected by shorter-term excursions over, say, a week or less. Accordingly, a long-term average may be the best measure of health risk.[(15)]

A continuum of critical exposure durations and appropriate averaging times for OELs is portrayed in Table 3.3.

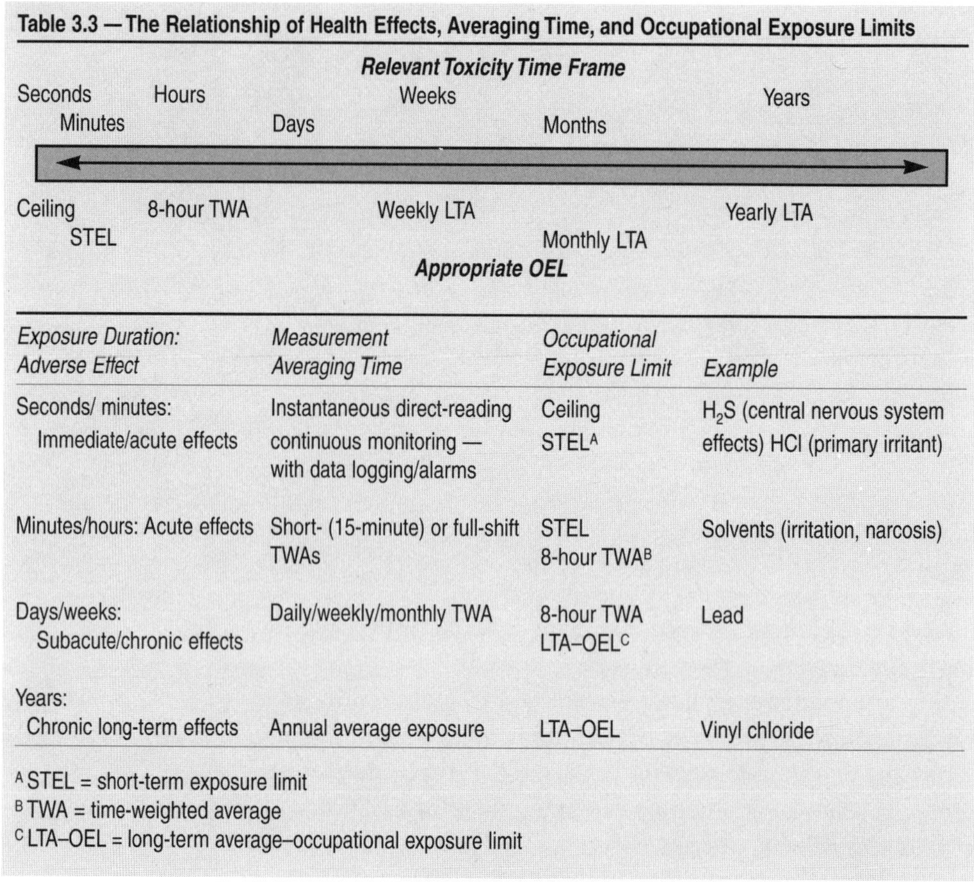

Table 3.3 — The Relationship of Health Effects, Averaging Time, and Occupational Exposure Limits

Relevant Toxicity Time Frame

Seconds — Minutes — Hours — Days — Weeks — Months — Years

Ceiling — STEL — 8-hour TWA — Weekly LTA — Monthly LTA — Yearly LTA

Appropriate OEL

Exposure Duration: Adverse Effect	*Measurement Averaging Time*	*Occupational Exposure Limit*	*Example*
Seconds/ minutes: Immediate/acute effects	Instantaneous direct-reading continuous monitoring — with data logging/alarms	Ceiling STEL[A]	H_2S (central nervous system effects) HCl (primary irritant)
Minutes/hours: Acute effects	Short- (15-minute) or full-shift TWAs	STEL 8-hour TWA[B]	Solvents (irritation, narcosis)
Days/weeks: Subacute/chronic effects	Daily/weekly/monthly TWA	8-hour TWA LTA–OEL[C]	Lead
Years: Chronic long-term effects	Annual average exposure	LTA–OEL	Vinyl chloride

[A] STEL = short-term exposure limit
[B] TWA = time-weighted average
[C] LTA–OEL = long-term average–occupational exposure limit

Acute Effects: For substances that act quickly to elicit their toxic response, it is important to control the dose across a single shift (8-hour TWA) or shorter period (e.g., 15 minutes for STELs and instantaneous for ceiling limits). A ceiling limit is warranted if the agent is fast-acting and especially if it is associated with irreversible health effects (e.g., hydrogen cyanide). The long-term average exposure may be less relevant if accumulation does not occur or is not important and there is complete recovery before the next shift (e.g., carbon monoxide).

Chronic Effects: For chronic disease agents it is important to limit the cumulative dose acquired by the employee. The relevant exposure parameter is the long-term average exposure. An exposure profile is deemed "acceptable" if the true long-term average exposure is less than an applicable long-term average OEL (LTA–OEL); however, few regulatory or authoritative LTA–OELs have been developed (examples are presented later). Instead, 8-hour TWA OELs have been used to limit cumulative dose for chronic disease agents. Properly implemented, single-shift limits will reduce the true long-term average exposure to a fraction of the 8-hour TWA–OEL. Rappaport, Selvin, and Roach showed, for example, that for a wide range of geometric standard deviations the true long-term average exposure will be less than half the 8-hour TWA–OEL when the true 95th percentile of the exposure distribution is less than the OEL.(16)

In the first edition of this book (published 1991) the AIHA Exposure Assessment Strategy Committee recommended, in the absence of a regulatory or authoritative LTA–OEL, setting an LTA–OEL for chronic disease agents at one-third the 8-hour TWA–OEL. Roach and Rappaport suggested that an LTA–OEL should be one-tenth to one-fourth the single-shift limit,(17) and this suggestion was endorsed by past chairs of ACGIH.(18)

Acute and Chronic Effects: Few substances result in purely acute or chronic effects. Many exhibit both acute effects related to single-shift or shorter exposures, and chronic disease from long-term exposure. For example, some aromatic organic compounds may exhibit acute neurotoxicity and chronic carcinogenicity. For these substances, the dose rate and cumulative dose are important, suggesting that both short-term OELs and long-term OELs are necessary to judge an exposure profile properly. The ceiling, STEL, or 8-hour TWA–OEL would be used to determine whether the exposure profile is currently controlled to prevent effects caused by single-shift or within-shift exposures. The LTA–OEL would be used to determine whether, over observation intervals of six months to a year, the long-term average exposure was adequately controlled to prevent chronic health effects.

Application of the OEL may affect whether exposures are classified as "acceptable," "unacceptable," or "uncertain." Given the temporal (hour-to-hour and day-to-day) variability in exposure levels, what exceedance of the OEL is permissible? The statistical application of the OEL should be defined by the standards-setting organization. Some OELs are defined as never-to-exceed values (e.g., ACGIH ceiling limits). Some OELs allow 5% exceedance, and some OELs may be defined as a long-term average value (LTA–OEL). Unfortunately, there are few statistically defined OELs, and each organization must decide how applicable regulatory and authoritative OELs should be applied. According to NIOSH, "in statistical terms, the employer should try to attain 95% confidence that no more than 5% of employee days are over the standard."(19)

The following examples illustrate instances when both single-shift and long-term goals have been identified. In the first example, NIOSH recommended a single-shift limit with the explicit goal of limiting long-term exposure below a specific value. In the second example, the European Commission standard for vinyl chloride has both single-shift and long-term average exposure limits.

NIOSH Respirable Coal Mine Dust Recommended Exposure Limit

In 1995, NIOSH issued an REL of 1 mg/m^3 for respirable coal mine dust.[(20)] This exposure limit was determined using a target long-term average exposure of 0.5 mg/m^3 and estimates of within-occupation variability for underground coal mining. NIOSH determined that the 95th percentile daily exposure (i.e., single-shift average exposure) for a miner whose long-term average exposure is 0.5 mg/m^3 will be approximately 1 mg/m^3. NIOSH then recommended an upper limit of 1 mg/m^3 for each single-shift average exposure.

European Long-Term Average OELs

In Europe, exposure limits with averaging times greater than eight hours have been developed for a small number of chemicals. When such limits are established, shorter-term exposure restrictions are also imposed. For example, a Long Term Technical Value (VTL) was established for vinyl chloride monomer (VCM) by an EC directive in 1978.[(21)] Implementation of this directive is illustrated with excerpts from a British employee awareness pamphlet:[(22)]

> *Employers must ensure that the exposure of employees to VCM in the air of working areas is as low as is reasonably practicable and that in any event it does not exceed the maximum exposure limits (MELs) for VCM. These are 3 parts VCM per million parts of air (ppm) averaged over a year (the annual limit) and 7 ppm (TWA) averaged over 8 hours.*

Summary

The first step in assessing occupational exposures in a workplace is "information gathering." Information is gathered on the workplace, work force, and environmental agents. This information is used to establish exposure groups and then assess worker exposures. At a minimum, the information gathered should include an understanding of:

- Operations, processes, and facilities;
- Work force, tasks, and division of labor;
- Chemical, physical, and biological agents in the workplace;
- How and when workers are exposed to the environmental agents;

- Exposure controls present in the workplace, including engineering controls, administrative controls, work practice controls, and personal protective equipment;
- Quantities of the environmental agents;
- Chemical and physical properties of the environmental agents; and
- Potential health effects of the environmental agents; mechanism of toxicity; and OELs associated with each agent.

References

1. **Burke, A.:** Under Your Skin. *Ind. Safety Hyg. News:*21-22 (July 1996).
2. "Work surface contamination." [Personal communication from Chris L. Packham, EnviroDerm Services, to Cathy Fehrenbacher, U.S. Environmental Protection Agency, 12/27/96 and 12/30/96.]
3. **Fenske, R.A., and J.J. van Hemmen:** Occupational Skin Exposure to Chemical Substances: Setting Limits. *Ann. Occup. Hyg. 38(4):*333-336 (1994).
4. **Occupational Safety and Health Administration:** "Appendix B to Subpart I — Non-Mandatory Compliance Guidelines for Hazard Assessment and Personal Protective Equipment Selection," *Federal Register 59:*16362 (April 6, 1994).
5. **Clayton, G.D., F.E. Clayton, R.L. Harris, L.J. Cralley, L.V. Cralley, and J.S. Bus (eds.):** *Patty's Industrial Hygiene and Toxicology,* Vols. I, II, and III. New York: John Wiley & Sons, 1994.
6. **American Conference of Governmental Industrial Hygienists:** *Documentation of the Threshold Limit Values and Biological Exposure Indices.* Cincinnati, Ohio: American Conference of Governmental Industrial Hygienists. [Published annually.]
7. **Klaassen, C.D. (ed.):** *Casarett and Doull's Toxicology — The Basic Science of Poisons,* 5th Ed. New York: McGraw-Hill, 1996.
8. Occupational Safety and Health Act of 1970: Public Law 91–596 (1970). OSHA PELs — *Federal Register 29* CFR 1910.1000.
9. Federal Mine Safety and Health Act of 1977 (FMSHAct): Public Law 91–173 (1977).
10. **Comité Européen de Normalisation:** *Workplace Atmospheres — Guidance for the Assessment of Exposure by Inhalation of Chemical Agents for Comparison with*

Limit Values and Measurement Strategy (EN 689). Brussels, Belgium: Comité Européen de Normalisation, 1995.

11. **American Conference of Governmental Industrial Hygienists:** *Threshold Limit Values (TLVs™) for Chemical Substances and Biological Exposure Indices (BEIs™).* Cincinnati, Ohio: American Conference of Governmental Industrial Hygienists. [Published annually or biannually.]
12. **American Industrial Hygiene Association:** *Workplace Environmental Exposure Level (WEEL) Guides.* Fairfax, Va.: American Industrial Hygiene Association. [Published annually.]
13. **National Institute for Occupational Safety and Health:** *Recommended Exposure Limits (RELs).* Cincinnati, Ohio: National Institute for Occupational Safety and Health. [Published periodically.]
14. **Paustenbach, D.J.:** Occupational Exposure Limits, Pharmacokinetics, and Unusual Work Schedules. In *Patty's Industrial Hygiene and Toxicology,* 3rd Ed., Vol. 3A (R.L. Harris, L.J. Cralley, and L.V. Cralley, editors). New York: John Wiley & Sons, 1994.
15. **Rappaport, S.M.:** Assessments of Long-Term Exposures to Toxic Substances in Air. *Ann. Occup. Hyg. 35(1):*61-121 (1991).
16. **Rappaport, S.M, S. Selvin, and S.A. Roach:** A Strategy for Assessing Exposures with Reference to Multiple Limits. *Appl. Ind. Hyg. 3:*310-315 (1988).
17. **Roach, S.A., and S.M. Rappaport:** But They Are Not Thresholds: A Critical Analysis of the Documentation of Threshold Limit Values. *Am. J. Ind. Med. 17:*727-753 (1990).
18. **Adkins, C.E., et al.:** Letter to the Editor. *Appl. Occup. Environ. Hyg. 5:*748-750 (1990).
19. **Leidel, N.A., K.A. Busch, and J.R. Lynch:** *Occupational Exposure Sampling Strategy Manual* (DHEW [NIOSH] Pub. No. 77–173). Cincinnati, Ohio: National Institute for Occupational Safety and Health, 1977. [National Technical Information Service (NTIS) Pub. No. PB274792.]
20. **National Institute for Occupational Safety and Health:** *Criteria for a Recommended Standard — Occupational Exposure to Respirable Coal Mine Dust* (DHHS [NIOSH] Pub. No. 95–106). Cincinnati, Ohio: National Institute for Occupational Safety and Health, 1995.
21. **Scheffers, T.M.L.:** "Testing Compliance with a One-Year Average Occupational Limit Value: An Example Based on

the European Community's Vinyl Chloride Legislation." Paper presented at the American Industrial Hygiene Conference & Exposition, Dallas, Texas, May 22, 1997.

22. **United Kingdom Health and Safety Executive:** "VCM and You." London: Her Majesty's Stationary Office Publications Centre, 1988.

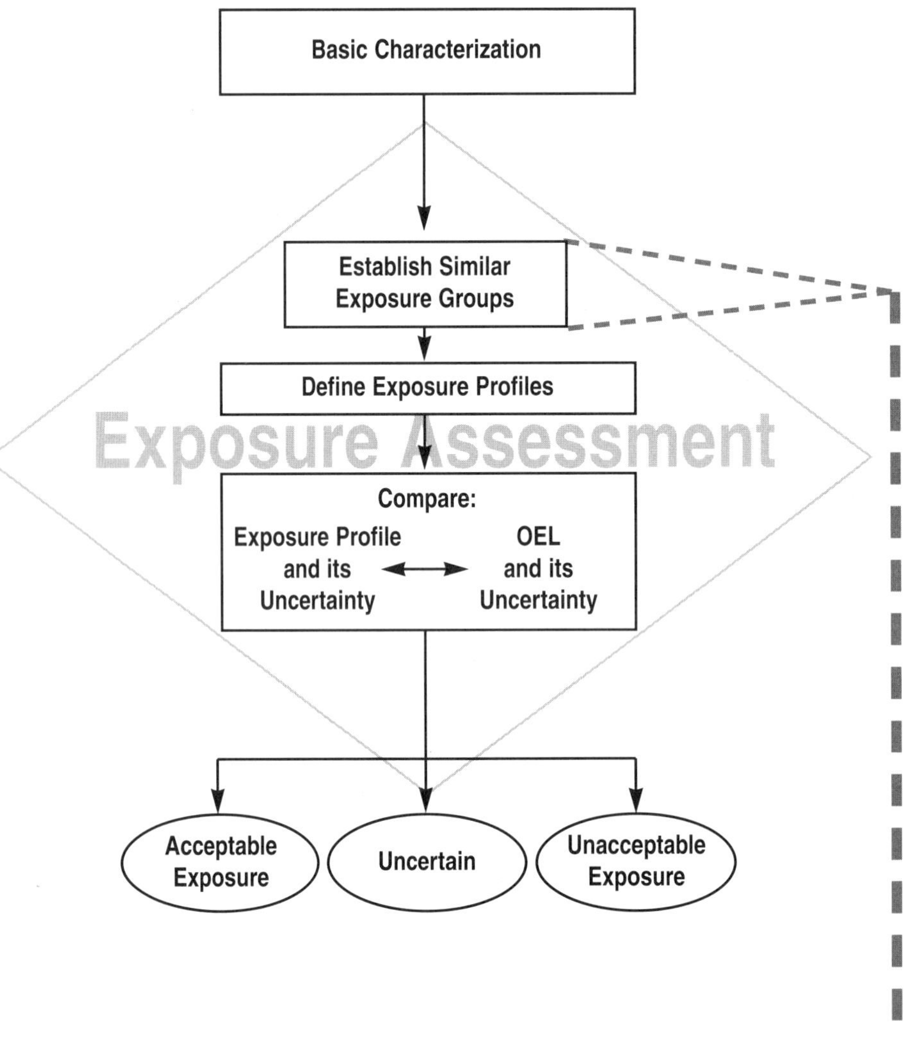

Purpose/Goals

Interpret available information to define exposure groups.

Tools

Criteria for establishing exposure groups:

- Observational approach —
  Process/job/task/environmental agents
- "Sampling" approach —
  Monitoring to define or refine groups

Outcome

- List of similar exposure groups
- Each worker is a member of at least one exposure group

4

Exposure Assessment: Establishing Similar Exposure Groups

Occupational exposure assessments are performed in workplaces employing a few, and up to, perhaps, thousands of workers. The magnitude of these exposures varies from minute-to-minute, hour-to-hour, and day-to-day. For the industrial hygienist, the primary goal is to assess the exposures and occupational health risks for all workers to all environmental agents on all days. The challenge is to do this accurately and efficiently, regardless of the diversity of exposures across workers and across time.

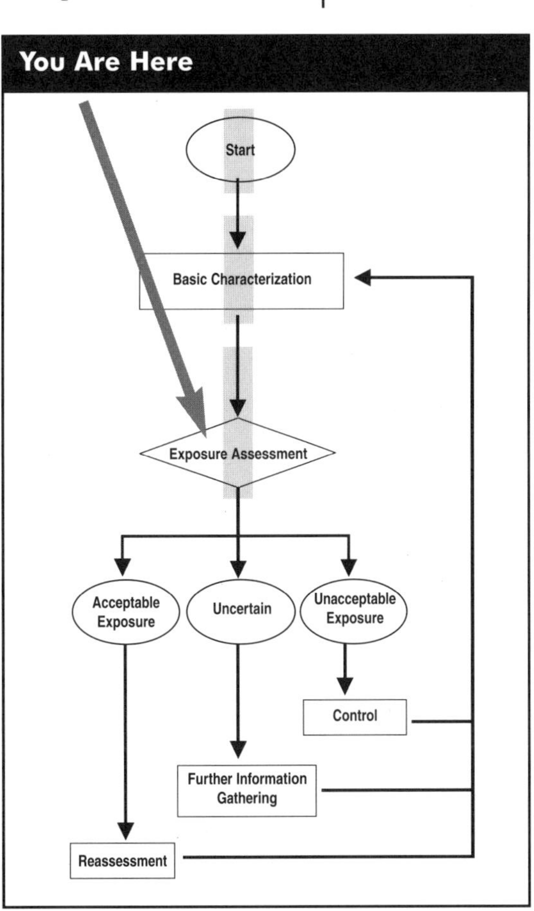

In most workplaces, it is difficult to measure exposures for every worker, and even if these assessments were practical, daily measurements are seldom possible. Although these difficulties may be overcome, for example, through the daily use of dosimeters that measure ionizing radiation exposure, measurement of each worker's exposure each day is seldom practical. The available resources in most workplaces and the current state of industrial hygiene instrumentation dictate that reality.(1)

Nothing new to industrial hygienists, one strategy for meeting these challenges is to assemble workers believed to have similar exposures into a group.(2) The qualitative or quantitative characterization of the exposure of one or a few in the group is then considered "representative" of the exposures of everyone in the group. This stratification of workers into "similar exposure groups" allows limited resources to be allocated better so that all of the exposures present in a particular workplace can be characterized.

In the first edition of this book, the term "homogeneous exposure group (HEG)" was used to describe this assemblage of like-exposed workers.[3] This tended to be confusing, however, because "homogeneous" has a rigorous statistical definition.[4-8] To avoid this misunderstanding, similar exposure group is used in this text. Similar exposure groups (SEGs) are groups of workers having the same general exposure profile because of the similarity and frequency of the tasks they perform, the materials and processes with which they work, and the similarity of the way they perform the tasks.

Two general methodologies are used to define SEGs: the observational approach and the sampling approach. In the traditional observational approach, workers are assigned to SEGs based on an examination of the activities they perform and a judgment on the expected similarity of their exposures. Exposure monitoring data are not needed. In the sampling approach, the exposures of many workers are measured and the individual workers are assigned to SEGs based on statistical analysis of the exposure data.[9]

Both approaches have advantages and disadvantages. Each has a place in this cyclic, continuously improving, comprehensive exposure assessment strategy:

1. Use the observational approach as the primary, default approach to defining SEGs.
2. Assess exposures for the SEGs formed by observation.
3. Identify critical SEGs for which the consequences of misclassifying an individual worker's exposure are very severe.
4. Use exposure monitoring and statistical analysis to check and refine critical SEGs using the sampling approach.

Establishing Similar Exposure Groups by Observation

Similar exposure groups are established by observation using the data gathered during the basic characterization of the workplace, work force, and environmental agents. The industrial hygienist reviews these data and uses his or her training and experience to group employees believed to have similar exposures. SEGs established by observation are generally described by the following determinants: process, job, task, and environmental agent.

Identifying the boundaries of processes, jobs, and tasks requires considerable judgment. Several hygienists independently assessing a workplace may not determine identical SEGs. With training, however, the differences should be insignificant.

The observational approach allows the industrial hygienist to make initial judgments about exposures to form SEGs and prioritize them for further action — either action in terms of exposure monitoring or action in terms of control. It also allows the industrial hygienist to use his or her training and experience to maximize limited monitoring resources to begin characterizing employee exposures. These limited resources for performing exposure assessments, coupled with the need to move quickly in prioritizing control and monitoring activities, practically forces an industrial hygienist to use an observational approach to form SEGs in a beginning program.

There are several suggested hierarchical strategies for establishing exposure groups by observation.[10] What must be stressed is the importance of a thorough basic characterization of the workplace using not only a review of records but also time on the production floor talking to workers and surveying the work process. This thorough understanding, coupled with sound professional judgment honed by training and experience, should help minimize the chance of misclassifying individual workers. The suggested strategies for establishing SEGs are:

- Classifying by process and environmental agent;
- Classifying by process, job, and environmental agent;
- Classifying by process, job, task, and environmental agent;
- Classifying by process, task, and environmental agent;
- Classifying work teams; and
- Classifying nonrepetitive work.

Classifying by Process–Environmental Agent

In the observational approach, the major work processes should be identified first. Frequently, workplaces are administratively organized into departments. The industrial hygienist's observational tour of the plant should help evaluate whether each department represents a unique process. If so, the administrative departments may be considered equivalent to the "process" element of the SEG. In some cases, an administrative department may contain two or more major processes — requiring further review and possible SEG refinement.

The other major input in identifying SEGs is the inventory of environmental agents compiled during the basic characterization process. The inventory should include each chemical mixture in use and its components. (Component information is usually available from material safety data sheets.) The inventory should be comprehensive and should include all production- and maintenance-related chemical agents, products, byproducts (e.g., off-gases), significant physical agents, and significant biological agents. Ultimately, every environmental agent identified in the basic characterization should be linked to one or more SEGs.

In some industrial operations, all employees working in a "process" are the SEG. An example of this equivalence is a process-oriented work team where each member of the team performs each task with approximately the same frequency. If the workers associated with the process are similarly exposed to the environmental agents, then each process–environmental agent combination is an SEG.

Unfortunately, seldom does classification of workers at the "process" level represent an SEG. The industrial hygienist must consider the division of labor and exposures among employees working in each process.

Classifying by Process–Job–Environmental Agent

The industrial hygienist should review the site's official job classification scheme available from the organization's human resources or personnel staff. Although the personnel job classification scheme is often a useful tool for identifying SEGs, these jobs (and associated environmental agents) should not be automatically accepted as SEGs. The similarity or dissimilarity of the jobs in each process should be considered carefully. In many workplaces, employees are assigned to personnel job classes for payroll purposes, and these job classes may not represent SEGs. There might be a need to establish a modified version of the personnel job class structure in order to have SEGs that accurately associate individual workers with exposures.

One personnel job class, for example, may include several distinct worker groups with substantially different exposure profiles. Workers on the day shift might have very different exposures from those doing the same job on the evening or night shift. The industrial hygienist should observe all work shifts and interview workers on each shift as needed.

The industrial hygienist must also ask whether the exposures for some personnel job classifications are unique. Personnel job classes, for example, may be organized around pay grades reflecting seniority rather than a discernible division of labor. Perhaps two or more personnel jobs can be merged into a single SEG because they have essentially equivalent exposures profiles.

Obviously, if a useful personnel job classification scheme is not available, the industrial hygienist will need to rely more heavily on the information gathered on the workplace, work force, and environmental agents. Generic job titles are used increasingly in industry. It is not unusual for perhaps all employees in a department to be identified as "technicians." The industrial hygienist must look beyond the organizational structure to the actual division of labor in the workplace. Normally, production and maintenance work is clearly organized and SEGs can be established from the observable division of labor.

Classifying by Process–Job–Task–Environmental Agent

More often than not, the classification scheme must be enhanced with identification of tasks. A task is a work element or series of work elements. "Maintenance," for example, is a common process in many industrial workplaces. Hypothetically, two job classifications can be identified in the maintenance process: electrician and maintenance mechanic. Welding is performed by maintenance mechanics, and the task "welding" links the maintenance mechanic job with the environmental agents associated with welding (such as welding fumes or ozone).

Since it is impractical to identify all tasks in most industrial operations, task characterization is important only when the additional detail will contribute significantly to understanding and managing the exposure(s).(10)

Assessing peak exposures is inherently task-related. A specific task must be identified as an element of the SEG (process–job–task–environmental agent) when assessing exposure relative to a ceiling (C) or short-term exposure limit (STEL). Furthermore, the specific task must be identified if the exposure is assessed as an 8-hour time-weighted average (TWA) and does not occur daily. An example would be a "welding" task that is performed only two days a week by a maintenance mechanic.

The basic characterization process should record relevant descriptive information on the significant tasks, including their frequency (e.g., days per year) and perhaps number of peak excursions occurring per day. This information is useful for prioritizing exposure groups for further information gathering and health hazard control.

Nonroutine Operations

For nonroutine operations, examination of work at the process–job–task level is often the easiest way to establish similar exposure groups. One proven observational approach is to use a work hierarchy, as is customary in a project management environment. Consider a nonroutine operation a "project" that can be divided into several steps, or what is commonly called a work breakdown structure. Each work element is further reduced to a set of smaller work tasks and these are further divided into detailed subtasks.

There are advantages and disadvantages to the project exposure assessment approach, of course. One advantage is that it relates well to a project management environment because it uses the language and structure to which project managers and engineers are accustomed. When performed using consistent procedures, the documentation is well-organized and leads to aggregation. Also, the exposure profile assumes the same beginning and end as the project. This means that worker exposures associated with a project can become part of the worker's historical exposure profile consisting of several project exposure profiles.

Disadvantages are that examination of work at this level of detail requires buy-in from the project manager, mainly because the industrial hygienist alone cannot adequately describe the work elements and tasks. It takes dedication and real persistence to implement this approach when projects are very short or very long in duration.

Classifying by Process–Task–Environmental Agent

The scheme for classifying workers by processes, jobs, tasks, and environmental agents can be used without identification of jobs. This strategy is effective when processes are strongly linked to manufacture of a product or application of a service (e.g., maintenance), and when tasks are strongly linked to identification and control of workplace exposure to environmental agents. Some organizations may choose to establish SEGs around the process, task, and environmental agent if classification of workers into jobs is difficult, or if adequate exposure histories are provided by linking workers to the SEG's process element. In practice it is very ambitious to create exposure histories in which workers are linked to specific tasks.

Classifying Work Teams

Some workplaces are organized around teams rather than job classifications. In operations in which teams are present, the industrial hygienist must carefully investigate the division of labor and use judgment when constructing SEGs.

Work teams may be assigned to production work in a department or process line, or to maintenance work in an area or facility. If that is the case, the work team may correspond to the process and job elements of the exposure group. If two or more teams are associated with a work area, then the work area is the process and each work team is a separate SEG.

Many industrial teams are true teams in the sense of shared responsibilities and flexible duties. Again, the division of labor must be carefully analyzed. The following criteria can be applied when classifying work teams:

- If workers are more or less permanently assigned to work positions, these positions are the SEG's job element.
- If workers rotate among positions but work the entire day at a given position, the work team is the SEG's job element and the position is the SEG's task element.
- If workers rotate among the positions and there is within-day rotation, the team is the SEG's job element and identification of tasks is important only when assessing exposure relative to a ceiling or STEL; such assessments are inherently task-related.

Classifying Nonrepetitive Work

Continuous change is a characteristic of some workplaces, such as job shop manufacturing, batch chemical synthesis, and research and development. It is difficult to establish SEGs in these workplaces. Meaningful exposure groups might exist one day and change the next.

When continuous change is a factor, the industrial hygienist must consider the objectives of the exposure assessment. If the objective is exclusively to assess compliance with OELs, the focus perhaps should be on identifying worst-case scenarios and then evaluating and controlling exposures accordingly. If the exposure assessment objectives include development of an historical database, perhaps for future medical or epidemiological purposes, the assessment is much more difficult. One approach may be to designate the product or project as the process or task, a strategy that could lead to an extensive number of exposure assessments. In any case, the industrial hygienist must apply considerable professional judgment while maintaining focus on the original exposure assessment objectives.

Example

The operations of a small metal manufacturing plant can be considered to illustrate the observational strategy for identifying similar exposure groups. Our example site manufactures resin-coated sheet metal. The product is manufactured and sold as coils which are shipped to other sites for further processing. Information on the workplace, work force, and environmental agents is used to identify SEGs. The strategy begins with identification of the site's major processes. Administratively the plant is organized into five departments:

- Casting;
- Rolling;
- Coil Coating;
- Shipping and Receiving; and
- Maintenance.

An observational tour of the plant reveals that the administrative departments correspond with the unique major processes of the plant. Moreover, in each department there is considerable opportunity to further stratify employees in view of their day-to-day exposures. (It is an unusual process that cannot be further subdivided — one example cited earlier might be a process-oriented work team.)

Let's consider the Coil Coating department of our metal products plant. Again, coil coating is deemed a unique process and therefore constitutes the "process" element of the SEG. There are three identical coil coating lines in the Coil Coating department. Each line produces the same product and production rates are similar.

Each coil coating line applies a single resin-coating system through roll application; there is no spraying or aerosol involved. The coating contains 2-butoxyethanol. The operation is noisy and positional measurements are in the range of 82–85 decibels (dB).

Although the coil coating process is unique, there is clear dissimilarity among worker exposures in the Coil Coating operation. There are three official jobs in the personnel job classification scheme: "Coil Feed Operator," "Discharge Operator," and "Helper." There is one Coil Feed Operator and one Discharge Operator per production line, and one Helper is shared by the Coil Coating and Casting departments. Each job is occupied by one employee per production line per shift and there are three eight-hour rotating shifts.

The Coil Feed Operator is responsible for loading the coating line; a small pendent mounted crane is used for this purpose and frequent reloads are required. This requirement limits the movement of the Coil Feed Operator to the feed end of the coil coating line. Besides maintaining the coiled metal supply, the Coil Feed Operator is responsible for filling the coating reservoir periodically during the workshift.

The Discharge Operator is responsible for removing the finished product from the coil coater and transporting the product to the Shipping and Receiving Department. The Discharge Operator is also responsible for a quality control step to determine the percent coating weight. A small piece of each coated roll is cut off, weighed, and then placed in a small degreaser containing methyl isobutyl ketone (MIBK). After the coating is removed, the piece is weighed again to determine its weight without the coating. This 15-minute task is conducted eight times per shift.

Although administratively assigned to Coil Coating, the Helper services both the Coil Coating and Casting processes. In Coil Coating, the Helper is responsible for identifying equipment problems and either remedying the problem herself, or contacting a Mechanic or Electrician from the Maintenance department for assistance. For example, it is not unusual for the Helper to apply the lubricant "Packing Grease 609" to bearings on the rolling equipment.

In Coil Coating, all three job classifications engage in a brief clean-up task at the end of each shift lasting no more than 15 minutes. The solvent "GenSol" is used during this task; the product contains 90% MIBK and 10% cyclohexanone.

The Helper is also assigned duties in the nearby Casting Department. The Helper will assist the Casting Operator in a metal purification task for approximately two hours each shift. The metal purification task is known as "fluxing." The Helper loads 65-kilogram bags of granular hexachloroethane into a pneumatic device that dispenses the chemical below the surface of the molten metal. The task is physically demanding and there is exposure to radiant heat emanating from the furnace. The noise levels are controlled below 80 decibels. However, there is potential for airborne exposure to hexachloroethane and the by-products of its reaction with the molten metal. The industrial hygienist's basic characterization of the process revealed that hydrogen chloride, hexachlorobenzene, and octochlorostyrene are produced when hexachloroethane reacts with the molten metal.

In Table 4.1 the SEGs in the Coil Coating operation are identified. This scheme is based largely on the personnel job class structure, although in most workplaces the official job class structure must be modified. For example, it would not be unusual in industry to find workers classified by the specific produc-

Table 4.1 — Similar Exposure Groups: Specific Job Descriptions

Process	*Job*	*Task*	*Environmental Agent*
Coil Coating	Coil Feed Operator	General	Noise
Coil Coating	Coil Feed Operator	General	2-butoxyethanol
Coil Coating	Coil Feed Operator	Cleanup	MIBK
Coil Coating	Coil Feed Operator	Cleanup	Cyclohexanone
Coil Coating	Discharge Operator	General	Noise
Coil Coating	Discharge Operator	General	2-butoxyethanol
Coil Coating	Discharge Operator	QC	MIBK
Coil Coating	Discharge Operator	Cleanup	MIBK
Coil Coating	Discharge Operator	Cleanup	Cyclohexanone
Coil Coating	Helper	General	Noise
Coil Coating	Helper	Lubricate	Packing Grease 609
Coil Coating	Helper	Cleanup	MIBK
Coil Coating	Helper	Cleanup	Cyclohexanone
Casting	Helper	Fluxing	Hexachloroethane
Casting	Helper	Fluxing	Hydrogen chloride
Casting	Helper	Fluxing	Hexachlorobenzene
Casting	Helper	Fluxing	Octochlorostyrene
Casting	Helper	Fluxing	Heat

tion line, rather than the work positions. Also, the hygienist's observation of the workplace might reveal significant differences in exposure across production lines. For example, if line 3 were adjacent to the Rolling department, the noise levels around line 3 might be significantly higher than lines 1 or 2. If that were the case, the Coil Feed Operator and the Discharge Operator for line 3 should be separate SEGs from workers in lines 2 or 3. The differentiation can be made at the process or job level of the SEG.

The list of SEGs in Table 4.1 is a simplified hypothetical example. In practice, every environmental agent identified in the basic characterization should be linked to a similar exposure group.

A significant feature of Table 4.1 is the identification of three SEGs exposed to MIBK during cleanup, and three SEGs exposed to cyclohexanone during cleanup. Essentially in this process there are workers in three jobs performing the same task. The industrial hygienist might choose to consolidate the six SEGs into two SEGs, one for each solvent. (Of course, if monitoring is needed, both solvents can be collected concurrently on one sampling media.) An organization that uses a process–task–environmental agent strategy toward the identification of SEGs would probably identify two SEGs from the start. Another organization might choose to retain the six SEGs in order to create and maintain exposure histories where individual workers are linked to the "job" element of the SEG.

As stated earlier, it would not be unusual to find a single

administrative job classification such as Coil Coat Operator, or to find administrative job classes based on seniority (e.g., Coil Coater I, Coil Coater II). The industrial hygienist must look beyond the personnel job structure and establish exposure groups in view of work practices and the similarity of exposures.

In our example, the "Cleanup" tasks were deemed significant in view of the volatility and toxicity of cyclohexanone and MIBK that were used in the cleaning solution. Perhaps in another facility using a less volatile and less toxic solvent, these tasks would not be deemed significant and the exposure grouping could be established at the chemical mixture level (e.g., the environmental agent is GenSol.)

Administrative reorganizations occur in most workplaces. In our example, perhaps management eliminates the job classification structure in the Coil Coating department and the two operators are merged into a single administrative job classification titled "Coil Coat Operator." The operators are now available to perform all work elements, but there is no change in the Helper's duties. What then is an appropriate update to the exposure grouping? The reclassification depends on how operators are actually deployed. If in practice nothing has changed (except on paper), then the SEGs in Table 4.1 remain valid. On the other hand, if there is a true change in worker deployment, this must be reflected in the SEGs.

If on a given day employees are dedicated to the same work positions that existed prior to the reorganization, the work positions can be designated as tasks. The SEGs that exist under this scenario are listed in Table 4.2.

If, however, there is within-day rotation across work positions, then the SEGs that exist under this scenario are listed in Table 4.3. The designation of task-based exposure groups remains valid for assessing compliance with the short-term exposure limits.

Table 4.2 — Similar Exposure Groups: General Job Descriptions

Process	*Job*	*Task*	*Environmental Agent*
Coil Coating	Coil Coat Operator	Coil Feed	Noise
Coil Coating	Coil Coat Operator	Coil Feed	2-butoxyethanol
Coil Coating	Coil Coat Operator	Discharge	Noise
Coil Coating	Coil Coat Operator	Discharge	2-butoxyethanol
Coil Coating	Coil Coat Operator	QC	MIBK
Coil Coating	Coil Coat Operator	Cleanup	MIBK
Coil Coating	Coil Coat Operator	Cleanup	Cyclohexanone

Table 4.3 — Similar Exposure Groups: Rotating Jobs

Process	*Job*	*Task*	*Environmental Agent*
Coil Coating	Coil Coat Operator	General	Noise
Coil Coating	Coil Coat Operator	General	2-butoxyethanol
Coil Coating	Coil Coat Operator	QC	MIBK
Coil Coating	Coil Coat Operator	Cleanup	Cyclohexanone
Coil Coating	Coil Coat Operator	Cleanup	MIBK

To create an accurate exposure history, it will be necessary to identify and record the task frequency (e.g., days per year), the "begin" and "end" dates of each SEG (i.e., similar exposure interval), and the date each worker joined and left the SEG.

Establishing Similar Exposure Groups by Sampling

In the sampling approach to forming similar exposure groups, the collection of monitoring data precedes the formation of SEGs.[11-14] The measured exposure values are then used to classify workers into SEGs. Provided that enough measurements are made, workers can be grouped with a given amount of homogeneity and a given amount of confidence using a statistical technique such as analysis of variance.

It has been suggested that a useful quantitative criterion is to group employees in a way that long-term average exposures of 95% of workers in a group differ by a maximum factor of two (see Figure 4.1).[11] Whether this criterion is appropriate depends on the nature of the exposures, the goals of the exposure assessment strategy, and the resources available. If the worker mean exposures differ by more than a factor of two in an SEG where exposures are rated as between half and one times the OEL, there might be an increased health risk for workers on the high end of the exposure distribution.

On the other hand, if worker mean exposures differ by as much as a factor of 10 in an SEG where the exposure profile is on the order of 1/100 times the OEL (e.g., 7 ppm acetone exposure relative to an OEL of 750 ppm), there still may be no cause for concern. Whether the industrial hygienist chooses to refine this SEG further in order to maintain a historical record of exposures for future epidemiological (or other) purposes will depend, for one, on the number of people in the group. It might not be productive to refine the SEG to the point at which there is only one person in the subset SEG. Other important factors are the resources available and the priorities of the exposure assessment and industrial hygiene program.

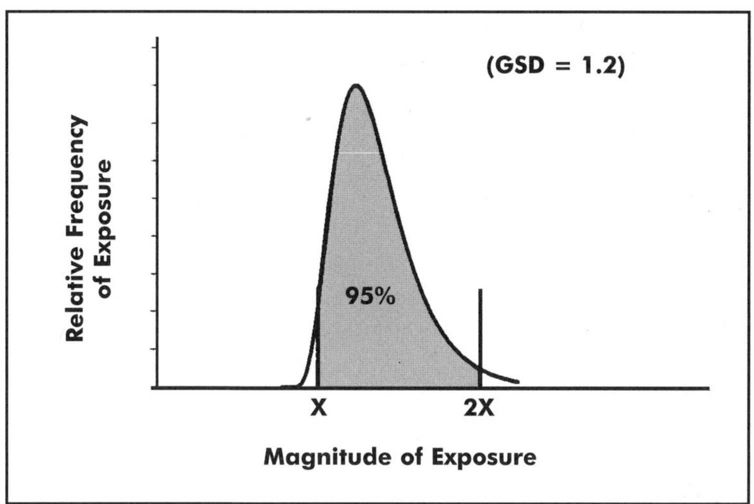

Figure 4.1 — Worker arithmetic mean exposures: factor of two maximum difference for 95% of workers in the group.

The sampling approach to forming SEGs has the advantage of objectivity; however, a large number of random measurements is required and multiple measurements must be made on individual workers in order to calculate the within-worker and between-worker components of exposure variability for accurate grouping. Under current practice, rarely are sufficient monitoring results available; however, advances in simple inexpensive personal monitoring devices (e.g., passive organic vapor monitors or diffusion indicator tubes) are beginning to make it easier to collect sufficient measurements.

Establishing similar exposure groups by sampling can be more accurate than classification by observation when individual work practices have a large effect on between-worker variability. Collecting monitoring data for many employees provides quantitative characterization of work practice variability and minimizes the misclassification of individual workers. Once sufficient data are collected to form SEGs in this fashion, however, the reason for forming the SEGs in the first place (to achieve economies in exposure characterization) is less important. With monitoring data collected for each worker there is less need to form groups since each individual's exposure has been quantitatively characterized.

Strict reliance on a sampling approach alone does not allow the industrial hygienist flexibility in prioritizing groups of workers for assessment or other action in the absence of quantitative data. Also, as will become apparent later in this text, quantitative data are often not necessary to resolve the exposure assessment (i.e., judge exposures acceptable or unacceptable).

Combining the Observational and Sampling Approaches

A practical and accurate exposure assessment program will combine both the observational and the sampling approaches to defining SEGs. Day-to-day variability in exposure for workers in an SEG has two sources: process or environmental conditions, and work practices. The observational approach is stronger when variability arises principally from the process; it is weaker when variability arises principally from individual work practices. These two components of variability must be evaluated through observation of the workplace, and careful investigation and follow-up on data acquired through exposure monitoring.

The observational approach is a practical methodology for identifying SEGs that allows the industrial hygienist to proceed with economical exposure assessment and management. This methodology is consistent with traditional industrial hygiene practice.

Determination of SEGs by observation requires fewer samples to judge exposures than the sampling approach. It also provides an opportunity to resolve the exposure assessment qualitatively, something not possible with a strict sampling approach. Moreover, the determinants used in the observational approach (i.e., process–job–task–environmental agent) are well-suited to focusing health hazard controls (e.g., engineering, hearing protection, etc.) when the assessment reveals an unacceptable exposure.

In the observational approach, errors in the expected similarity of exposures can lead to misclassification of individual exposures. The chance of misclassification is affected by a variety of factors, including the thoroughness of the information gathering, the training and experience of the industrial hygienist, and the degree to which individual work practices influence individual exposures.

The risks associated with this misclassification will vary from one SEG to another. It is important for the industrial hygienist to recognize those SEGs for which misclassifications present a significant risk. He or she must then make an effort to generate exposure monitoring data to check the homogeneity of the grouping and refine worker exposure classifications as appropriate. Chapter 7 of this book presents recommendations for using ANOVA to refine these critical SEGs.

Summary

Similar exposure groups are needed for efficient exposure assessment of each worker each day. These SEGs usually are described by the determinants "process," "job," "task," and "environmental agent."

An exposure assessment and management program will be forced by the breath of the challenge and limited resources to take advantage of the economies offered by the observational approach for grouping workers into SEGs. In doing so, the industrial hygienist will accept the risk of possibly misclassifying some workers.

As the organization's exposure assessment program matures, the industrial hygienist will be able to identify those SEGs in which the risk posed by individual misclassification is a concern. Those critical SEGs can be targeted for more extensive exposure monitoring. Statistical analysis of the monitoring data can then be used to check the homogeneity of the SEGs formed by observation, and if necessary individuals can be assigned to a new SEG.

References

1. **Damiano, J.:** A Guideline for Managing the Industrial Hygiene Sampling Function. *Am. Ind. Hyg. Assoc. J. 50(7):*366-371 (1989).
2. **Corn, M., and N. Esmen:** Workplace Exposure Zones for Classification of Employee Exposures to Physical and Chemical Agents. *Am. Ind. Hyg. Assoc. J. 40(1):*47-54 (1979).
3. **Hawkins, N.C., S.K. Norwood, and J.C. Rock:** *A Strategy for Occupational Exposure Assessment.* Akron, Ohio: American Industrial Hygiene Association, 1991.
4. **Rappaport, S.M., H. Kromhout, and E. Symanski:** Variation of Exposure Between Workers in Homogeneous Exposure Groups. *Am. Ind. Hyg. Assoc. J. 54(11):*654-662 (1993).
5. **Scheffers, T.M.L.:** Letter to the Editor. *Am. Ind. Hyg. Assoc. J. 55(9):*873-874 (1994).
6. **Cole, C.J.:** Letter to the Editor. *Am. Ind. Hyg. Assoc. J. 55(9):*874-875 (1994).
7. **Gómez, M.R.:** Letter to the Editor. *Am. Ind. Hyg. Assoc. J. 55(9):*875 (1994).
8. **Rappaport, S.M.:** Letter to the Editor. *Am. Ind. Hyg. Assoc. J. 55(9):*875-877 (1994).
9. **Rappaport, S.M.:** Assessments of Long-Term Exposures to Toxic Substances in Air. *Ann. Occup. Hyg. 35(1):*61-121 (1991).

10. **Damiano, J.:** Quantitative Exposure Assessment Strategies and Data in the Aluminum Company of America. *Appl. Occup. Environ. Hyg. 10(4):*289-298 (1995).
11. **Rappaport, S.M., R.H. Lyles, and L.L. Kupper:** An Exposure Assessment Strategy Accounting for Within- and Between-Worker Sources of Variability. *Ann. Occup. Hyg. 39:*469-495 (1995).
12. **Kromhout, H., E. Symanski, and S.M. Rappaport:** A Comprehensive Evaluation of Within- and Between-Worker Components of Occupational Exposure to Chemical Agents. *Ann. Occup. Hyg. 37:*253-270 (1993).
13. **Heederik, D., and F. Hurley:** Workshop Summary — Occupational Exposure Assessments: Investigating Why Exposure Measurements Vary. *Appl. Occup. Environ. Hyg. 9(1):*71-73 (1994).
14. **Lyles, R.H., L.L. Kupper, and S.M. Rappaport:** A Lognormal Distribution-Based Exposure Assessment Method for Unbalanced Data. *Ann. Occup. Hyg. 41(1):* 63-76 (1997).

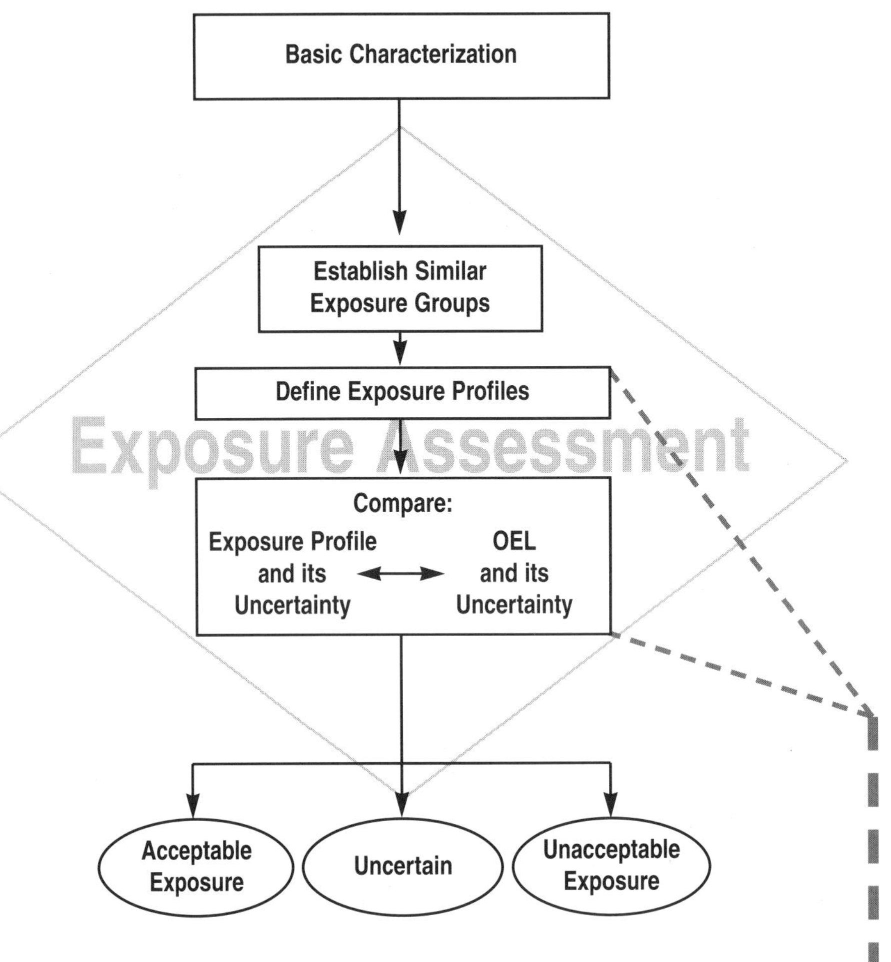

Purpose/Goals

- Define exposure profiles for the exposure groups.
- Make judgments about the acceptability of the exposure profiles.

Tools

Exposure judgment based on the interpretation of available qualitative and quantitative data

- Exposure profile
- Exposure rating
- Training and experience
- Exposure modeling tools
- Monitoring data

Outcome

- Exposure profile for each exposure group
- Judgment about the acceptability and the uncertainty of the exposure profile for each exposure group

5

Exposure Assessment: Defining and Judging Exposure Profiles

Experienced industrial hygienists assess exposures using subjective principles. When visiting a workplace or thinking about exposure conditions, the industrial hygienist will consciously or subconsciously picture the exposure profile and decide whether the exposures are acceptable. In this chapter, a systematic framework for this process is provided so it can be conducted consistently and can be better documented.

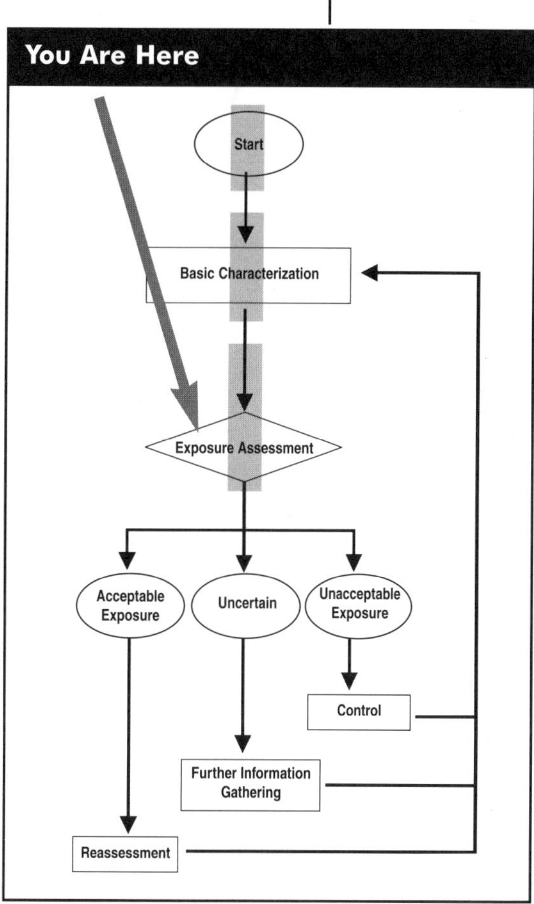

Overview

The process for defining and judging exposure profiles is illustrated in Figure 5.1. As described in Chapter 4, available information on the workplace, work force, and environmental agents is used to establish SEGs and these data are then used to define the exposure profiles for each SEG and to select appropriate OELs.

Once the exposure profile is defined, it should be compared with the OEL to determine the acceptability of its risk. In other words, the exposure profile (and its associated uncertainty) is compared with the OEL (and its associated uncertainty) and the industrial hygienist must judge whether the risk posed by the

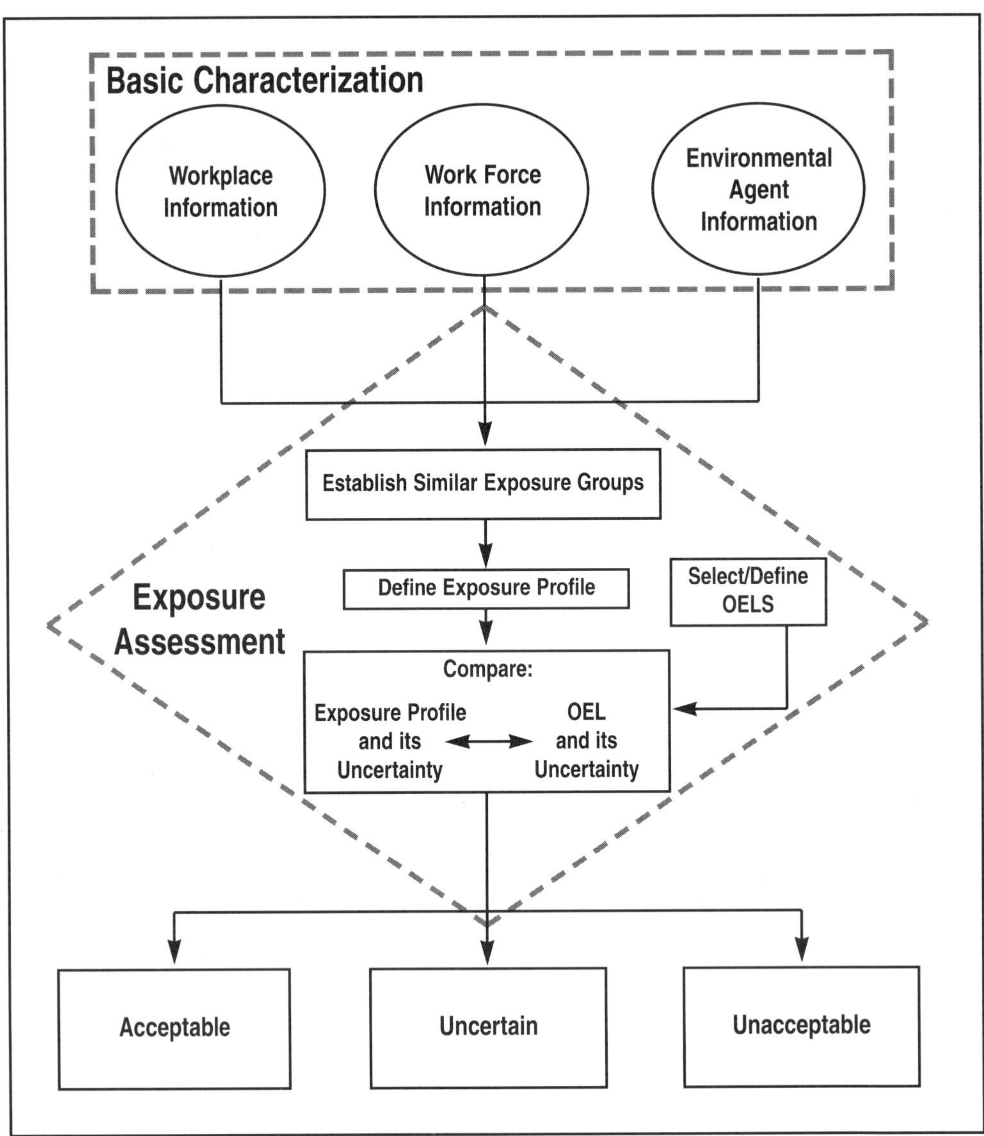

Figure 5.1 — Defining and judging exposure profiles.

exposure situation is acceptable. It should be noted that separate exposure assessments should be performed for each OEL. If, for example, an environmental agent has both an 8-hour time-weighted average (TWA) OEL and a peak OEL (short-term exposure limit [STEL] or ceiling limit), two evaluations are appropriate.

Initially, each SEG should be classified as "acceptable," "unacceptable," or "uncertain." Exposures judged acceptable are documented as such, but they should be reassessed periodically to verify that their status continues as acceptable. Exposures judged unacceptable must be controlled. Ultimately, as the exposure assessment cycle continues, "uncertain" exposures should be resolved through further information gathering to reduce the uncertainty in the exposure profile or the uncertainty in the OEL. Moreover, further information may be gathered on acceptable exposures to verify the acceptability judgment, and further information may be gathered on unacceptable exposures to guide the selection of health hazard controls.

In conducting an exposure assessment, the industrial hygienist should evaluate all available information to determine a best-estimate picture of the exposure profile, based on professional judgment. Generally, this exposure information will vary in quantity and quality: it may be comprised almost entirely of descriptive information, or it may be high grade quantitative exposure measurements. The OEL might have been set by a reputable organization based on comprehensive toxicological mechanisms, or it might be a "working OEL" established on limited health effects data. In either case, to resolve the exposure judgment, the industrial hygienist must compare the exposure profile (and its uncertainty) with the OEL (and its uncertainty) to evaluate the exposure's risk.

Defining the Exposure Profile

An exposure profile is a characterization of the temporal (e.g., day-to-day) variability of exposure levels for an SEG. Characterizing an exposure profile requires an estimate of the exposure and its variability, in addition to some judgment about how good those estimates are. The exposure profile estimate may be highly quantitative — complemented by exposure means, standard deviations, and formal statistical confidence limits — or it may be more qualitative, relying on knowledge, experience and professional judgment as described in this chapter.

An industrial hygienist, for example, may be confident that a judgment about lead (Pb) exposures for a group of hand soldering workers is accurate based on previous experience with a different hand soldering operation. The past experience presents the industrial hygienist with data and information that, even without air monitoring data, the upper extreme exposures of the exposure profile are well within acceptable limits. Indeed, judgments of this sort are made every day. The exposure assessment strategy outlined in this book simply asks that the industrial hygienist at least take the time to explain and document those judgments.

The precision of the exposure profile characterization must be "good enough" to meet the needs of the acceptability judgment.

Those needs will be defined in large measure at the outset of the assessment process when particular objectives of the strategy are defined. The accuracy of the exposure characterization increases not only with more monitoring results but also with more and better qualitative information (i.e., knowledge of how exposures are affected by workplace, work force, and environmental agent factors). If epidemiology is a consideration, the assessment characterization must be specific enough to be useful in future epidemiological work.

Initial Exposure Assessments

As shown in Figure 5.2, exposure assessment is a tiered, cyclic process. During each cycle, the industrial hygienist should use all available data to make exposure assessments. Initial assessments in the first cycle, however, usually are made using a knowledge base that generally lacks in quantitative data — a notion illustrated in Figure 5.3.

A low level of quantitative information on the exposure is often associated with a high level of uncertainty about the specific level of exposure. One way to deal with this is to develop an estimated range of exposures based on worst-case assumptions and use the highest estimate of exposure from this relatively large range of possible exposures (known as an uncertainty band). Thus, the exposure is purposely overestimated, and if this overestimate is acceptable when compared with an OEL, the exposure may be judged acceptable (i.e., it is possible to have an estimated rating that is highly uncertain but still acceptable).

The initial assessment will be able to resolve many of the low and trivial exposure profiles as acceptable and many of the gross overexposures as unacceptable. Because of a lack of data, however, there might be a number of exposures that cannot be resolved. Subsequent cycles through the exposure assessment process will allow the industrial hygienist to generate additional information (e.g., monitoring or health effects data) or use more sophisticated exposure models to better characterize these unresolved exposures.

Exposure Ratings

The exposure profile is a vehicle for summarizing and judging exposures to environmental agents in the workplace. A useful tool for beginning to characterize the exposure profile is the exposure rating. An exposure rating is an estimate of exposure level relative to the OEL. Suggested categorization schemes for

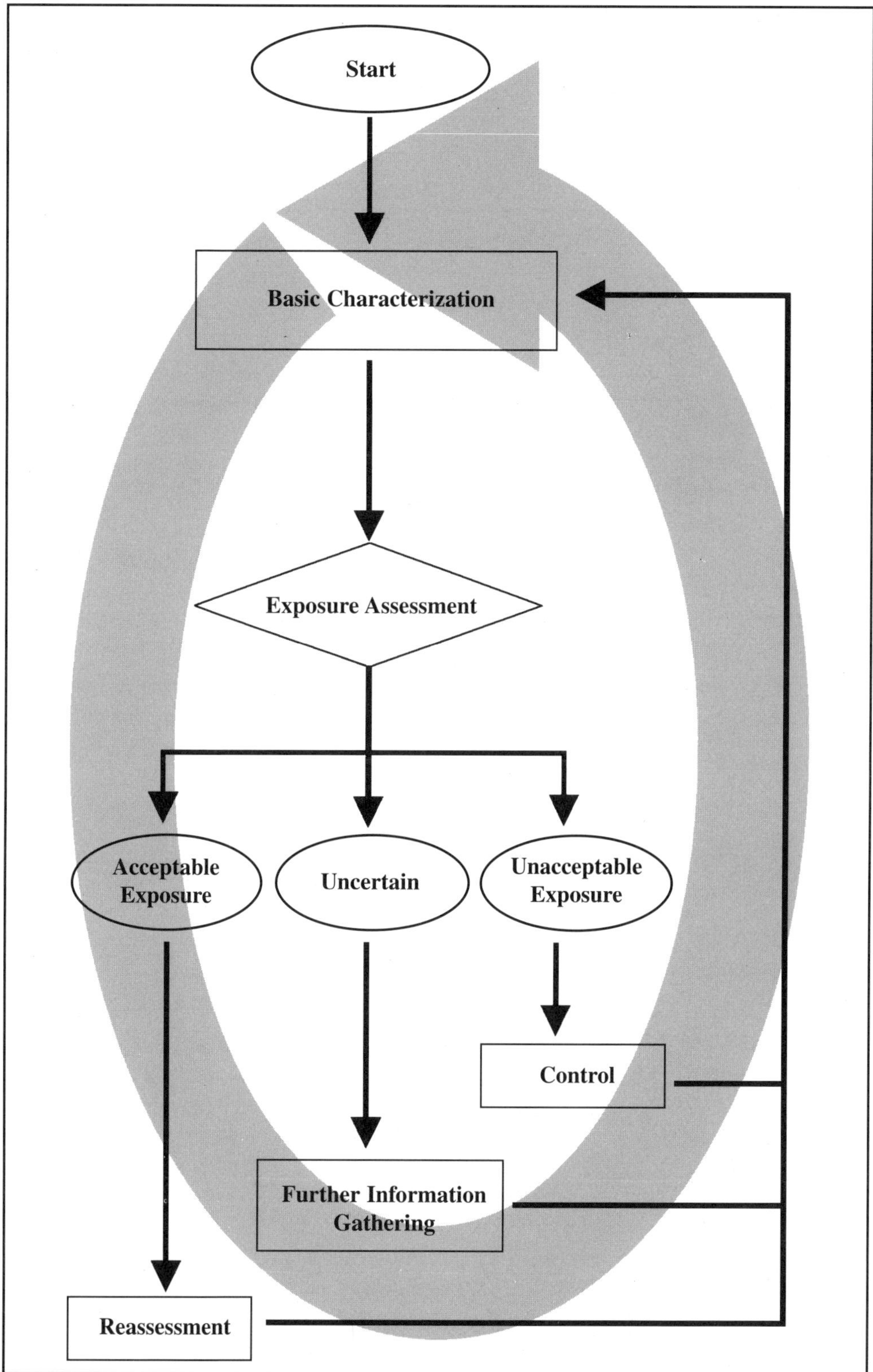

Figure 5.2 — Cylic, continuous improvement, exposure assessment process.

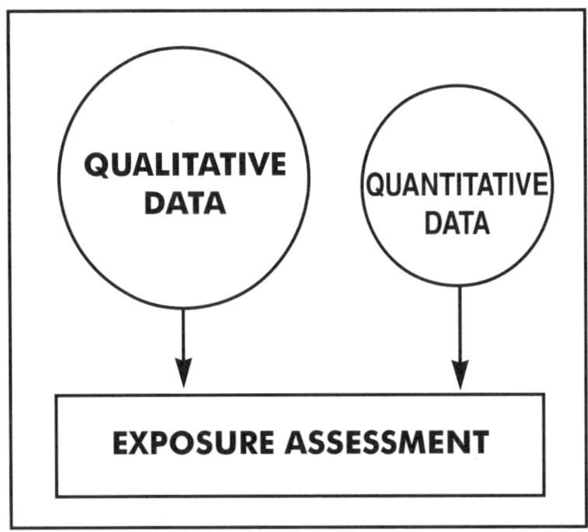

Figure 5.3 — Initial exposure assessment.

rating exposures are depicted in Tables 5.1 and 5.2. The industrial hygienist should find that exposure ratings streamline the assessment process, particularly during initial assessments when monitoring data often are sparse. Table 5.1 is based on an estimate of the arithmetic mean of the exposure profile relative to the LTA–OEL; Table 5.2 is based on an estimate of the 95th percentile of the exposure profile relative to the OEL. The industrial hygienist's choice of rating schemes should depend on how OELs are defined by regulatory and authoritative standards-setting organizations and on how they are applied in the exposure assessment.

When rating dermal exposure potential, it may be helpful to categorize the magnitude of exposure using descriptive terms such as "incidental contact," "routine contact," and "immersion of hands." Dermal exposure assessments are addressed in Appendix II.

In performing the initial exposure rating, the industrial hygienist should assume the absence of personal protective equipment (PPE) used to control exposures (such as respirators, hearing pro-

Table 5.1 — Exposure Rating Categorization: Based on an Estimate of the Arithmetic Mean of the Exposure Profile

4	>LTA–OEL
3	50%–100% LTA–OEL
2	10%–50% LTA–OEL
1	<10% LTA–OEL

NOTE: A long-term average–occupational exposure limit (LTA–OEL) is the acceptable average concentration of an environmental agent exhibiting cumulative adverse health effects.

Table 5.2 — Exposure Rating Categorization: Based on an Estimate of the 95th Percentile Relative to the OEL

4	>5% exceedance of the OEL (95th percentile > OEL)
3	>5% exceedance of 0.5 x OEL (95th percentile between 0.5 x OEL and 1.0 x OEL)
2	>5% exceedance of 0.1 x OEL (95th percentile between 0.1 x OEL and 0.5 x OEL)
1	Little to no exceedance of 0.1 x OEL (95th percentile <0.1 x OEL)

Applying Information Gathered During the Basic Characterization

To define the exposure profile, information on the workplace, work force, and environmental agents is gathered.

Workplace information:

- Observation of the workplace, providing data on the processes. For example:
  - Continuous vs. batch process;
  - Sources of release and contamination;
  - Environmental temperature, humidity, and wind velocity;
  - Pressure and temperature of the process;
  - Historical data on fugitive emissions;
  - Surface area of vaporizing sources;
  - Production or throughput rate;
  - Frequency, duration, and intensity of spills or other process upsets; and
  - Housekeeping;
- Review of the engineering controls in place (e.g., noise abatement features, exhaust ventilation, etc.). and their reliability in maintaining adequate control of worker exposures.

Work force information:

- Information on the division of labor, and observation of the jobs and tasks and the associated frequency and duration of exposures.
- Work schedules and worker rotation.
- Review of prescribed work practice controls, worker training, personal protective equipment, and their reliability in maintaining adequate control of worker exposures through enforcement of required work practices.
- Observations, comments, and data from workers, safety staff, medical staff, and others on the conditions of exposure and health effects (e.g., prevalence of dermatitis).

Environmental agent information:

- The location's materials inventory and material safety data sheets (MSDSs), providing information on the quantities of materials in use, their chemical and physical properties, and their warning properties.
- Review of the health effects associated with the environmental agents, including routes of exposure, adequacy of the toxicological data, and reported rationale for the OELs.
- Available exposure data, including positional measurements of exposure and exposure assessment findings from other workplaces with similar operations.

tectors, and chemically protective gloves). This approach will allow the industrial hygienist to determine precisely where and to what degree workers depend on PPE — generally the least desirable method of controlling a health hazard.

Exposure ratings can be made on the basis of:

Monitoring data

- Personal monitoring data
- Screening measurements

Surrogate data

- Exposure data from another agent
- Exposure data from another operation

Modeling

- Predictive modeling based on physical and chemical properties
- Predictive modeling based on process information

Each of these approaches is discussed below.

Monitoring Data

Personal monitoring data: If exposure measurements have been performed, the results may be valuable, especially if the process has not changed significantly. It can help to plot past data over time to determine exposure trends. If exposures are trending higher or lower, the industrial hygienist may choose to use only the most recent exposure data in the assessment. Perhaps, conditions have changed: the previous monitoring data can then serve as a point of reference in estimating current exposures. Further information on generating and interpreting quantitative exposure data is provided in Chapters 6 and 7. Control charts that can help evaluate data trends are addressed in Appendix X.

Screening measurements: If there are suitable direct-measurement methods, screening level measurements may be used to guide the rating process. Techniques such as using detector tubes, photoionization detectors, respirable aerosol monitors, or sound level meters can provide quick results that help calibrate the industrial hygienist's judgment. These screening tools may be used to check "worst case" tasks, or typical exposure levels. Measurement data can clarify work practice variability between workers and between work groups. Screening measurements can lessen or eliminate the need for more costly personal monitoring data. For example, the noise levels in the hypothetical coil coating operation described in Chapter 4 ranged from 82 to 85 dB. If the criteria in Table 5.2 are used with an OEL of 85 dB, an exposure rating of "3" (50%–100% of the OEL) can be assigned to the SEGs in the coil coating operation.

Surrogate Data

Exposure data from another agent: With caution, an industrial hygienist might be able to estimate exposure based on measured data for another agent used similarly in the workplace. Even if exposure conditions have changed, the monitoring data can provide some basis for estimating potential exposures to workers in SEGs. Adjustments based on professional judgment may be made using the following criteria:

- relative quantities of the environmental agent in use;
- frequency and duration of exposure;
- work practices;
- physical and chemical properties of the environmental agents; and
- operating conditions and control devices in use.

Surrogate data are sometimes used when estimating exposures associated with a mixture. The exposure estimate for a selected component (marker substance) may provide a basis for estimating exposures to other components of the mixture. This method, however, should only be used if the industrial hygienist has knowledge and experience regarding the behavior of the individual components in the mixture.

In our hypothetical coil coating operation, exposure data for methyl isobutyl ketone (MIBK) may reasonably be used as surrogate data for assessing exposure to cyclohexanone. Employees use a solvent containing 90% MIBK and 10% cyclohexanone during short duration clean-up tasks. The ACGIH STEL for MIBK is 75 ppm, but there is no ACGIH STEL for cyclohexanone. The industrial hygienist may choose to use a conservative working STEL of 35 ppm, which is 1.5 times the 8-hour time-weighted average–threshold limit value (TWA–TLV). The vapor pressure for MIBK is 16 mmHg and the vapor pressure for cyclohexanone is 5 mmHg. If the measured exposures to MIBK are rated a "2" in accordance with the criteria in Table 5.2, the exposure to cyclohexanone may conservatively be rated a "2" as well.

Exposure data from another operation: The exposure estimate can be based on experience with use of the agent in another operation. For example, in our hypothetical coil coating operation, the Helper's exposure rating for heat stress may be based in part on a prior assessment of the nearby Casting

Operator's exposure to heat. Another example would be the case of an agent with good warning properties (e.g., odor, irritation) with which the industrial hygienist has experience from another operation. Those warning properties might be enough for the industrial hygienist to make an acceptability judgment in the present operation.

Modeling

Predictive modeling based on physical and chemical properties: Models are one way to estimate exposure to chemical, physical, and biological agents.[1-6] The physical properties of electromagnetic radiation, for example, are commonly used to estimate a variety of potentially harmful exposures (such as gamma radiation and laser radiation). Also, it is not unusual to assess heat stress through the use of models based on selected parameters of heat exposure (e.g., wet bulb globe temperature) and the metabolic demands of the task (e.g., kilocalories per hour).

Models are not limited to predicting present-day exposures. They can be used to estimate historical exposures that cannot be recreated, as well as possible future exposures in hypothetical situations. Equipment noise emissions are frequently modeled to assess prospectively the noise exposures associated with the introduction of new equipment into a workplace.

Industrial hygienists must keep in mind that all scientific models, including occupational exposure models, are more or less generalized — crude representations of actual conditions. Thus, predictions from physical–chemical inhalation models to estimate exposures to chemical agents should be interpreted with caution. Results tend to be "order-of-magnitude" estimates rather than fine characterizations of exposures.

Those using physical–chemical models to predict workplace exposures to airborne chemical agents need to recognize and appreciate that the sources of air contaminants, removal mechanisms, transfer mechanisms, and worker interactions are all distributed through time and space. This recognition and understanding, however, does not mean all of these factors have to be treated explicitly or included in every model. Indeed, physical–chemical modeling — like all other aspects of exposure and risk assessment — operates best when used in a tiered approach.

Relatively simple and uncomplicated models are used first and are replaced with more sophisticated tools only if needed. Elementary models are relatively easy to use and require only a minimum of input data. This means they render answers quickly and with fairly low cost; however, they are relatively crude and, if properly constructed, overestimate the exposure and risk. For example, simple models assume steady-state concentrations (e.g., dilution or even no ventilation models) rather than try to describe the time dependence of concentration. Every simplifying assumption reduces the ability of a model to predict fine details of the workplace concentration and exposure gradients. As long as the industrial hygienist confirms that the simplifying assumptions tend to overestimate exposures, the models can be an effective tool for evaluation of worker exposure. Comparing the OEL with this purposeful overestimation of exposure should allow an industrial hygienist to quickly conclude that the exposure is "acceptable" or that more work is needed. The additional work might mean use of a more sophisticated physical–chemical model that requires expanded resources and data to run but renders better (i.e., less overestimating) exposure predictions.

Specific details of modeling tools used in this approach are presented in Appendix I.

Example: Modeling Exposure Estimate

The Discharge Operator knows that the small degreaser uses about 50 mL MIBK in each shift. The degreaser is located in a small QC laboratory (10 ft × 9 ft × 10 ft) adjacent to the coating bay. This lab is ventilated with about 125 cfm of fresh air. A simple equilibrium ventilation model can be used to estimate the MIBK (MW = 100, Sp. Gr. = 0.8) concentration in the room. Since the Discharge Operator never spends longer than 15 minutes in the room every hour, the MIBK STEL of 75 ppm is an appropriate OEL.

$$C = \frac{G}{(Q)(m)} \quad (1)$$

where:
C = concentration
G = generation rate
Q = ventilation rate
m = mixing factor between 0 and 1

Conservative estimates of the MIBK generation rate (G) and the effective ventilation rate (Q)(m) are required for an initial estimate of concentration using this model. A conservative estimate of effective ventilation rate is found by adjusting the mechanical ventilation rate Q by a value of mixing factor m that represents poor mixing (typically 0.1–0.3).

Since use of the degreaser by the Discharge Operator probably accounts for most of the vapor generation, a conservative estimate of G would be one that is based on activity at the degreaser. For this example, we assume the vapor is generated only when the Discharge Operator is in the room. The vapor, therefore, is emitted for only 15 minutes every hour and the activity is repeated eight times per shift.

G = 50 mL/(15 minutes per use)(8 uses) = 0.417 mL/min

0.417 mL/min × 0.8 g/mL = 0.334 g/min

0.334 g/min × 1 mole/100 g × 24.45 L/mole = 0.082 L/min

Q = 125 ft^3/min

125 ft^3/min × 28.3 L/ft^3 = 3537.5 L/min

Choose m = 0.1 as conservative

$$C = \frac{0.082 \text{ L/min}}{(3537.5 \text{ L/min})(0.1)} \times 10^6 = 232 \text{ ppm:}$$

about 309% of the STEL–OEL of 75 ppm

Successful (i.e., protective) application of the tiered modeling approach depends on realistically conservative model inputs. Careful reasoning by the industrial hygienist and documentation of the rationale is necessary before these exposure estimates should be accepted with confidence.

Predictive modeling based on process information: Information management systems that estimate and track multimedia releases to the ambient environment are often used at larger plants and work sites. They represent an opportunity for the industrial hygienist to use an existing system for data relevant to the exposure assessment process. These information systems include process models containing parameters (e.g., material volumes, production times, temperatures, pressures) used to predict air emissions, water discharges, and other waste stream estimates. An enterprising industrial hygienist can leverage this resource, adopting it as a tool for exposure assessment and thereby saving time and money. It could, for example, be useful to examine fugitive emission estimates from a process to see the impact on worker exposure in that process area. This may be a good way to corroborate observations in the absence of industrial hygiene monitoring data, or to identify likely locations of potential exposures.

Physical–Chemical Exposure Models

The construction and use of models is not mysterious; it's simply science. In the context of modeling inhalation exposures for industrial hygiene, we can consider this effort as investigating and seeking to understand the determinants of airborne contaminant source generation and control. As we discern and size the critical variables governing the generation and control of airborne toxicants, we can form the tools that will build our knowledge base and confidence to predict actual concentrations and exposures in the real world with simulated scenarios. As such, model development consists of formulating hypotheses about the predictors of exposure and then testing these hypotheses with data from experiments; it is the scientific method.

As we understand why and how physical–chemical models are developed, we will see that they represent a structural basis for exposure assessment. Physical–chemical exposure models, along with statistical analysis of monitoring data, form the scientific foundation for characterizing worker exposures. Comparing the exposure profile with the OEL provides the basis for risk assessment.

By using a model, an industrial hygienist's insight to possible exposures is enhanced, even if the model is not perfectly accurate. The noted statistician G.W.E. Box has been attributed with the following profound observation, "All models are wrong, but some are useful." Even remarkably elegant and presumably complete and correct basic scientific models such as those devised by Sir Isaac Newton to describe the laws of motion are wrong under certain conditions as described by Albert Einstein. Thus, predictions from physical–chemical inhalation models, which at this point are far from elegant or complete, should be interpreted cautiously.

Most models have not been validated, but limited evaluation of models has demonstrated that model predictions — when carefully constructed (and designed to be overestimating) — can generate results that are within an order of magnitude of measured exposures.

Exposure Rating in the Absence of an OEL

An exposure rating is an estimate of exposure relative to the OEL. In the absence of an established OEL, the industrial hygienist will need to approximate a "working OEL" to rate exposures and ultimately differentiate acceptable from unacceptable exposures. This working OEL can be based on the toxicological information collected during the basic characterization phase.

In our hypothetical coil coating plant, airborne exposures to octochlorostyrene were associated with the fluxing task in the casting process. A formal OEL is not available, and a literature review reveals that octochlorostyrene exhibits a low order of

Table 5.3 — Manufacturing Plant Exposure Ratings

Process	*Job*	*Task*	*Agent*	*Exposure Rating*	*Basis for Exposure Rating*
Coil Coating	Coil Feed Operator	General	Noise	3	Screening measurements
Coil Coating	Coil Feed Operator	General	2-butoxyethanol	2	Modeling
Coil Coating	Coil Feed Operator	Cleanup	MIBK	3	Personal monitoring data
Coil Coating	Coil Feed Operator	Cleanup	Cyclohexanone	3	Exposure data from another agent
Coil Coating	Discharge Operator	General	Noise	3	Screening measurements
Coil Coating	Discharge Operator	General	2-butoxyethanol	2	Modeling
Coil Coating	Discharge Operator	QC	MIBK	4	Modeling
Coil Coating	Discharge Operator	Cleanup	MIBK	3	Personal monitoring data
Coil Coating	Discharge Operator	Cleanup	Cyclohexanone	3	Exposure data from another agent
Coil Coating	Helper	General	Noise	3	Screening measurements
Coil Coating	Helper	Cleanup	MIBK	3	Personal monitoring data
Coil Coating	Helper	Cleanup	Cyclohexanone	3	Exposure data from another agent
Coil Coating	Helper	Lubricate	Packing grease 609	1	Modeling
Casting	Helper	Fluxing	Heat	4	Exposure data from another operation
Casting	Helper	Fluxing	Hexachloroethane	1	Exposure data from another operation
Casting	Helper	Fluxing	Hydrogen chloride	4	Screening measurements
Casting	Helper	Fluxing	Hexachlorobenzene	3	Exposure data from another operation
Casting	Helper	Fluxing	Octochlorostyrene	3	Exposure data from another agent

acute toxicity. Nevertheless, the industrial hygienist decides to take a conservative approach because of the chemical similarity of octochlorostyrene to other slowly metabolized and biologically persistent compounds; a working OEL of 25 $\mu g/m^3$ as an 8-hour TWA is set, by analogy with hexachlorobenzene.

How exposures for each SEG were rated in our coil coating operation is summarized in Table 5.3.

Selecting Occupational Exposure Limits

All exposure assessments are predicated on the availability of an OEL. By providing an abridged answer to the question "How much is too much?" the OEL provides a rational criterion for differentiating acceptable from unacceptable exposures. Accordingly, an exposure assessment cannot be completed in the absence of an OEL unless exposure to the agent is eliminated.

Ostensibly, exposure ratings within the OEL are acceptable and ratings exceeding the OEL are unacceptable. Of course, exposure assessments are not that simple because the quality of OELs varies. Some OELs are formed from a wealth of laboratory and epidemiological data, while others are based on analogy, extrapolation, and judgment. The industrial hygienist must consider the quality of the data supporting the OEL in judging whether to use the regulatory or authoritative OEL, or to adopt a more conservative internal OEL or working OEL. Although regulatory agencies and organizations specify the use of OELs, industrial hygienists frequently have the latitude to use a more conservative standard, or to define an OEL when one is not available (i.e., working OEL). With this freedom, of course, comes accountability for the choice.

In every occupational exposure assessment, in fact, the industrial hygienist must identify the appropriate OEL. He or she might choose to use a regulatory or authoritative OEL, or choose to modify a standing limit by some safety factor if there are weaknesses in the standard's underlying toxicological basis. If an OEL is not available, the industrial hygienist must use available data to establish an internal OEL or set a working OEL. Fortunately, few situations are so devoid of data that an internal or working OEL cannot be formulated. (See sidebar on "Setting Occupational Exposure Limits" on page 77.)

In cases in which few toxicological data are available, working OELs may be only rough guidelines and highly uncertain. In our hypothetical example, the working OEL for octochlorostyrene is highly uncertain. Such uncertainty must be considered when judging the exposure. If the uncertainty in the OEL is high, the industrial hygienist can use appropriately large safety factors to gain confidence that the risk is not underestimated. The safety factors can be applied explicitly in the determination of the working OEL, and they can be factored into the exposure evaluations in the form of worst case modeling. The point here is that the industrial hygienist's "professional judgment" needs to be somewhat visible and based in explainable fact. This can be done by incorporating this judgmental foundation into our best estimate of toxicity and exposure for any scenario for which we are responsible.

There may be situations, hopefully rare, when a working OEL cannot be assigned because enough data are not available. A normal precaution would be that the exposure is too risky and should be controlled aggressively.(7) Exposures could be judged "unacceptable" and then in the absence of an OEL controlled through the maximum use of engineering controls (e.g., enclosed process), work practice controls, and personal protective equipment (e.g., respiratory and dermal protection). Some organizations use this strategy when it is difficult to establish the character or toxicity of the potential workplace exposures: organizations such as research and development, hazardous waste processing, and emergency response activities (e.g., fire fighting).

An interesting approach is the one sometimes used in the pharmaceutical industry when it is difficult to identify the no observable effect level (NOEL) of some drugs and organic byproducts synthesized in production processes. It often is not feasible to fully characterize the toxicity for each ingredient and byproduct, but there is still reason to believe that the chemical agents are biologically active. One system uses basic toxicity information to classify compounds into one of five hazard categories known as "Performance-Based Exposure Control Limits (PB–ECL)."(8) Exposures are then controlled to below rough "exposure control limits" using standard control practices for each category.

The following are considered when setting performance-based exposure control limits:

- Potency (mg/day);
- Severity of acute effects (life-threatening);
- Acute warning properties;
- Onset of warning symptoms;
- Medical treatability;
- Need for medical intervention;
- Acute toxicity;
- Sensitization;

Table 5.4 — General Containment Levels Used in One Pharmaceutical Company (Adapted from Naumann et al.[8])

Category for Performance-Based Exposure Control Limit	General Corresponding Numerical "Exposure Control Limit" 8-Hour TWA	General Corresponding Wipe Test Criteria	Containment Level
1	In the range of 1–5 mg/m^3	In the range of 100 mg/100 cm^2	Good manufacturing practices
2	In the range of 0.1–1 mg/m^3	In the range of 1 mg/100 cm^2	Good manufacturing practices (with more stringent controls)
3	In the range of 1–100 μg/m^3	In the range of 100 μg/100 cm^2	Essentially no open handling (closed systems should be used)
4	In the range of <1 μg/m^3	In the range of 10 μg/100 cm^2	No open handling (closed systems must be used)
5	In the range of 0.1 μg/m^3	In the range of 1 μg/100 cm^2	No manual operations, no human intervention (robotics/remote operations encouraged)

- Alteration in quality of life (disability);
- Likelihood of chronic effect (e.g., cancer, reproductive toxicity, systemic toxicity);
- Severity of chronic effects (life-shortening);
- Cumulative effects; and
- Reversibility.

Once classified, the control practices shown in Table 5.4 should be applied.

Judging Exposures

Following the definition of the exposure profile and the selection of the OEL, each SEG must be judged acceptable, unacceptable, or uncertain. As stated earlier, to resolve the exposure assessment, the industrial hygienist must compare the exposure profile (and its uncertainty) with the OEL (and its uncertainty) to evaluate the risk posed by the exposure (see Figure 5.4).

Early in the assessment process, the initial best guess likely will be based on little or no quantitative data (e.g., monitoring results). Consequently, there may be a great deal of uncertainty in the best guess estimate. This uncertainty may be expressed as

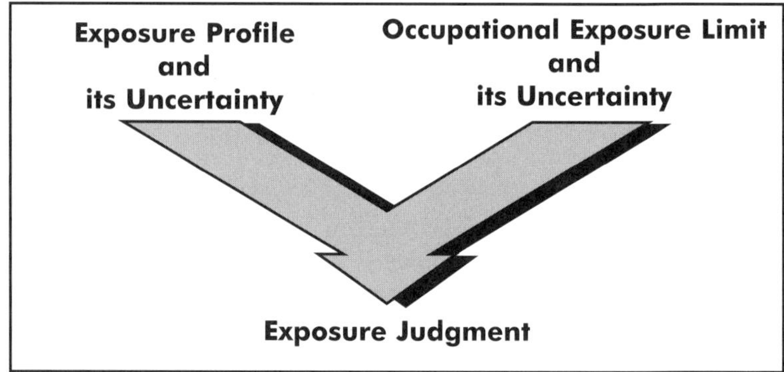

Figure 5.4 — Judging exposures.

a subjective range or intentional overestimate upper boundary — or, in the case of monitoring data, a statistical confidence limit.

Conceptually, we could construct an uncertainty band around the OEL. Given an OEL of 10 mg/m³ as a TWA, for example, we may determine that the real OEL is in the range of 5–50 mg/m³, based on our review of the supporting information and newly developed data.

We could also construct an uncertainty band around the exposure. If the uncertainty band for the exposure is below the uncertainty band for the OEL, the exposure usually will be judged acceptable (see Figure 5.5), and if the uncertainty band for the exposure is above the uncertainty band for the OEL, the exposure usually will be judged unacceptable. If, however, the uncertainty band for the exposure is within the same range as the OEL's uncertainty band, we might not be able to determine whether the exposure is acceptable or unacceptable (see Figure 5.6). In that case, the industrial hygienist must decide whether there is enough concern to classify the exposure as unacceptable and initiate a control program, or whether the existing exposure can continue while additional data are gathered. Further information gathering should reduce the uncertainty bands for the SEG exposure and/or the OEL.

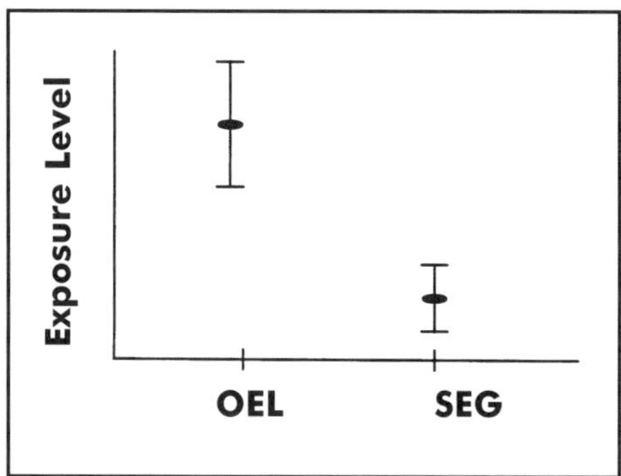

Figure 5.5 — Acceptable exposure.

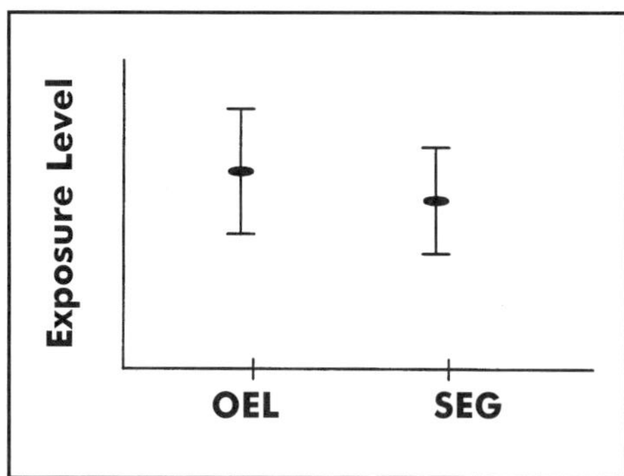

Figure 5.6 — Uncertain or unacceptable exposure.

Setting Occupational Exposure Limits

Some organizations have established procedures for developing OELs when there are no TLVs, WEELs, MAKs, or other exposure limits.[9-11] The development of an OEL can be challenging, especially for organizations with limited resources. Nevertheless, when a formal or working OEL is absent, the exposure assessment cannot be completed.

The health effects information collected during the basic characterization will be used in establishing an OEL. The industrial hygienist should seek technical input from colleagues in toxicology, occupational medicine, epidemiology, etc. — and, if possible, these colleagues should be actively involved in establishing the OEL. Moreover, the OEL should be the driving force for developing the technology needed to assess exposures and comply with the limit. In other words, the OEL should be established without regard to whether an analytical method exists at the sensitivity required by the OEL, or whether the current engineering technologies are sufficient to adequately control exposures below the OEL.

For carcinogens, mathematical models generally are applied to dose-response data and the fitted models are used to predict the risk at a given dose. The probability of observing tumors is believed primarily to be a function of cumulative dose. Many occupational health professionals are familiar with acceptable risk values (developed via cancer risk assessments) ranging from 1 in 1000 to 1 in 10 million.

For noncarcinogens, the likelihood of observing an adverse health effect depends principally on the daily dose. The approach for non-cancer risk assessments generally involves making a qualitative determination that the substance poses an adverse health effect risk and then using an uncertainty (i.e., safety) factor to determine the level of exposure below which that adverse health effect is unlikely to be induced in humans. This approach typically is used when animal toxicity data are available, but it can also be used when human epidemiological data are available. Generally, a NOEL is the value of interest. A NOEL represents the highest exposure level that does not induce the toxicologically significant health effect at a statistically significant rate. If a NOEL cannot be defined, then a lowest observable effect level (LOEL) becomes the value of interest.[12,13]

Depending on the toxicological study and whether a NOEL or LOEL is selected, uncertainty factors are selected to predict the level of exposure at which humans are unlikely to experience adverse health effects. Uncertainty factors are selected to account for uncertainties associated with the experimental design of the toxicological study as well as extrapolation from animals to humans. The U.S. Food and Drug Administration (FDA) developed the uncertainty factor approach and recommends using a 100-fold uncertainty factor as a general method of dealing with lack of extrapolation knowledge.[12,13] This 100-fold uncertainty determinant incorporates a safety factor of 10 when extrapolating from animals to humans and an additional factor of 10 to account for differing sensitivities within the human population. An uncertainty factor of 100 is commonly used with NOELs derived from chronic toxicity studies.[14] In selecting the uncertainty factor to be used with a LOEL, the EPA recommends use of an additional uncertainty determinant (usually between 1 and 10) to account for the fact that no NOEL could be derived, for a total uncertainty factor of 1000 for a LOEL.[13] When setting OELs using a risk assessment approach, consultation with qualified toxicologists and risk assessors is recommended.

When there are no toxicity data on which to base an OEL, one might develop a working OEL based on toxicity data for one or more chemically analogous substances and appropriate safety factors. The safety factor reflects the uncertainty associated with using data on chemical similarity instead of on the compound itself.[15]

Nonroutine Operations

Industrial hygienists often rely more on direct-reading measurement tools to make judgments on nonroutine operation exposures. Contrary to routine operations, for which there may be relatively luxurious amounts of planning and preparation time, the short notice and duration of some nonroutine operations propel us into what could be called "just-in-time" industrial hygiene. That is, we have to rapidly recognize, evaluate, and control the exposure in a matter of a few minutes or hours. Most, if not all, industrial hygienists are more comfortable making these judgments with the assistance of equipment such as direct-reading instruments.

We must anticipate that quick judgments on exposure acceptability will have to be made as the nonroutine operation unfolds. It may be wise to identify "hold points" (i.e., logical breaks in the operation) where the industrial hygienist can collect data or assimilate already collected data. These hold points should be discussed and agreed on with the work crew before starting the operation. This strategy allows an opportunity to assess the effectiveness of engineering controls, prescribed work practices, and personal protective equipment. It provides for a near real-time assessment on the acceptability of the operation's exposures.

Ultimately, the exposure must be judged acceptable or unacceptable, or the cost associated with further information gathering is not worthwhile. In the latter case, the exposure should be classified as unacceptable and controlled as a health hazard.

Acceptable Exposures

An SEG's exposure profile should be found acceptable if its exposure and variability are low enough that risks associated with the exposure profile are low. Whether the average exposure, upper extremes of the exposure — or both — are the important characteristics on which to base the exposure rating depends on the particulars of the situation.

To classify an exposure as acceptable, the industrial hygienist should be confident the probability of adverse health effects is minimal. High confidence in the exposure profile and/or the OEL might permit exposures close to the OEL to be classified acceptable, while less confidence in the exposure profile or the OEL might require exposures to be a small fraction of the OEL in order to have the exposure classified acceptable.

Exposures judged acceptable might not need further immediate action; however, the industrial hygienist may choose to measure the exposure to verify the acceptability judgment and ensure that the exposure does not go out of control.

In our hypothetical manufacturing plant, workers in the coil coating process use a solvent containing methyl isobutyl ketone (MIBK) during a clean-up task. Personal monitoring data are available from a previous exposure assessment and worker interviews indicated that the clean-up has not changed significantly since the samples were collected. Five personal samples were collected to measure short-term (i.e., 15 minute) exposures to MIBK. Four of the five samples were less than 10% of the 75 ppm STEL; one sample measured 20 ppm. The industrial hygienist judges the MIBK exposures to be acceptable; however, there is some uncertainty in the exposure profile because of the low number of samples.

Unacceptable Exposures

Determination of unacceptable exposures is sometimes easier. Usually an exposure would be judged unacceptable if the average exposure (e.g., TWA) or the upper extremes of exposure (peak) were high enough to present an unacceptable risk (i.e., the exposure exceeds the OEL).

Certainly, if there is evidence of adverse health effects associated with the environmental agent, the SEG's exposures should be classified as unacceptable. Consider the example of our coil coating plant. Perhaps the exposure assessment revealed that one heat-related illnesses had occurred among the Helpers engaged in the fluxing task. This history of an illness combined with the observable exposure to radiant heat and the physical demands of the task should lead the industrial hygienist to judge the heat exposure as unacceptable.

The observable presence of skin contact when dermal absorption is a significant route of exposure could suggest an "unacceptable" exposure. The same is true for an observable potential for inadvertent ingestion when ingestion is a significant route of exposure. If, on the other hand, there is an accepted method for assessing exposure through biological monitoring, the industrial hygienist might classify the exposure uncertain and resolve the assessment through a quantitative evaluation of a biomarker. Another option is to consider dermal exposure monitoring.

Obviously, subjective values play a role in judging the acceptability of exposures. A health risk acceptable to one person might be unacceptable to another. The acceptable risk, for example, could vary with the potential health effects. Greater risk may be permitted for an environmental agent associated with transient health effects, while a more conservative approach could be applied to environmental agents associated with severe chronic or irreversible health effects. Risk can be interpreted broadly to include the risk of adverse health effects as well as other exposure-related risks. These might include community concerns, legal liability, regulatory compliance or even aesthetics — many of which could be quite different from an assessment of health risk.

In any event, the industrial hygienist should strive to establish and communicate explicit criteria for acceptable risk. In general, these value-laden judgments should be incorporated into determination of an OEL, and in setting a limit on the proportion of exposures (normalized to the OEL's averaging time) above which the exposure is considered unacceptable.

Uncertain Exposures

An assessment is uncertain when the SEG cannot be classified as acceptable or unacceptable. Enough data might not be available to make a decision with which the industrial hygienist is comfortable. This might occur because the exposure profile is not adequately characterized (i.e, the magnitude and variability of exposure are not well understood and cannot be predicted). It might also occur because a lack of health effects data makes it difficult or impossible to establish an OEL. Both factors impact the amount of uncertainty in the assessment.

In some operations the available data may be so sparse the industrial hygienist is forced to use worst case assumptions to estimate exposure. When this purposely overestimated exposure is well below the OEL, the industrial hygienist should categorize the exposure as acceptable. When the overestimation is greater than the OEL, the industrial hygienist has two options: The situation can be resolved through further information gathering (e.g., exposure monitoring) or the exposure can be declared unacceptable if a decision is made not to investigate further.

In our coil coating plant, significant exposures to 2-butoxyethanol vapor should be unlikely given the chemical's low vapor pressure of 0.8 mmHg. On the other hand, the coating is manually dispensed into a reservoir and skin contact is possible. Skin absorption is a significant route of exposure for 2-butoxyethanol. The exposure is judged uncertain pending the collection of air and/or biological monitoring data.

Managing Uncertainty

The magnitude of the uncertainty associated with exposure assessments is an important consideration when judging exposures. Knowledge that the assessment has integrity or significant gaps in data is critical for exposure assessment.

The importance of uncertainty can be minimal if the agent exhibits low-level toxicity and the likelihood of exposure is low. When the outcome of the exposure is extreme (e.g., irreversible harm), the importance of uncertainty may be high. The industrial hygienist must decide what level of uncertainty he or she is willing to accept.

Scientific uncertainty about exposure has two sources: exposure variability and lack of knowledge. When knowledge or data are nonexistent, the uncertainty may be of such magnitude that the temporal variability is overshadowed. There are many methods of evaluating uncertainty, ranging from a simple subjective estimate to a complicated probabilistic analysis. In general, simple techniques are used initially and more sophisticated techniques (such as Monte Carlo analysis) are used for complicated or critical exposure assessments.(16,17) Uncertainty analysis is addressed in Appendix III.

Approaches using classical statistical analysis can be used to evaluate uncertainty in measured exposure values. For example, the measured values may be used to calculate confidence estimates for percentiles of the exposure distribution. Additional information on statistical approaches is found in Chapter 7.

Resolving Uncertain Exposure Assessments: Cycling Through the Exposure Assessment and Management Process

Uncertain exposures can be resolved in two ways: Additional data can be gathered or the exposure can be categorized as unacceptable and further controlled. The type of necessary data will vary among SEGs. The exposure profile for one SEG may be well understood, but few toxicity data may be available. If so, it is important to collect — or even generate — the needed data. Another SEG may have few available data on which to base an exposure profile estimate. In that case, it is important to generate data to better characterize the exposure profile through modeling; air, noise, or biological monitoring; or other means. If the decision is made not to do further investigation, the exposure must be categorized as unacceptable and controlled below a level that protects workers.

The exposure assessment process derives much of its strength from its cyclic nature. Cycling through the process will tend to strengthen the designation of SEGs, increase confidence in exposure judgments, expand the exposure database, and reduce exposure levels — thus improving employee health protection. The cyclic nature of the assessment process is consistent with

Trigger for Exposure Measurements: 10% of the OEL

Under most exposure conditions, the probability of exceeding the OEL can be held to less than 5% if measured exposures are held to less than 10% of the OEL.[(21)] The exposure conditions include 1) a geometric standard deviation of 2 representing between-day and within-worker variability; 2) a coefficient of variation of 0.1 reflecting random error in the sampling and analytical methodology; and 3) a fairly stable work environment. Trigger levels for other parameters can be determined using the methodologies cited in Figure L-1 in Leidel et al. 1977[(22)] and Equation A-19 in Rock 1982.[(23)] [Please note that there is a typographic error in Equation A-19. The first plus sign should have been published as a negative sign.]

the continuous improvement features of the industrial hygiene management system published by the American Industrial Hygiene Association.[(18–20)]

Threshold for Exposure Monitoring

A threshold of 10% of the OEL is suggested as a trigger for beginning to collect exposure monitoring or modeling data to support the exposure judgment. Whether a particular evaluation that falls between 10% and 100% of the OEL is judged acceptable or uncertain, there is a discernible risk for unacceptable exposure conditions, and this risk escalates with increasing exposure level estimates. Accordingly, generating exposure or modeling data is suggested in this range in order to establish adequate confidence in the exposure assessment.

This exposure monitoring threshold will help drive accrual of data and validate acceptable exposure judgments. To validate the full assessment process, the industrial hygienist should consider randomly measuring a small percentage of SEG exposures (5%–10%) that were rated "<10% of the OEL," in addition to those SEGs for which ratings exceeded the "10% of the OEL" criterion. In judging whether this criterion is exceeded, an estimate of the arithmetic mean or of percent exceedance can be used. Exposure ratings 2, 3, and 4 in Tables 5.1 and 5.2 would exceed the 10% of the OEL threshold.

An example is provided in our hypothetical coil coating operation. The noise exposures were rated a "3" in accordance with Table 5.2. The basis for this rating was positional noise measurement data that revealed levels in the range of 82–85 dB. In many industrial operations, of course, there is significant variability in noise levels during the workday, and frequently there is signifi-

Table 5.5 — Manufacturing Plant Exposure Judgments

Process	*Job*	*Task*	*Agent*	*OEL*	*Exposure Rating*	*Exposure Judgment*
Coil Coating	Coil Feed Operator	General	Noise	85 dBA – 8-hour TWA	3	Acceptable
Coil Coating	Coil Feed Operator	General	2-butoxyethanol	25 ppm – 8-hour TWA, skin	2	Uncertain
Coil Coating	Coil Feed Operator	Cleanup	MIBK	75 ppm – STEL	3	Acceptable
Coil Coating	Coil Feed Operator	Cleanup	Cyclohexanone	35 ppm – STEL, skin	3	Acceptable
Coil Coating	Discharge Operator	General	Noise	85 dBA – 8-hour TWA	3	Acceptable
Coil Coating	Discharge Operator	General	2-butoxyethanol	25 ppm – 8-hour TWA, skin	2	Uncertain
Coil Coating	Discharge Operator	QC	MIBK	75 ppm – STEL	4	Unacceptable
Coil Coating	Discharge Operator	Cleanup	MIBK	75 ppm – STEL	3	Acceptable
Coil Coating	Discharge Operator	Cleanup	Cyclohexanone	35 ppm – STEL skin	3	Acceptable
Coil Coating	Helper	General	Noise	85 dBA – 8-hour TWA	3	Acceptable
Coil Coating	Helper	Cleanup	MIBK	75 ppm – STEL	3	Acceptable
Coil Coating	Helper	Cleanup	Cyclohexanone	35 ppm – STEL skin	3	Acceptable
Coil Coating	Helper	Lubricate	Packing grease 609	5 mg/m^3 – 8-hour TWA	1	Acceptable
Casting	Helper	Fluxing	Heat	Varies with metabolic demands	4	Unacceptable
Casting	Helper	Fluxing	Hexachloroethane	9.7 mg/m^3 – 8-hour TWA	1	Acceptable
Casting	Helper	Fluxing	Hydrogen chloride	5 ppm – ceiling limit	4	Unacceptable
Casting	Helper	Fluxing	Hexachlorobenzene	25 µg/m^3 – 8-hour TWA	3	Uncertain
Casting	Helper	Fluxing	Octochlorostyrene	25 µg/m^3 – TWA working OEL	3	Uncertain

cant day-to-day variability in noise exposures. In view of the uncertainty associated with this variability and the exceedance of the suggested 10% of the OEL trigger for exposure monitoring, the industrial hygienist should consider collecting at least several full-shift noise dosimeter samples through personal monitoring as the next step toward reducing assessment uncertainty. (Note that the OEL for noise in this example is 85 dBA as an 8-hour TWA [3 dB doubling rate].)

Another SEG in our coil coating operation involved application of the heavy lubricant "Packing Grease 609." This exposure was rated little to no exposure above 10% of the OEL. Application of the lubricant involves little to no exposure to hydrocarbon vapors and mist, and the industrial hygienist's workplace observations confirmed little to no opportunity for significant skin contact.

In Table 5.5, the exposures judged for each SEG in our coil coating plant are summarized.

Strategies for gathering and using monitoring data are described in Chapters 6 and 7. These strategies are based on a starting minimum of 6 to 10 exposure measurements per SEG. Initially, it might not be necessary to collect the recommended minimum number of measurements. A smaller number may be adequate to resolve the exposure assessment and judge the risk acceptable or unacceptable. This opportunity will occur with SEGs initially judged uncertain, and when a few exposure measurements reveal levels far below or above the OEL.

Summary

Inputs to the exposure assessment include all available data. This typically means an information base of varying quality and type. The available data may be composed almost entirely of descriptive information with a low level of quantification or it may consist of high grade quantitative exposure data. To make a decision about the exposure profile and its acceptability, the industrial hygienist should analyze and interpret data using professional judgment. Early in the assessment process the level of available quantitative data might be poor and the hygienist will need to base the exposure profiles on professional judgment and make appropriately conservative assumptions to fill in the blanks.

Assessment outcomes are 1) an estimate and understanding of the SEGs exposure profile, and 2) a judgment of the risk posed by the exposure profile (acceptable, unacceptable, or uncertain).

References

1. **Jayjock, M.A., and N.C. Hawkins:** A Proposal for Improving the Role of Exposure Modeling in Risk Assessment. *Am. Ind. Hyg. Assoc. J. 54(12):*733-741 (1993).
2. **Jayjock, M.A.:** Assessment of Inhalation Exposure Potential from Vapors in the Workplace. *Am. Ind. Hyg. Assoc. J. 49(8):*380-385 (1988).
3. **Nicas, M., and R.C. Spear:** Application of Mathematical Modeling for Ethylene Oxide Exposure Assessment. *Appl. Occup. Environ. Hyg. 7(11):*744-748 (1992).
4. **Fehrenbacher, M.C., and A.A. Hummel:** Evaluation of the Mass Balance Model Used by the Environmental Protection Agency for Estimating Inhalation Exposure to New Chemical Substances. *Am. Ind. Hyg. Assoc. J. 57(6):*526-536 (1996).
5. **Nicas, M.:** Estimating Exposure Intensity in an Imperfectly Mixed Room. *Am. Ind. Hyg. Assoc. J. 57(6):*542-550 (1996).
6. **American Conference of Governmental Industrial Hygienists:** *Industrial Ventilation: A Manual of Recommended Practice,* 22nd Ed. Cincinnati, Ohio: American Conference of Governmental Industrial Hygienists, 1995.
7. **United Nations:** "United Nations Conference on the Environment and Development (UNCED)." Rio de Janeiro, Brazil, June 1992.
8. **Naumann, B.D., E.V. Sargent, B.S. Starkman, W.J. Fraser, G.T. Becker, and G.D. Kirk:** Performance-Based Exposure Control Limits for Pharmaceutical Active Ingredients. *Am. Ind. Hyg. Assoc. J. 57(1):*33-42 (1996).
9. **American Conference of Governmental Industrial Hygienists:** *Threshold Limit Values (TLVs®) for Chemical Substances and Physical Agents and Biological Exposure Indices (BEIs®).* Cincinnati, Ohio: American Conference of Governmental Industrial Hygienists. [Published annually.]
10. **American Industrial Hygiene Association:** *Workplace Environmental Exposure Level (WEEL) Guides.* Fairfax, Va.: American Industrial Hygiene Association. [Published annually.]
11. **Deutsche Forschungsgemeinschaft:** *List of MAK and BAT Values: Report No. 32.* Commission for the Investigation of Health Hazards of Chemical Compounds in the Work Area. 1996.

12. "Occupational Exposure to 2-Methoxyethanol, 2-Ethoxyethanol and their Acetates — Section VI. Risk Assessment," *Federal Register 54:* (23 March 1993). pp. 15526–15632.
13. "Air Contaminants. Final Rule," *Code of Federal Regulations* Title 29, Part 1910.54. January 19, 1989. pp. 2332–2929.
14. **U.S. Environmental Protection Agency:** *Guidelines for Reproductive Toxicity Risk Assessment* (EPA 630/4–96/00). Washington, D.C.: U.S. Environmental Protection Agency/Office of Research and Development, 1996.
15. **Fairhurst, S.:** The Uncertainty Factor in Setting of Occupational Exposure Standards. *Ann. Occup. Hyg. 39(3):*375-385 (1995).
16. **Hawkins, N.C., M.A. Jayjock, and J. Lynch:** A Rationale and Framework for Establishing the Quality of Human Exposure Assessments. *Am. Ind. Hyg. Assoc. J. 53(1):*34-41 (1992).
17. **Jayjock, M.A.:** Uncertainty Analysis in the Estimation of Exposure. *Am. Ind. Hyg. Assoc. J. 58(5):*380-382 (1997).
18. **American Industrial Hygiene Association:** *Occupational Health and Safety Management System: An AIHA Guidance Document.* Fairfax, Va.: American Industrial Hygiene Association, 1996.
19. **Redinger, C.F., and S.P. Levine (eds.):** *New Frontiers in Occupational Health and Safety: A Management Systems Approach and the ISO Model.* Fairfax, Va.: American Industrial Hygiene Association, 1996.
20. **Dyjack, D.T., and S.P. Levine:** Critical Features of an ISO 9001/14001 Harmonized Health and Safety Assessment Instrument. *Am. Ind. Hyg. Assoc. J. 57(10):*929-935 (1996).
21. **Roach, S.:** *Health Risks from Hazardous Substances at Work — Assessment, Evaluation, and Control.* New York: Pergamon Press, 1992. pp. 318, 326, 327.
22. **Leidel, N.A., K.A. Busch, and J.R. Lynch:** *Occupational Exposure Sampling Strategy Manual* (DHEW [NIOSH] Pub. No. 77–173). Cincinnati, Ohio: National Institute for Occupational Safety and Health, 1977. [National Technical Information Service (NTIS) Pub. No. PB274792.]
23. **Rock, J.C.:** A Comparison Between OSHA-Compliance Criteria and Action-Level Decision Criteria. *Am. Ind. Hyg. Assoc. J. 43(5):*297-313 (1982).

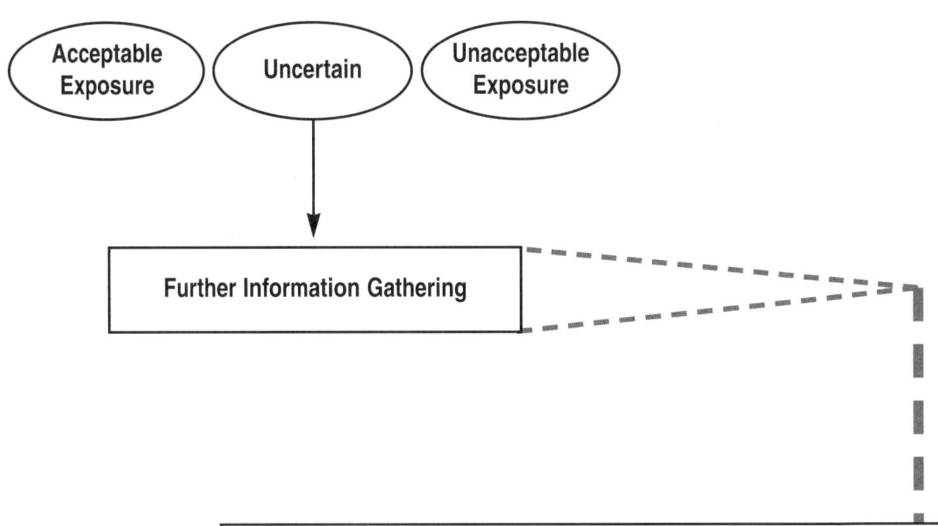

Purpose/Goals

- Prioritize exposure groups for further information gathering.
- Gather or generate additional qualitative or quantitative information so that exposure groups can be better characterized and/or the risk posed by the exposure better understood.

Tools

- Prioritization
  Exposure rating
  Toxicity rating
  Uncertainty rating
- Information gathering
  Qualitative:
  – Exposure modeling
  – Further process/task/job characterization
  – Further health effects data collection

  Quantitative:
  – Air exposure monitoring
  – Dermal exposure monitoring
  – Biological monitoring
  – Epidemiology
  – Toxicology testing
- Validation of exposure assessments
- Diagnostic evaluation of control
- Evaluation of control use and maintenance

Outcome

Information and/or data that can be used to enhance the basic characterization and better define exposure groups, their exposure profile, and the risk posed by the exposure profile

6 Further Information Gathering

In this chapter, the strategies used to resolve uncertain exposure assessments are described. Generally, information gathering is a learning process. The industrial hygienist must continually assess his or her knowledge of the operation, the environmental agent, and the exposure potential in order to determine what additional information is needed to make a confident decision about the exposure profile and its acceptability.

The additional information needed may be about the magnitude and variation of exposures or the toxicity or properties of the agent, the operation being performed, or the work practices. Although this chapter focuses on techniques for quantifying the exposure profile, the reader is cautioned not to overlook the importance of this additional information in the exposure assessment

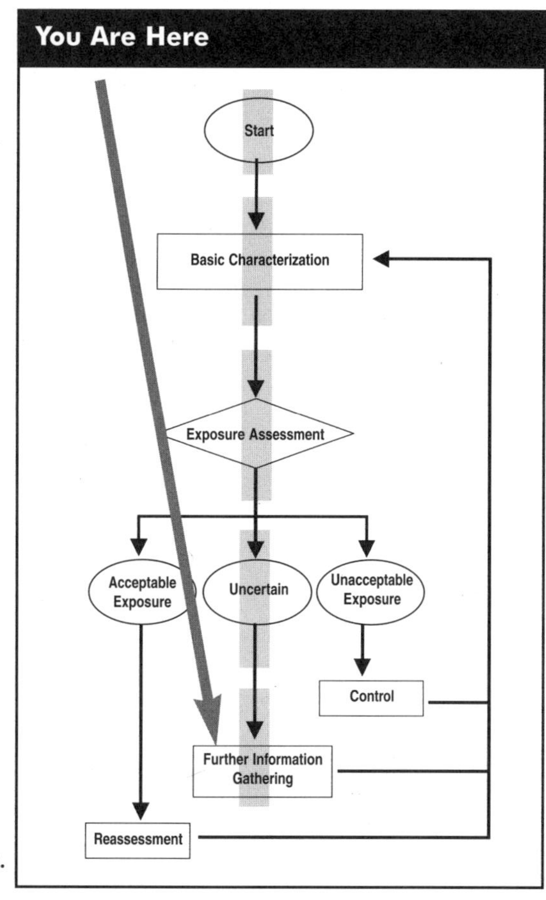

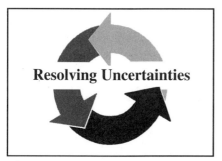

Figure 6.1 — Resolving uncertainties.

process. After all, exposure monitoring might not answer the most important questions for judging uncertain exposures as acceptable or unacceptable.

Prioritizing SEGs for Information Gathering

Some organizations have hundreds, even thousands, of SEGs. Significant time and resources are often required to generate the toxicological and monitoring data needed to resolve exposure assessments that have been judged uncertain. Substantial resources might also be needed to verify the exposure assessments judged acceptable in which the exposure rating exceeds the "10% of the OEL" threshold for exposure monitoring. Prioritization of the SEGs for information gathering is important to ensure that efforts are being focused on those that might present the highest health risk.

Health risk is a function of the exposure level and the severity of the health effect for a given amount of exposure (toxicity). This can be displayed graphically, as shown in Figure 6.2. This simple model allows SEGs to be ranked from low to high potential health risk so they can be assigned priority for action. SEGs ranked so they fall in the northeast corner (upper right side) will

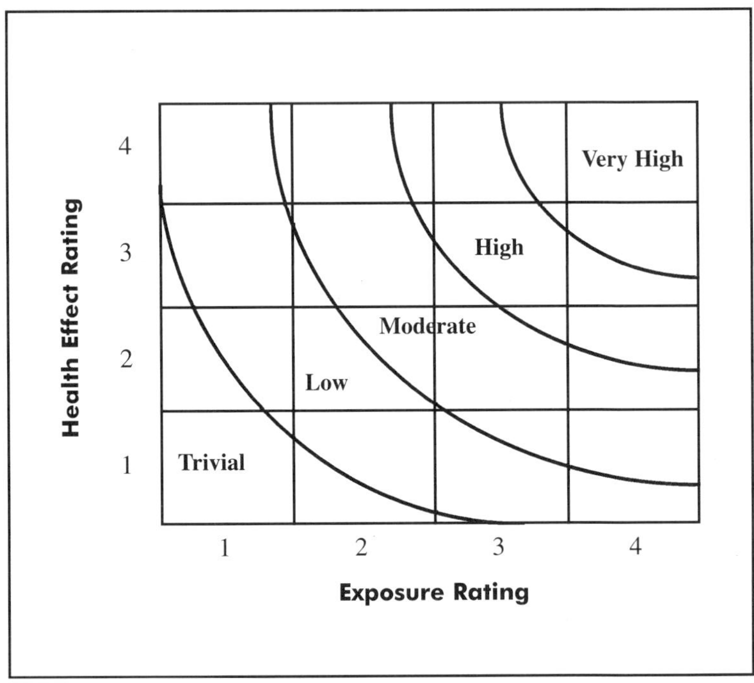

Figure 6.2 — Health risk.

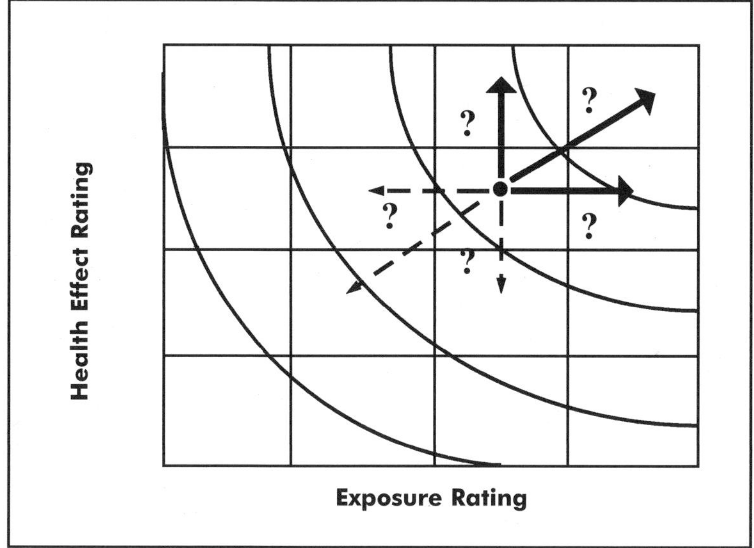

Figure 6.3 — Influence of uncertainty on health risk.

be given highest priority because they represent the highest health risk. SEGs ranked so they fall in the southwest corner of the figure (lower left side) will be given lowest priority for action.

Whether the appropriate action for an SEG is further information gathering or control depends on several factors. Two of the most important are 1) uncertainty associated with the health risk ranking, and 2) resources required either to gather additional information or to control the exposure better. If exposure control is inexpensive relative to the cost of information gathering, the best course may be to reduce the exposure without spending resources on information gathering.

Of course, if the true exposure and the true toxicity associated with each SEG were known, there would be no need for information gathering. Exposure control programs could be prioritized and defined based directly on the health risk defined by the exposures and potential health effects. In the real world, however, estimates of exposure and toxicity are often uncertain — particularly early estimates in a beginning exposure assessment and management program.

Uncertainty adds additional risk because either the exposure or the toxicity may be higher than stated (see Figure 6.3). (They may also be lower than stated, but the precautionary principle demands that the worst-case estimates be used in the absence of complete information.) SEGs with uncertain health risk ratings should be given priority for information gathering. If the health risk rating is not uncertain, then resources should not be spent gathering additional information.

Several schemes have been developed to estimate exposure and toxicity so that health risk can be estimated. These vary from simple descriptive categories and mathematical relationships to elaborate predictive models as typified by some large corporate programs.[1-4] It should be remembered that priority rating schemes are not strictly qualitative nor quantitative; in fact, they generally lie somewhere on a continuum between the two extremes.

A prioritization scheme is nothing more than a "tool" for helping to rank-order SEGs for further information gathering. In Chapter 5, the "exposure rating" was identified as a vehicle for categorizing the exposure associated with a single SEG. However, the context here is not judging the acceptability of exposures for SEGs, but rather prioritizing SEGs for further information gathering. The additional information collected thereafter is then used to resolve uncertain SEGs as acceptable or unacceptable, or it is used to verify SEGs initially judged to be acceptable or unacceptable.

Prioritization schemes are not foolproof reflections of relative risk. The industrial hygienist is cautioned not to overanalyze the prioritization scheme or overinterpret its results. Numerous real world factors cannot be captured by even the most sophisticated schemes. The industrial hygienist should apply his or her full knowledge of exposures in the workplace toward appropriately adjusting the SEG rankings produced by the organization's prioritization scheme.

Which priority-ranking mechanism is used will depend on the particular needs and capabilities of the organization. Perhaps most important is that a standard mechanism be agreed on and used consistently throughout the organization.

A Note on Prioritization Schemes

The methods presented in this text for prioritizing information gathering and control efforts are not perfect or foolproof. They will not place every SEG in its proper rank for follow-up with exact precision. What they will do is provide a first suggestion for priority that will handle large numbers of SEGs in a manner that is both simple and generally representative of risk. In perhaps a more important role, they also serve to illustrate an important message of this text: that exposure assessment results must be used to prioritize industrial hygiene programs and follow-up. We hope they prove to be a catalyst for your own thinking about prioritization mechanisms and are a starting point for developing prioritization mechanisms that work well for your needs.

In this book, a simple three-variable scheme will be used to prioritize information gathering. The three variables are exposure, health effects, and uncertainty. Individual organizations may want to design different ranking schemes that include other variables. These might include:

- Number of workers in the SEG;
- Frequency of exposure (e.g., days per year);
- Frequency of peak exposures; and
- Type of exposure controls.

One Scheme for Prioritizing Information Gathering

Step 1: Assess exposure as a component of risk and determine an exposure rating.

This exposure rating is the output from the assessment step discussed in Chapter 5. As detailed, the industrial hygienist reviews all available information (both qualitative and quantitative) to make a judgment about the exposure profile and to assign it to a category in the exposure rating scheme defined in the assessment program (see Tables 5.1 and 5.2 on page 64).

Step 2: Assess health effects as a component of risk and determine a health effects rating.

Each SEG is assigned a health effects rating based on the toxicity of the environmental agent. Categorizations that were originally published in the first edition of A Strategy for Occupational Exposure Assessment are provided in Table 6.1.[5] Industrial hygienists have several other health effects rating schemes available.[6-9] They should choose a scheme that works well in their own organization. When a scheme is selected, it should be documented in the written exposure assessment program.

Table 6.1 — Health Effects Rating Scheme: AIHA Health Effects Rating

Category	*Health Effect*
4	Life-threatening or disabling injury or illness.
3	Irreversible health effects of concern.
2	Severe, reversible health effects of concern.
1	Reversible health effects of concern.
0	Reversible effects of little concern, or no known or suspected adverse health effects.

The health effects of nonchemical environmental agents (such as noise, radiation, or even biological agents) can also be rated. Classification schemes have been developed for rating the virulence and severity of disease for biological agents.[10] Similarly, the American National Standards Institute (ANSI) has established a rating scheme for lasers.[11]

In the absence of toxicological or epidemiological data for the environmental agent, the health effects rating should be based on the agent's chemical or physical properties and its similarity to other agents with known health effects.

Step 3: Compute health risk rating.

As discussed earlier, health risk is a function of the potential health effect caused by the agent (toxicity) and the potential exposure. After rating health effect and exposure, a health risk rating can be calculated using Equation (1). This is displayed graphically in Figure 6.4.

$$\text{Health Risk Rating} = \text{Health Effect Rating} \times \text{Exposure Rating} \qquad (1)$$

Health Effect Rating				
4	**4**	**8**	**12**	**16**
3	**3**	**6**	**9**	**12**
2	**2**	**4**	**6**	**8**
1	**1**	**2**	**3**	**4**
	1	2	3	4
	Exposure Rating			

Figure 6.4 — Potential health risk (health risk rating = health effect rating × exposure rating).

Health Effects Rating Systems

Many health effects rating systems have been established to provide standardization in hazard labeling of chemical agents and standardization of health risk phrases in material safety data sheets.[12] The European Union (EU) has established standard toxicity classifications for use on labels.[15] Popular rating schemes developed in the United States are NFPA 704 by the National Fire Protection Association[7] and the "Hazardous Materials Identification System (HMIS)" by the National Paint and Coatings Association.[8,9] In the HMIS, chemical agents are categorized into four groups: Classes 0 through 3, with Class 3 the most toxic.

In general, the classification criteria in these systems have more basis in acute, rather than chronic, health effects. The acute health effect criteria are based on lethality (e.g., acute oral LD_{50}, acute dermal LD_{50}, and acute LC_{50} data); however, the American National Standards Institute in ANSI Z129.1 uses a rating scheme for cancer, mutagenicity, and teratogenicity.[13]

A pharmaceutical industry health effects rating scheme known as the "Performance-Based Exposure Control Limits" was discussed in Chapter 5. Health effects rating schemes for occupational exposure assessments have also been developed at Pfizer,[3,14] Union Carbide,[9] and other organizations. Union Carbide uses a health effects rating known as the "Bodily Impact Rating (BIR)." The BIR is assigned to a specific chemical agent, mixture, or process stream. It indicates the material's potential for causing adverse health effects. BIRs range from 0 to 4, with 0 applying to materials that are relatively harmless and 4 applying to materials that are extremely toxic.

The BIR is assigned using specific criteria that emphasize:

- Chronic adverse health effects over acute effects;
- Toxicity over OELs; and
- Toxicity of decomposition products, as appropriate.

Step 4: Assess uncertainty as a component of risk and determine an uncertainty rating.

Uncertainty is a function of 1) confidence in health effects data; 2) confidence in exposure rating; and 3) reliability of existing controls. Just as there are several schemes for rating exposure and toxicity, various other schemes can be envisioned for rating uncertainty — again, ranging from simple descriptive categories to elaborate models that provide a rating based on a variety of inputs:

- Has the operation been observed?
- Has ventilation been measured?
- Are monitoring data available?
- Is there a well-established OEL?

- Is the frequency and duration of the operation known?
- Is information on exposure variability available?
- Is there information on how work practices contribute to exposures?

Each organization should agree on a standard procedure and use it consistently. In this text, a simple three-category qualitative scheme for rating uncertainty is delineated (see Table 6.2). Each SEG's exposure assessment will be placed into one of the three uncertainty categories: 2-Highly Uncertain, 1-Uncertain, and 0-Certain.

In general, SEGs judged acceptable or unacceptable are rated "0-Certain," or perhaps "1-Uncertain," but usually not "2-Highly Uncertain." The 2-Highly Uncertain rating usually corresponds to uncertain judgments made when significant information on the exposure profile or health effects is missing. An exception might be the case in which a decision was made to reclassify an uncertain SEG as unacceptable and implement control procedures because the relative cost of control was much less than the cost of further information gathering.

SEGs are rated 1-Uncertain when there is enough information to make a judgment but further information gathering is warranted to verify the exposure assessment. For example, exposure monitoring data are needed to verify the exposure assessment when the exposure rating is based on no monitoring data and the rating is within 10%–100% of the OEL.

The 0-Certain rating is applied to SEGs judged acceptable or unacceptable. Further information gathering is not needed for the exposure profile or health effects. The industrial hygienist's confidence in the exposure judgment is based on data or conservative models. Knowledge of the exposure profile is based on monitoring data collected on the SEG, or another SEG having similar exposures. Confidence in the OEL is based on toxicological data for the environmental agent or a similar agent.

Table 6.2 — Uncertainty Rating

2	*Highly Uncertain* — The acceptability judgment was made in the absence of significant information on the exposure profile and/or health effects.
1	*Uncertain* — There is enough information to make a judgment, but further information gathering is warranted to verify the exposure assessment.
0	*Certain* — The environmental agent's exposure profile and health effects are well-understood. The industrial hygienist has high confidence in the acceptability judgment.

Step 5: Compute Priority ranking for information gathering. Once the Health Risk Rating and Uncertainty ratings have been established, an information gathering priority rating or index can be calculated for each SEG in the workplace. Simply multiplying the two parameters (see Equation [2]) is sufficient to scale the SEGs for a first cut from low to high priority (see Figure 6.5). Setting priorities for information gathering is particularly valuable when the workplace consists of many SEGs.

$$\text{Information Gathering Priority Rating} = \text{Health Risk Rating} \times \text{Uncertainty Rating} \quad (2)$$

Of course, because the Health Risk Rating is a function of the Exposure Rating and the Health Effect Rating, Equations 6.1 and 6.2 can be combined into one step (Equation [3] and Figure 6.6)

$$\text{Information Gathering Priority Rating} = \text{Exposure Rating} \times \text{Health Effects Rating} \times \text{Uncertainty Rating} \quad (3)$$

Because rating systems can oversimplify the degree of concern, the industrial hygienist should be alert to other factors that may affect an SEG's priority rank. For example, concurrent exposures to two or more environmental agents with additive, or perhaps synergistic, health effects could affect prioritization for

Health Risk Rating	Certain 0	Uncertain 1	Highly Uncertain 2
16	0	16	32
12	0	12	24
9	0	9	18
8	0	8	16
6	0	6	12
4	0	4	8
3	0	3	6
2	0	2	4
1	0	1	2

Uncertainty Rating

Figure 6.5 — Information gathering priority (information gathering priority = health risk rating × uncertainty rating).

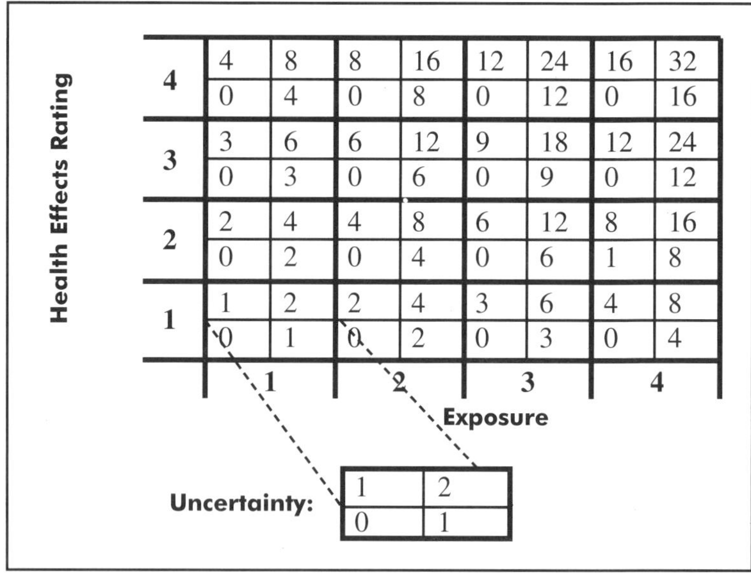

Figure 6.6 — Information gathering priority: an alternative view (information gathering priority = health effect rating × exposure rating × uncertainty).

further information gathering. The industrial hygienist should make a judgment to adjust the initial ranking of SEGs in a manner that is internally consistent and seems reasonably appropriate in light of all the relevant information collected during the basic characterization. When there is uncertainty, conservative decisions erring on the side of health and safety should be made.

At this point it should be noted that exposure control is always an option. If it is believed that considerable time will be needed to gather sufficient information to resolve an uncertain, high risk exposure, then a short-term control (such as respiratory protection) should be recommended in the interim.

There is a point at which controlling uncertain exposures may be a better strategy than further information gathering. It might, for example, be more cost-effective to implement health hazard controls than to generate the additional toxicological data needed to resolve an uncertain exposure. There may also be times when it is more cost-effective to immediately control uncertain exposures than to spend resources attempting to characterize the exposure profile further.

Application of this prioritization scheme in our hypothetical coil coating plant is illustrated in Table 6.3. The Helper's exposure to octochlorostyrene, and the Discharge Operator's exposure to MIBK during the QC task are the highest priority for information gathering.

Table 6.3 — Manufacturing Plant Prioritization for Information Gathering

Process	Job	Task	Agent	OEL	Exposure Rating	Health Effects Rating	Health Risk Rating	Uncertainty Rating	Information Gathering Priority Rating	Information Needed
Coil Coating	Coil Feed Operator	General	Noise	85 dBA – 8-hour TWA	3	3	9	1	9	Noise dosimetry
Coil Coating	Coil Feed Operator	General	2-butoxyethanol	25 ppm – 8-hour TWA, *Skin*	2	2	4	2	8	Air and/or biological monitoring
Coil Coating	Coil Feed Operator	Cleanup	MIBK	75 ppm – STEL	3	2	6	1	6	Air monitoring
Coil Coating	Coil Feed Operator	Cleanup	Cyclohexanone	35 ppm – STEL, *Skin*	3	2	6	1	6	Air monitoring
Coil Coating	Discharge Operator	General	Noise	85 dBA – 8-hour TWA	3	3	9	1	9	Noise dosimetry
Coil Coating	Discharge Operator	General	2-butoxyethanol	25 ppm – 8-hour TWA, *Skin*	2	2	4	2	8	Air and/or biological monitoring
Coil Coating	Discharge Operator	QC	MIBK	75 ppm – STEL	4	2	8	2	16	Air monitoring
Coil Coating	Discharge Operator	Cleanup	MIBK	75 ppm – STEL	3	2	6	1	6	Air monitoring
Coil Coating	Discharge Operator	Cleanup	Cyclohexanone	35 ppm – STEL, *Skin*	3	2	6	1	6	Air monitoring
Coil Coating	Helper	General	Noise	85 dBA – 8-hour TWA	3	3	9	1	9	Noise dosimetry
Coil Coating	Helper	Cleanup	MIBK	75 ppm – STEL	3	2	6	1	6	Air monitoring
Coil Coating	Helper	Cleanup	Cyclohexanone	35 ppm – STEL, *Skin*	3	2	6	1	6	Air monitoring
Coil Coating	Helper	Lubricate	Packing Grease	5 mg/m^3 – 8-hour TWA	1	1	1	0	0	None
Casting	Helper	Fluxing	Heat	Varies with metabolic demands	4	2	8	0	0	None
Casting	Helper	Fluxing	Hexachloroethane	9.7 mg/m^3 – 8-hour TWA	1	2	2	1	2	Air monitoring
Casting	Helper	Fluxing	Hydrogen chloride	5 ppm – ceiling limit	4	1	4	0	0	None
Casting	Helper	Fluxing	Hexachlorobenzene	25 μg/m^3 – 8-hour TWA	3	4	12	1	12	Air monitoring
Casting	Helper	Fluxing	Octochlorostyrene	Working OEL: 25 μg/m^3 – 8-hour TWA	3	4	12	2	24	Toxicological

It is of interest to note that the Helper's exposures to heat and hydrogen chloride during fluxing were judged unacceptable. Rather than collect more information on exposures or health effects, the fluxing task should be given high priority for health hazard controls and low priority for information gathering.

Information Gathering: Acquiring More Toxicology/Process/Worker Information

If the exposure assessment for an SEG is uncertain, additional information on the workplace, work force, or the environmental agents — or all three — is needed.

Traditionally, industrial hygienists have used monitoring data to better understand the exposure profile and help reduce the uncertainty in the exposure assessment. However, a better understanding of the profile alone may not be the most important information needed for resolving some assessments.

The need for additional health effects data probably will occur most frequently, simply because of the extensive number of chemicals used in the workplace and the scarcity of toxicological data on many of them. Complicating matters are questions about additive or synergistic effects posed by concomitant exposures to environmental agents. Epidemiological studies can also be performed to gather more health effects data and resolve uncertain exposure assessments.

As an example, we might consider in our coil coating plant that after further review and discussion it was decided a formal OEL was needed for octochlorostyrene because the fluxing process was also present in several other sites. Toxicologists were consulted, and they recommended a long-term average–OEL of 10 $\mu g/m^3$ in consideration of the slow metabolism and long-term risks of octochlorostyrene exposure. *(The OEL for octochlorostyrene listed in Table 6.3 is therefore changed from a working OEL of 25 $\mu g/m^3$ [8-hour TWA] to an internal LTA–OEL of 10 $\mu g/m^3$.)*

The industrial hygienist may also need to gather more information about the workplace and work force — including information on work practices, frequency and duration of exposures, quantities of materials in use, and exposure controls in place.

Types of needed data include:

- *Material data:* What, for example, happens when you heat this material to 200°C?
- *Control data:* Does the laboratory fume hood have an adequate face velocity?

- *PPE data:* What is the filtration efficiency and service life of the respirator cartridge?
- *Work force data:* Have workers been trained in how to operate the control system?
- *Process data:* How many kilograms of the material are added to each batch?

Exposure modeling may be used to resolve some uncertain exposure assessments. Gathering the information needed for the model parameters might be more cost- and time-effective than exposure monitoring.

Information Gathering: Acquiring More Monitoring Data

Monitoring data are used to help resolve, refine, or confirm the exposure assessment. Monitoring is the measurement of exposure concentrations during a given period. This includes personal monitoring of air contaminants in a worker's breathing zone, noise dosimetry, radiation dosimetry, biological monitoring, and dermal pad monitoring.

Monitoring Objectives

Monitoring objectives or strategies can be broadly grouped into three categories: baseline, compliance, and diagnostic.

- *Baseline:* What is the SEG's exposure profile (i.e., exposure magnitude and variability)? Are the exposures acceptable or unacceptable?
- *Compliance:* Are the workplace exposures in compliance with OELs?
- *Diagnostic:* What are the exposure sources? How do the sources and tasks contribute to the exposure profile?

Blindly hanging a pump on a worker is both inefficient and ineffective for evaluating and controlling critical exposures. Careful thought and implementation of the monitoring program pays large dividends in information gathered and cost-effectiveness.

Baseline Monitoring

Baseline monitoring is used to evaluate exposure levels and their variability (minute-to-minute, day-to-day, etc.) for agents to which workers in an SEG are exposed.(17) Although the exposure profile can (and generally will) be compared with an OEL, the focus should be on obtaining an accurate estimate of the profile. In baseline monitoring, a random sampling strategy to determine the profile for a given period generally is used. If documented properly, baseline monitoring data can be useful for future epidemiological studies.

Compliance Monitoring

Compliance monitoring is used to assess adherence to OELs, often focusing on worst-case conditions. The NIOSH compliance strategy is commonly used.(18) This methodology is based on monitoring the worst case or "most exposed worker." If the worst-case condition or worker exposure cannot be identified by observation, random sampling of workplace exposures can be performed, and statistical analysis can be used to characterize the upper tail of the exposure profile.

Compliance monitoring data collected when a worst-case strategy is used does not characterize the exposure profile. Worst-case monitoring data must be interpreted carefully because these data do not reflect the SEG's "true" exposure profile and, therefore, might not reflect the actual health risk for workers in the SEG.

Diagnostic Monitoring

When trying to identify the exposure source and understand how sources, tasks, and other variables (e.g., production rates) contribute to worker exposure, diagnostic monitoring should be conducted. The results can help the industrial hygienist devise the most appropriate and efficient control strategies for unacceptable exposures.

If the source is from a fixed piece of equipment, area monitoring techniques are appropriate. If the source moves with a worker or depends on individual work practices, personal monitoring techniques are appropriate. In most cases, measurement averaging times should reflect process cycle times rather than OEL averaging times. Using a longer averaging time will simply average out the actual data required for problem identification.

Wipe testing is a form of diagnostic monitoring. The quantity of a chemical agent or radioisotope per unit surface area can be used as a measure of contamination.(19) Surface wipe monitoring and use of colorimetric skin patches can help particularly in evaluating the effectiveness of controls or work practices implemented to reduce dermal exposures.

Choosing the Measurement Method Based on Exposure Pathways

Because of the complexity of the workplace environment, all possible exposure pathways must be considered before a monitoring method and strategy can be selected. The model por-

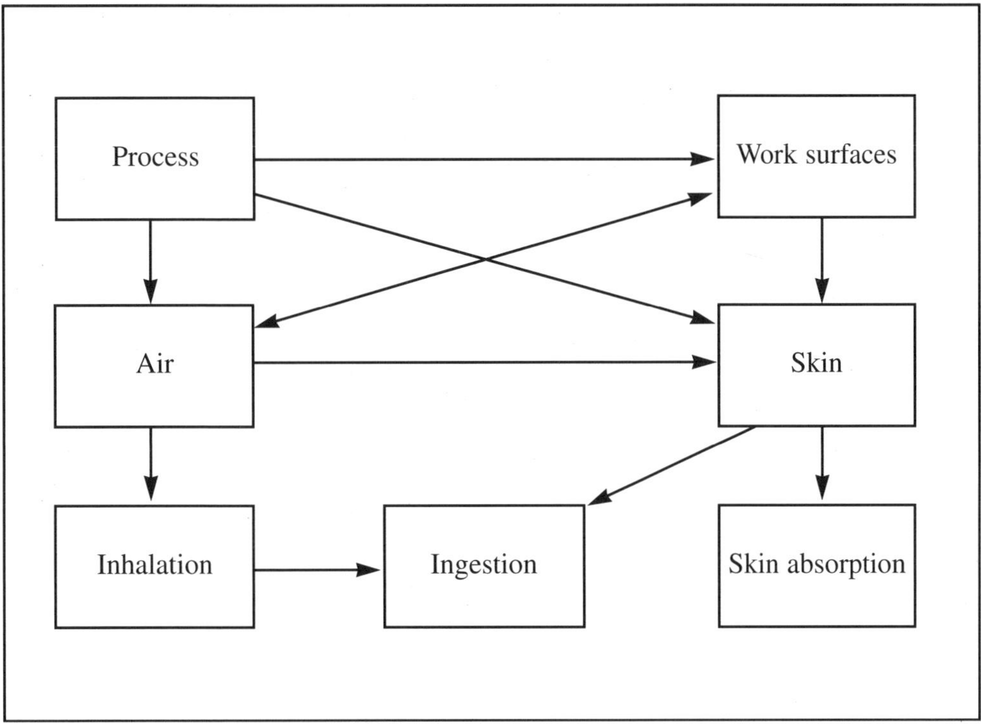

Figure 6.7 — Exposure pathway model.

trayed in Figure 6.7 highlights the potential pathways leading from the process to the worker and provides a framework for evaluating the pathways of each environmental agent. Once an agent is airborne, comes into contact with the skin, or settles onto work surfaces, exposure can occur via inhalation, skin or eye absorption, or ingestion. A model such as the one in Figure 6.7 should be considered carefully for each situation since identification of all critical exposure routes is fundamental when selecting appropriate monitoring methods. For physical and biological agents, similar consideration of exposure pathways is also important (e.g., whole body exposures). Without considering all pathways, an industrial hygienist may overlook a critical exposure pathway.

Inhalation

Inhalation exposure is often the most significant route of workplace exposure. Agents that are released directly into the air may be transported directly into a worker's breathing zone, or settle out and later be resuspended from a surface. Knowledge of the agent's physical properties is essential since the agent may occur in different chemical states at different temperatures and pressures. For highly volatile (high vapor pressure) solvents, it is critical to evaluate inhalation exposure. On the other hand, if an agent has low volatility (low vapor pressure), the primary exposure pathway may be skin absorption or ingestion. Also, physical disturbance of a low volatility agent might result in generation of an aerosol and exposure via inhalation.

Skin or Eye Absorption

For many agents, an important route of exposure is through the skin or eyes. Some chemical agents are able to pass through the dermal barrier and add to any exposures occurring via inhalation or ingestion; some are destructive or irritating to the skin tissue itself. This exposure pathway generally involves contact with the agent directly, or secondarily from a surface that has been contaminated. Biological monitoring may be indicated if there is significant skin contact and skin absorption is a significant route of exposure. Methods for measuring dermal exposure are addressed in Appendix II.

Ingestion

For some agents, such as lead, ingestion can be a significant exposure route. It is, however, usually a relatively minor route of exposure in the workplace, particularly when employees follow a reasonable level of personal hygiene and eating areas are kept clean of contamination. Identification of this pathway as a potential exposure route is usually based on workplace observations.

Exposure Monitoring

Area Monitoring

Area measurements are collected at fixed positions and, therefore, usually do not accurately reflect the exposure of individuals. They can be used to measure emissions from process equipment or background levels of an environmental agent. Area monitoring can be used to determine concentration contours or gradients of agents (such as sound pressure levels) in a room. Real-time area monitoring can be used for a variety of purposes, including the detection (via measurement and alarm) of peak concentrations of acutely toxic agents — particularly those with poor warning properties (i.e., carbon monoxide, hydrogen sulfide). Area measurements can be used in time trend analyses to detect seasonal variation, process cycling, or changes in efficiency of ventilation controls. They also are used principally to support diagnostic monitoring.

More often than not area monitoring is inadequate for exposure assessment, because for area or positional measurements to truly represent exposure workers must be almost stationary (nonmobile). In most SEGs a significant portion of the exposure originates from tasks and the associated near-field exposures. Even in those SEGs in which the exposure originates in the far-field (background), fixed positional measurements are usually inaccurate.

Personal Monitoring

The goal of personal monitoring is to estimate the dose of an environmental agent a worker receives during some period of interest. The actual dose is seldom measurable, so surrogates must be measured for an estimate. The most common surrogates are the worker breathing zone agent concentrations and hearing zone noise levels. The industrial hygienist measures the average level of the agent near the worker's mouth and nose or, in the case of noise dosimetry, near the ear. The measured concentration represents the potential exposure, and the effective exposure is lower if personal protective equipment is worn.

Averaging Times

Measurements should be collected integratively over the OEL's averaging period (eight hours for 8-hour TWAs, 15 minutes for STELs, etc.). If the monitoring duration is less than the OEL's integration period, or less than the full length of exposure in a workday, the industrial hygienist may not acquire an accurate measure of exposure. Extreme care must be taken when extrapolating partial-shift exposure values to full-shift exposures. A significant portion of the 8-hour average exposure may have occurred during the period not included in the monitoring. Short-term monitoring strategies have been developed for assessing compliance with 8-hour OELs.[20,21]

Determining the Number of Measurements Required

The ideal strategy for defining the exposure profile for an environmental agent would be to monitor each worker's exposure each day. Since that generally is not possible, a subset of workers and days (or other appropriate periods) is chosen for monitoring and the results are used to estimate the exposure profile inferentially. Industrial hygienists have long struggled to come up with an acceptable answer to the question: "How many measurements are necessary?" Even today, professional judgment is the predominant way to determine the measurement number. In fact, the number of measurements needed depends on a variety of factors, including the monitoring goal and the SEG's exposure profile. If one measurement result is far below 10% of the OEL threshold or well above 100% of the OEL, that may be all the monitoring required to judge the exposure acceptable or unacceptable. If the exposure profile is highly variable or positioned within the range of 10% to 100% of the OEL, then more samples might be needed to adequately characterize the exposure profile.[22,23]

In the realm of statistical sampling strategies for baseline monitoring, however, a sufficient number of random measurements must be taken to adequately estimate the exposure profile. Monitoring data can then be used to estimate exposure profile parameters such as the arithmetic mean (measure of central tendency) and the standard deviation (measure of dispersion about the mean value).

A review of statistical sampling theory reveals that there is a point of diminishing returns (that is, a certain minimum number of measurements are needed to estimate the parameters with acceptably small uncertainty). Further measurements may provide successively less information, an idea illustrated by the charts in Figure 6.8. These charts were developed using a t-table and an assumed population distribution that is normal. Under those conditions a plateau is reached in estimating the mean and standard deviation after about six to 10 measurements. Fewer than six measurements leaves a great deal of uncertainty about the exposure profile. More than 10 measurements provides additional refinement in estimates, but the marginal improvement may be small considering that cost per measurement is essentially constant. The plateaus indicate that at least six random measurements should be taken for each SEG monitored, unless measured exposures are much less than the OEL (<10%) or greater than the OEL, in which case it may be possible to reach a decision with fewer measurements. A reasonable approximation of an exposure distribution often is possible with about 10 measurements; however, for rigorous goodness-of-fit testing for a distribution, 30 measurements or more might be needed. This is particularly important for exposures near an OEL.

Random sampling

The six (or more) measurements taken to characterize an exposure profile should be acquired randomly from the SEG in order to help ensure an accurate estimate. All commonly used statistical tests assume random sampling.

For a sample to be truly random it must be collected so there is equal probability of selecting any exposure period for any worker in the SEG during the interval of the assessment. A statistically

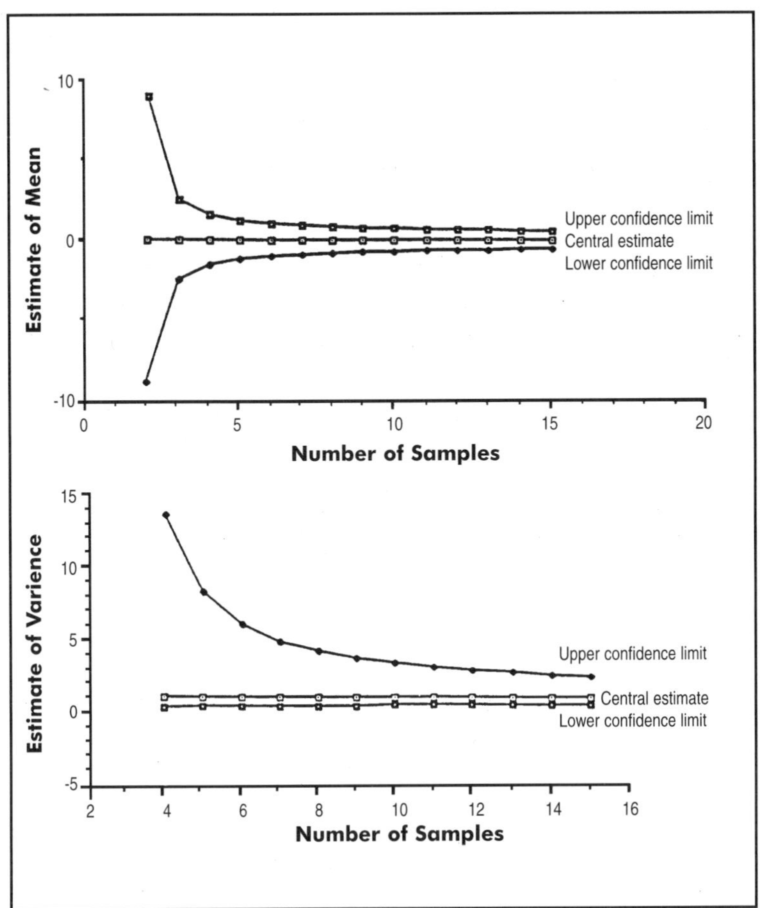

Figure 6.8 — Effect of sample size on estimating population mean and standard deviation.

valid random sampling strategy would use a source of random numbers to select monitoring dates, work shifts, and individual workers in the SEG.

Unfortunately, there are numerous real world constraints that affect monitoring schedules and priorities, thereby making true random sampling in a statistical sense very difficult. The real world constraints that may preclude random sampling include business schedules, logistical problems, limitations in the availability of technicians for sample collection, holidays, and even the weather.

One step-by-step approach to random sampling for exposure monitoring would proceed as follows:

1. Identify the appropriate interval for the exposure assessment.
2. Identify the OEL's appropriate averaging time.
3. Randomly choose dates from the exposure interval during which monitoring will be performed.

4. Randomly choose work shifts from each date for monitoring.
5. Randomly choose workers from the SEG for monitoring during the chosen shift.
6. If appropriate to the OEL's averaging time (e.g., STEL or ceiling limit), randomly choose high-exposure tasks during the shift for monitoring.

In baseline monitoring, the exposure assessment interval is the time span during which the SEG's exposure profile remains largely unchanged (i.e., it is "stationary.") Certainly there is minute-to-minute, hour-to-hour, and day-to-day variation in exposure levels. Over the long term, however, the average exposure level and variability remain constant. The interval over which the exposure profile remains constant will depend on many factors and could last for only a few hours to several years.

Sometimes the industrial hygienist is unable to predict how long the exposure profile will remain unchanged, especially if there are no plans to change the process, tasks, engineering controls, etc. Accordingly, the exposure assessment interval should be long enough to accurately measure exposure level variability; however, the period should not be so long as to unreasonably delay identification of unacceptable exposures.

Within the interval over which the profile remains stationary many exposure periods relevant to the OEL averaging time are possible. For an OEL with an 8-hour averaging time, there should be several possible 8-hour exposures of interest to the exposure assessment. When using a random sampling approach to decide which of those possible 8-hour exposures will be measured, each potential combination must be just as likely to be chosen as any other.

The industrial hygienist should strive to randomize sample collection as much as possible. Although it might not be possible to select dates randomly over the exposure assessment interval, monitoring dates should be designated with little to no regard for operating conditions and events that would directly bias the results. The industrial hygienist should also strive to avoid clustering the samples over a short period (e.g., one week), especially when there are exposure variations caused by production rates and other factors.

Selection of work shifts follows selection of monitoring dates. The selection process is easy if there is only one work shift per day, but in many places the employees in a SEG may work two or three different shifts during a 24-hour period. Again, the ideal strategy would be to use a source of random numbers to select the shifts for monitoring; however, technician resources for sample collection generally are more available on the day shift. It might be reasonable to collect samples on the day shift and assume these samples also represent the evening and night shifts — if there is no discernible difference between operations across shifts and if employees work a rotating shift schedule. Be extremely careful when making these decisions, however. Even changes in the supervision level from shift to shift can significantly impact employee behavior and exposures.

Day shift-only monitoring is not sufficient if there are significant differences between shifts that might affect exposure levels. In this case the industrial hygienist should try to schedule monitoring in a way that allows each work shift to have an equal likelihood of being selected for monitoring.

In many workplaces, employees work "straight" shifts (that is, those on the day shift remain on the day shift, and those on the evening shift remain on the evening shift; workers do not rotate across work shifts). The industrial hygienist should be especially cautious in the presence of a straight shift work force. At the least, each work shift should be given an equal likelihood of being selected for monitoring. It is not uncommon for ostensibly identical operations to be performed differently on the evening or night shift, perhaps as a result of differences in production rates or work practices. Accordingly, it might be determined by observation or by sampling that each work shift is a separate SEG.

Selection of individual workers usually follows selection of monitoring dates and work shifts. Again, the ideal strategy would be to use a source of random numbers to select individual workers for monitoring. A good practice is to randomly select workers before the beginning of the work shift so interested and disinterested workers do not bias the assessment. It is important to avoid selection practices that might bias the exposure values. Volunteers who are too interested or zealous might bias the assessment, especially if work practices can significantly affect exposure levels.

It is even more difficult to collect random samples when the exposure occurs intermittently (i.e., it does not occur daily). Despite the limitations, insight into the temporal variation in exposure levels is just as important for intermittent tasks as it is for daily tasks.

If the OEL is an STEL with a 15-minute averaging time, then there will be many possible 15-minute worker exposures within the time interval of interest to the SEG exposure assessment. When other information is absent to help the industrial hygienist focus his or her monitoring efforts, a random monitoring approach would demand that every 15-minute period have an

Nonroutine Operations

Exposure assessment during nonroutine operations usually means collecting the minimum number of measurements required to support the industrial hygienist's judgment on the acceptability of exposures. Random sampling is usually not part of the plan when assessing nonroutine operations, but there are opportunities for the astute industrial hygienist to use random sampling. If a task is going to last for a sufficient number of days, you may choose to perform random sampling and collect a satisfactory number of measurements so you can perform statistical analyses. For example, you may be evaluating an operation in which workers are using a plasma arc cutting torch to dismantle a stainless steel exhaust ventilation system that will take several weeks to complete. Based on monitoring with a direct-reading instrument for several days, you know that carbon monoxide is present in the 10–20 ppm range. A random sampling scheme can be designed and implemented to collect enough 8-hour TWA data so that the mean and variability can be depicted.

equal likelihood of being chosen for monitoring.

Fortunately, it usually is possible for the industrial hygienist to use professional judgment to predict which of the tasks performed during the day are most likely to result in the highest 15-minute exposure. However, within the interval of the exposure assessment (which could be days or many months) that task will probably occur many times. A random sampling approach would ensure that each of the many repetitions of the high-exposure task was just as likely to be monitored as any other and that each worker performing the task at the time chosen was just as likely to be monitored.

In maintaining an exposure database, it is critical to segregate monitoring data collected by a baseline random sampling strategy from exposure data collected by worst-case and diagnostic strategies. Mixing randomly collected data with nonrandomly collected data will result in a distorted exposure profile.

Biological Monitoring

When available, toxicokinetic models and validated biological monitoring techniques permit the collection of biological specimens (e.g., urine, blood, or exhaled air) for the detection of the chemical agent or its metabolite. These provide an indication of past or current chemical exposure.

Biological monitoring results can reflect the integrated exposure of all pathways and thereby give a more accurate indication of absorbed dose than air contaminants measured in a worker's breathing zone.[24] Biological monitoring should be considered when skin absorption or inadvertent ingestion are significant routes of exposure, or when available air monitoring metrics are weak or not established.[24] Biological monitoring should not supplant workplace environmental monitoring. In general, the worker should not be used to assess the work environment.

The confidentiality of biological monitoring data should be considered. If biological monitoring data are collected to support an industrial hygiene exposure assessment, they may be considered exposure data and generally not subject to medical confidentiality. (Some governmental laws and regulations require that confidentiality practices be applied to industrial hygiene exposure data.) To avoid an expectation of confidentiality, when biological samples are collected by an organization's medical staff or the laboratory results are reported by the medical staff, workers should be advised that the data are not medical records per se and are not subject to confidentiality.

Records that disclose the nature of a worker's health (e.g., audiometric data, pulmonary function data, etc.) are medical records and are subject to medical confidentiality. If health care providers collect biological monitoring data to help assess an individual worker's health condition, they should be considered medical data — subject to the customary confidentiality practices.

Biological monitoring should be performed only with validated methods so that results can be compared with biological OELs.[25] Validated methods specify appropriate collection times based on the chemical agent's toxicokinetics. If the agent's biological half-life is short (e.g., less than 5 hours) then collection should be performed prior to the shift and at the end of the shift. If the agent or its metabolites accumulate over the course of a workweek, collection should be conducted at both the beginning and end of the week.[24]

Dermal Monitoring

Dermal exposure pads can be used to measure the amount of a chemical agent deposited on the skin. Dermal monitoring pads can be used for quantitatively assessing exposure to nonvolatile liquids. For dermal exposure to pesticides, however, whole body (whole garment) assessments are considered superior to pad sampling techniques,[26] based on the uncertainty in extrapolating the amount collected on the pad to the surface area of skin.

Other dermal exposure assessment techniques include rinsing the hands or gloves with water or another collection media and then measuring the amount rinsed from the hands.[27]

Fluorescent methods have also been used to estimate the potential for dermal contact.[28] Data interpretation can be complicated because the measured chemical is a surrogate for the actual exposure.

Wipe tests are also used to assess indirectly the potential for skin contact with work surfaces. Wipe tests are a quantitative means for determining trends in work practices and housekeeping procedures (e.g., cleanliness of lunchroom areas).[19,29,30] Wipe tests can be used diagnostically to measure the relative concentration of surface contamination throughout a workplace and to measure trends in the concentration of contamination on a given surface over time. More information on dermal exposure assessment is provided in Appendix II.

Summary

The prioritization of SEGs for further information gathering is based on exposure, potential health effects, and uncertainty. The additional information needed to resolve an uncertain exposure might include information about the exposure profile as well as information on potential agent health effects. For cases where further information is needed on the exposure profile, monitoring strategies are selected and applied in view of the underlying exposure assessment objectives and critical exposure pathways. The outcome is the prioritized collection of information needed to resolve uncertain exposure assessments. The next step is to examine the information for decision making, perhaps using statistical tools to help evaluate monitoring data. Described in Chapter 7 are decision-aiding tools that can be applied to exposure monitoring data in order to assist in evaluating whether exposures (and, therefore, health risks) are acceptable or unacceptable.

References

1. **Norwood, S.K., M.G. Ott, C.N. Park, and G.C. van Beck:** "Optimizing Sampling Strategies by Combining Traditional and Statistical Approaches." Paper presented at the American Industrial Hygiene Conference, Philadelphia, Pa., May 1983.
2. **Nelson, T.J., and S.W. Dixon:** "Management of Air Sampling Results." Paper presented at the American Industrial Hygiene Conference, Philadelphia, Pa., May 1983.
3. **Tait, K.:** The Workplace Exposure Assessment Expert System (WORKSPERT). *Am. Ind. Hyg. Assoc. J. 53(2):*84-98 (1992).

4. **Holzner, C.L., R.B. Hirsh, and J.B. Perper:** Managing Workplace Exposure Information. *Am. Ind. Hyg. Assoc. J. 54(1):*15-21 (1993).
5. **Hawkins, N.C., S.K. Norwood, and J.C. Rock:** *A Strategy for Occupational Exposure Assessment.* Akron, Ohio: American Industrial Hygiene Association, 1991.
6. **Wass, T.L.:** "An Approach to the Process Characterization — Exposure Risk Assessment and Prioritization." Paper presented at the American Industrial Hygiene Conference & Exposition, Kansas City, May 1995.
7. **National Fire Protection Association:** *Standard System for the Identification of the Fire Hazards of Materials* (NFPA 704), Quincy, Mass.: National Fire Protection Association, 1994.
8. **National Paint and Coatings Association:** "Hazardous Materials Identification System (HMIS)." National Paint and Coatings Association, 1500 Rhode Island Avenue, N.W., Washington, DC 20005.
9. **Henry, B.J., and K.L. Schaper:** PPG's Safety and Health Index System: A 10-Year Update of an In-Plant Hazardous Materials Identification System and Its Relationship to Finished Product Labeling, Industrial Hygiene and Medical Programs. *Am. Ind. Hyg. Assoc. J. 51(9):*475-484 (1990).
10. **Centers for Disease Control and Prevention:** *Classification of Etiologic Agents on the Basis of Hazard.* Atlanta, Ga.: Centers for Disease Control and Prevention/Office of Biosafety, 1976.
11. **American National Standards Institute:** *American National Standard for the Safe Use of Lasers* (ANSI Z136.1–1993). New York: American National Standards Institute, 1993.
12. **Ignatowski, A.J., J.D. Hamilton, and E.D. Weiler:** Review of International Criteria and Mixture Rules for Health Hazard Classification. *Regul. Toxicol. Pharmacol. 22:*231-242 (1995).
13. **Sowinski, E.J., et al.:** Criteria for Identifying and Classifying Carcinogens, Mutagens and Teratogens. *Regul. Toxicol. Pharmacol. 7:*1-20 (1987).
14. **Tait, K.:** The Workplace Exposure Assessment Workbook. *Appl. Occup. Environ. Hyg. 8(1):*55-68 (1993).
15. **The Council of the European Communities:** "Council Directives on the Minimum Safety and Health Requirements Regarding the Protection of Workers from Risks Related to Exposure to Biological, Chemical and

Physical Agents" (Directive 80/1107/EEC [O.J. L 327]). *Off. J. European Communities,* 27 November 1980.
— 67/548/EEC (27 June 1967)
— 88/379/EEC, Council Directive (7 June 1988)
— 88/379/EEC (7 June 1988)
— 91/155/EEC (5 May 1991)
— 91/115/EEC, Annex V 3.1.1 (1 March 1991)
— 91/115/EEC, Supplemental Council Directive (5 March 1991)
— 92/32/EEC (1993)

16. **Booher, L.E.:** "Exposure Assessment — Hurdling the Barriers." Paper presented at the American Industrial Hygiene Conference & Exposition, Washington, D.C., May 1996.
17. **Damiano, J.:** A Guideline for Managing the Industrial Hygiene Sampling Function. *Am. Ind. Hyg. Assoc. J. 50(7):*366-371 (1989).
18. **Leidel, N.A., K.A. Busch, and J.R. Lynch:** *Occupational Exposure Sampling Strategy Manual* (DHEW [NIOSH] Pub. No. 77–173). Cincinnati, Ohio: National Institute for Occupational Safety and Health, 1977. [National Technical Information Service (NTIS) Pub. No. PB274792.]
19. **Klingner, T.D., and T. McCorkle:** The Application and Significance of Wipe Samples. *Am. Ind. Hyg. Assoc. J. 55(3):*251-254 (1994).
20. **Nicas, M., and R.C. Spear:** A Task-Based Statistical Model of a Worker's Exposure Distribution: Part I — Description of the Model. *Am. Ind. Hyg. Assoc. J. 54(5):*211-220 (1993).
21. **Nicas, M., and R.C. Spear:** A Task-Based Statistical Model of a Worker's Exposure Distribution: Part II — Application to Sampling Strategy. *Am. Ind. Hyg. Assoc. J. 54(5):*221-227 (1993).
22. **Hewett, P.:** Sample Size Formulae for Estimating the True Arithmetic or Geometric Mean of Lognormal Exposure Distributions. *Am. Ind. Hyg. Assoc. J. 56(3):*219-225 (1995).
23. **British Occupational Hygiene Society:** *Sampling Strategies for Airborne Contaminants in the Workplace* (Technical Guide No. 11) by I.G. Guest, J.W. Chessie, R.J. Gardner, and C.D. Money. Leeds, United Kingdom: H & H Scientific Consultants Ltd., 1993.
24. **American Conference of Governmental Industrial Hygienists:** *Topics in Biological Monitoring.* Cincinnati, Ohio: American Conference of Governmental Industrial Hygienists, 1996.

25. **American Conference of Governmental Industrial Hygienists:** *Documentation of the Threshold Limit Values and Biological Exposure Indices*. Cincinnati, Ohio: American Conference of Governmental Industrial Hygienists, 1995.
26. **Chester, G.:** Evaluation of Agricultural Worker Exposure to, and Absorption of, Pesticides. *Ann. Occup. Hyg. 37(5):*509-523 (1993).
27. **Fenske, R.A., and C. Lu.:** Determination of Handwash Removal Efficiency: Incomplete Removal of the Pesticide Chlorpyrifos from Skin by Standard Handwash Techniques. *Am. Ind. Hyg. Assoc. J. 55(5):*425-432 (1994).
28. **Fenske, R.A.:** Dermal Exposure Assessment Techniques. *Ann. Occup. Hyg. 37(6):*687-706 (1993).
29. **McArthur, B.:** Dermal Measurement and Wipe Sampling Methods: A Review. *Appl. Occup. Environ. Hyg. 7(9):*599-606 (1992).
30. **Ness, S.A.:** *Surface and Dermal Monitoring for Toxic Exposures.* New York: Van Nostrand Reinhold, 1994.

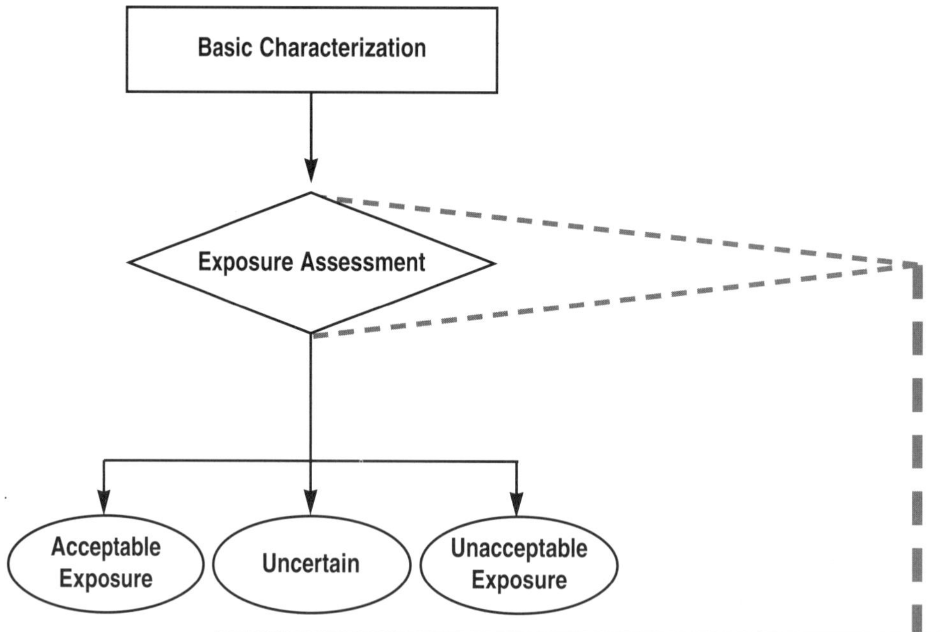

Purpose/Goals

- Make judgment about the acceptability of the exposure profile.
- Refine SEGs and their exposure profiles.

Tools

- Exposure judgment based on the interpretation of available qualitative and quantitative data:
  - Exposure profile
  - Exposure rating
  - Training and experience
  - Monitoring data
  - Statistical tools
    - Descriptive statistics
    - Probability plots
    - Tolerance limits
    - Exceedance fraction
    - Confidence limits on the mean exposure
    - Nonparametric tolerance limits
    - Control charts
- Refining SEGs:
  - ANOVA analysis of within- and between-worker variability

Outcome

- Refined SEGs
- Exposure profile for each exposure group
- Judgment about the acceptability and the uncertainty of the exposure profile for each exposure group

7

Quantitative Exposure Data: Interpretation, Decision Making, and Statistical Tools

The information gathered for the exposure assessment must be interpreted to make two decisions:

- Is the SEG's exposure profile (exposure and its variability) adequately characterized?
- Is the exposure profile acceptable?

Information needed to make these decisions will change depending on the purpose of the exposure assessment. A baseline exposure assessment requires characterization of the SEG's exposure profile. A compliance-based program will focus efforts on exposures near OELs.

As has been noted in previous chapters, not all exposure assessments require collection of quantitative data. If monitoring data are collected, however, statistical tools can help aid in understanding the monitoring data to form a better "picture" of the exposure profile. This better understanding of the data is then used, along with other factors, to aid in judging the exposure profile's acceptability.

If a well-planned strategy is followed for gathering the data needed to assess exposures, interpretation is usually not difficult. The difficult part is setting up good SEGs, gathering the appropriate information to

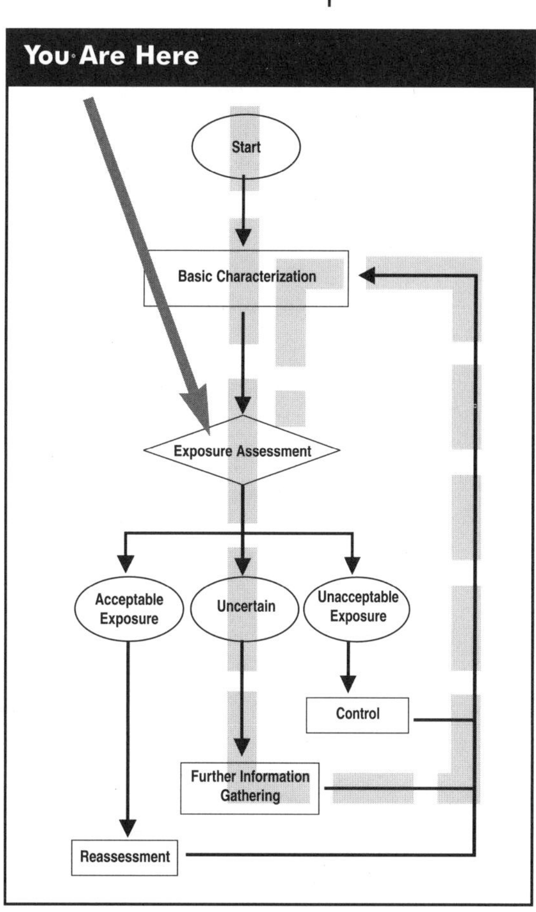

aid the judgment, and — if quantitative data are needed — developing a monitoring strategy that will answer the appropriate questions. Done properly, this "up front" work makes the interpretation process more straightforward and unbiased. The industrial hygienist must have basic knowledge of the qualitative and quantitative data limitations, statistical tools, and other aids to judgment that will be included in the assessment.

Exposure Profile

An exposure profile is a summary "picture" of the exposures experienced by an SEG. This would include an understanding of the central tendency of the exposures (such as the mean exposure) and some understanding of the breadth, or variability, of the exposures (such as the minimum and maximum exposures, or the frequency with which the exposures exceed the OEL).

Just as an industrial hygienist's confidence in a professional judgment increases with process experience, confidence in monitoring results increases as more measurements are made. The fewer the measurements, the less confident we are that the limited "picture" of the exposure profile really represents the true distribution. Exposure variability is particularly hard to estimate with few measurements, and trying to make a good and useful estimate about the extremes of the distribution (e.g., the upper tail of the exposure profile) is nearly impossible with only a few measurements unless they are conducted using a strategy of monitoring "worst-case" conditions. Identifying the worst-case conditions requires judgment based on a qualitative understanding of exposures and factors that influence their variability.

Exposure "Acceptability"

The characterized exposure profile is used to determine whether the risk posed by the exposure is acceptable. Risk can be interpreted broadly to include other exposure-related risks in addition to the risk of adverse health effects. These may include employee or community concerns, legal liability, or even regulatory compliance — which can be quite different from a good assessment of health risk.[1]

It should be noted that the original exposure assessment objectives, the decisions defining acceptability, and the chosen monitoring strategies will influence the types of risks that can be assessed. If the exposure assessment objectives were limited to determining compliance or noncompliance with governmental standards, then the information collected might not have much use for evaluating other types of industrial hygiene-related risks.

Exposure Acceptability Judgments

As discussed in Chapter 5, three judgments can be made about the acceptability of an SEG's exposure profile: 1) It is acceptable; 2) It is unacceptable; or 3) The exposure assessment is uncertain because there is not enough information available to make a judgment (e.g., the exposure profile has not been adequately characterized, or there is limited toxicity data on the agent).

Inputs to Judgment

A variety of tools are available for aiding the judgment — with varying degrees of sophistication and cost. Good exposure assessment uses the right combination of tools needed to efficiently make an adequate characterization of the exposure profile to answer the relevant questions of risk.[2] Among the tools and factors available to aid and influence the judgment are:

- Process experience;
- Material characteristics;
- Toxicity knowledge;
- Work force characteristics;
- Frequency of task;
- Frequency of peak excursions;
- Monitoring results;
- Statistical tools;
- Confidence in exposure limit;
- Modeling techniques;
- Biological monitoring; and
- Availability and adequacy of engineering controls.

The application and importance of most of these elements should be familiar to practicing industrial hygienists. They are discussed elsewhere in this book and in other basic industrial hygiene texts.

Professional judgment is critical for interpretation and use of these factors and tools. Even the statistical tools require professional judgment to be used and interpreted properly. Judgment is needed to set up the sampling strategy, choose appropriate statistical tools, and interpret the results of the statistical analysis.

Statistics often rely on assumptions and rules. Judgments must be made on how well those assumptions and rules have been met by the data being interpreted. The constraints for formal reliance on statistics alone can be difficult to meet when typical industrial hygiene methods are used. The requirements of randomization can be especially challenging.

Judgment and consideration of other factors such as material toxicity, confidence in the OEL, and process characteristics must also be used to determine the difference between statistical and practical significance. It may be possible to determine that an average exposure to chemical "X" (LTA–OEL = 100 ppm) was 95 ppm with a statistical 95% upper confidence limit of 98 ppm. You would then be 95% sure that the average exposure was below the 100 ppm exposure limit. From a practical standpoint, however, you might find the risk unacceptable because of concerns about the lack of an adequate safety factor in the exposure limit.

It is therefore incumbent on the industrial hygienist to be familiar with the uses and limitations of statistical tools so they can be properly chosen to assist in good judgment of risk rather than used improperly to make bad judgments.

Much of the remainder of this chapter focuses on the proper use of statistical tools for summarizing and interpreting data. It should be noted, however, that this is not a statistics primer. References are provided to help industrial hygienists fulfill their obligation to become more statistically literate.

Statistical Considerations

Statistical tools are powerful only if their theoretical bases and limitations are understood by the person using them. The practicing industrial hygienist must know statistical fundamentals well. Without knowing these fundamentals (e.g., confidence interval, tolerance limit, basic probability distribution characteristics) the industrial hygienist cannot evaluate the basic assumptions underlying statistical tools and might end up using them incorrectly.

Statistical issues must be considered early in the assessment process. They should be included in the development of the exposure assessment strategy and when determining a monitoring strategy.

The rules for applying statistical analysis techniques to data are fairly strict and, as a practical matter, may be more difficult to meet in industrial hygiene than in other scientific endeavors. The requirements for random sampling, in particular, may present severe roadblocks. Also, typical industrial hygiene data sets can be said to be approximated by a particular distribution, but usually there is insufficient data to verify the true distribution.

Nevertheless, our goal should be to ensure as much as possible that measurements are collected randomly and that data reasonably conform to the appropriate distribution. Inferences made with statistical tools must be considered carefully. Professional judgment must be applied along with the statistical data analysis. The judgment must include a consideration of how well the data fulfill the requirements for applying inferential statistics.

Another practical consideration when applying statistics to industrial hygiene data is the expense that may be involved in generating the large numbers of air or noise measurements needed to evaluate a particular operation. When exposures are near the OEL the number of measurements needed to prove adherence (with a high level of confidence using a formal statistical test) can be excessive. Table 7.1 shows that for SEGs with moderate to high exposure variability and mean exposures near the LTA–OEL (true mean ≥0.5 × LTA–OEL) 41 or more measurements might be needed to achieve high confidence that the mean exposure is less than the LTA–OEL. In some of those cases, it may be best to use resources to reduce the SEG's exposures rather than spend them on the additional monitoring that will be needed to prove that exposures are below the LTA–OEL.

In spite of their limitations, statistical tools are useful because they help form a picture of the exposure profile that would otherwise be difficult to obtain. If their limitations are understood, they will greatly enhance knowledge of the exposure profile.

It is especially important for industrial hygienists to develop an intuitive "feel" for exposures that are lognormally distributed. People generally have a great deal of experience with objects and distributions (especially the normal distribution) that are symmetrical. Therefore, our first impulse is to visualize a distribution of data as though it is symmetrical — even though it may better conform to an asymmetrical distribution (such as the lognormal distribution). Statistical tools can help us overcome this bias toward symmetry that can interfere with an accurate interpretation of data from lognormal and other right-skewed distributions.

This book does not provide an exhaustive review of statistical tools. Instead we present those tools we believe strike a good

Table 7.1 — Approximate Sample Size Requirements to be 95% Confident that the True Mean Exposure is less than the LTA–OEL (Power = 90%)

	SAMPLE SIZE (n)				
Ratio: true mean/OEL	Low variability (GSD* = 1.5)	GSD* = 2	Moderate variability (GSD* = 2.5)	GSD* = 3	High variability (GSD* = 3.5)
0.75	25	82	164	266	384
0.5	7	21	41	67	96
0.25	3	10	19	30	43
0.1	2	6	13	21	30

*GSD = geometric standard deviation
Source: British Occupational Hygiene Society[3]

balance between usefulness, ease of use, precision, and statistical power. Because of limitations inherent in the application of statistics to industrial hygiene data, this text often makes a choice for simpler analysis techniques even though more precise yet more complicated statistical methods may be available. For readers who are interested, reference to these more complicated techniques is provided.

Population vs. Sample

In statistical terms, the population is every possible member of a distribution and the sample is a subset of the population that has been drawn for observation or measurement. Suppose we had a simple example of a three-person SEG that ran a degreasing tank in a three-shift (one person per shift) five-days-a-week operation. In assessing a year's worth of eight-hour shift exposures for that SEG, the population would be every eight-hour shift exposure occurring during that year — about 780 eight-hour exposures. The sample would be the few eight-hour shift exposures that were actually monitored (maybe 10 different full-shift exposures). We rely on these few monitored full-shift exposures (the sample) to summarize and infer things about exposures on all the shifts (the exposure population).

You can see that those 10 shifts in the statistical sample must be chosen properly, and the monitoring results interpreted carefully, if they are to give an accurate picture of what is occurring in the entire population of 780 eight-hour shift exposures. Even with sound sampling and analysis techniques, the estimate we make will be uncertain because we have only "looked" at about 1.3% of the full-shift exposures in the population.

As industrial hygiene exposure scenarios get more complex due to increasing numbers of workers, materials, processes, and tasks, the importance of careful sampling strategy and data analysis becomes even more apparent. Simply changing the example above to one that has nine employees in the SEG (three employees per shift) increases our population of full-shift exposures in a year to about 2340. If we take only 10 air samples during the year to evaluate this operation, we are "observing" less than 0.5% of the full-shift exposures in the population.

Exposure Distributions and Parametric or Nonparametric Statistical Tools

A population distribution is a description of the relative frequencies of the elements of that population. The most powerful statistical tools (parametric statistics) require knowledge or assumptions about the population's distribution. This understanding of the population's underlying distribution is what gives parametric statistics their great power. Just as we can efficiently say many things about a specific object once we know it has the underlying shape of a sphere, so too can we efficiently say many things about a population distribution once we know its basic shape.

If we know nothing about the underlying distribution of exposures, nonparametric statistics can help. These statistical tools tend to focus on robust measures such as the distribution median or other percentile because they are less sensitive to outliers and spurious data. Unfortunately — as attractive as the nonparametric statistics are for minimizing assumptions — these methods have lower statistical power and usually require many more measurements for statistically based decision making.

Common Distributions in Industrial Hygiene

Two distributions are particularly important to industrial hygiene data: the normal and the lognormal distribution. The random sampling and analytical error associated with an air monitoring result is usually presumed to be normally distributed. The random fluctuations in exposure from shift to shift or within shifts tend to be lognormally distributed.[4] Of these, exposure fluctuations (either from shift to shift or within a shift) account for the vast majority of an exposure profile's variability.[1,5]

This has important ramifications for sampling strategies trying to "do more with less." As discussed earlier, a few measurements (6–10) usually assess only a minute percentage of the exposures of interest. Therefore, we would not expect the fluctuations of exposures in that population to be well-characterized; yet, that fluctuation in exposures accounts for the vast majority of the exposure profile's variability (usually more than 85%).[5] Whatever we can do to better characterize those exposure fluctuations will increase our confidence in the estimate of the exposure profile. If we have resources to commit to exposure monitoring, usually the most efficient approach would call for putting resources into more measurements (i.e., generate more data to better characterize exposure fluctuations) rather than into more precise sampling methods (i.e., have better confidence in each datum).[1]

Distribution Verification

The lognormal distribution model is often a reasonable model when there is a physical lower limit for possible values (such as zero), large values sometimes occur, and the processes that gen-

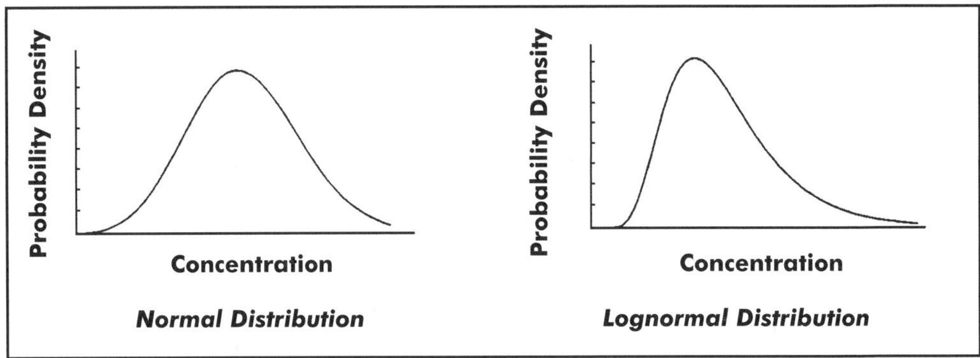

Figure 7.1 — Normal and lognormal distributions.

erate or control exposures tend to interact in a multiplicative manner.[6] It is reasonable to presume that the underlying distribution for workplace exposure data is the lognormal distribution unless there is a compelling reason to believe otherwise; however, the assumption of lognormality should be checked. It is always important that the underlying distribution of any data set be verified prior to statistical analysis so that appropriate statistical tools can be selected.

Checking the presumption of distribution lognormality also allows review of SEGs to determine whether they have been set up appropriately or if they should be adjusted.[1] Because a lognormal distribution is usually expected, having data that are not lognormally distributed is one factor that might make the industrial hygienist review the original classification of workers into SEGs.

Methods for verifying whether data are lognormally distributed include logprobability plots,[3] a Ratio Metric calculation,[7] a W-test,[8] or a test developed by Filliben.[10]

A logprobability plot is the simplest and most straightforward way to check data for lognormality. These plots have the added advantage of providing a beginning picture of the exposure distribution. If the data form a straight line on the logprobability plot — signifying lognormality — then the line can be used to estimate the distribution's geometric mean (GM = the 50% point) and geometric standard deviation (GSD = the 84% point divided by the 50% point). It also provides a rough idea of upper percentiles.

The W-test is the most rigorous test for lognormality, but it also is the most complicated to perform. (Using a computer package, such as HYGINIST,[9] eliminates that roadblock.) The use of probability plotting and the W-test for verifying the lognormality of data sets is demonstrated in Appendix V.

Sampling Randomly from Stationary Populations

Using statistical tools to make accurate estimates of a population of exposures requires that the sample used be drawn randomly from a population of exposures that does not change over the period of interest.

Random Sampling

For the sample to be random, there must be no systematic or preferential selection of a population's elements. As discussed in Chapter 6, each element in the population must have equal likelihood of being observed.

We can refer again to the simple degreaser example with 780 possible full-shift exposures in a year's population of SEG exposures. The need to sample randomly would require that every one of the possible 780 full-shift exposures have an equal chance of being included in the 10 exposures that were actually monitored. Most industrial hygienists would probably admit that monitoring the night-shift exposures is more difficult than monitoring the day-shift exposures, yet to use statistical tools properly and "fairly" to get an unbiased characterization of the population of exposures this random sampling requirement must be met.

Practical considerations of travel constraints, weather, process operation parameters, budgetary limits, and the need to characterize multiple exposure profiles make statistically randomized sampling extremely difficult in the real world. Nevertheless, industrial hygienists must develop monitoring strategies that choose days and workers for monitoring in a manner that is as close to random as possible. Avoid known bias in the selection of workers or periods to be monitored. If possible, avoid clustering your monitoring into consecutive periods. Monitor during different seasons to avoid biases introduced by factors that change with weather conditions. Make a point to understand process cycles and avoid biases they might introduce.

The tendency in industrial hygiene practice is to focus monitoring efforts on "typical" events, which, of course, can bias the exposure profile results. In theory, unusual events should not be excluded if they occur naturally in the workplace. By excluding these rare but natural events, a bias is built into the monitoring data.

Autocorrelation

Autocorrelation occurs when the contaminant concentration in one time period is related to the concentration in a previous period. Clustering all the samples in one period when autocorrelation occurs will result in an underestimate of variability in the exposure profile and an imprecise estimate of the mean exposure.[11,12] In the context of a room with a low ventilation rate, it makes sense that if the contaminant concentration is high during one five-minute period it will be high during the next five-minute period simply because ventilation systems have finite mixing periods for exchanging air. Thus, on average, five-minute periods of low contaminant concentration will tend to be followed by another five-minute period of low concentration and five-minute periods of high concentration will tend to be followed by other periods of high concentration. Collecting a series of five-minute samples during consecutive five-minute periods will tend to "grab" either a low concentration cycle or a high concentration cycle. In addition to underestimating the concentration variability, the results of the monitoring will underestimate or overestimate the true degree of exposure — depending on whether a high or low concentration cycle happened to have been grabbed.

Although there is evidence that strict statistical autocorrelation is less likely to occur in consecutive day-to-day exposure measurements than in shorter periods (e.g., minute to minute),[12-14] there may be systematic influence caused by known or unknown environmental or process parameters operating on those consecutive days. Clustering all measurements into consecutive days will lessen the likelihood of identifying the unknown systematic bias. Known systematic bias must be accounted for in the data analysis (e.g., choice and interpretation of statistical tools) and interpretation.

When interpreting the monitoring data, judgment must be used to determine how well the monitoring strategy has met the statistical requirement of random sampling. Ask yourself, "Within the SEG was there a systematic selection of workers, dates, or times for monitoring?" In very obvious nonrandom cases, simple descriptive statistics can be useful, but the ultimate decisions should be made on the basis of a professional judgment that recognizes the selection bias. If there is a good faith effort to acquire a near-random sample, the industrial hygienist may choose to use statistical methods. Interpretation of the outcomes, however, should be tempered with a judgment about the "randomness" of the sampling protocol. In any case, good industrial hygiene practice calls for investigating and evaluating any exposure measurement above the OEL.

Stationary Population

If statistical tools are to be applied appropriately, the underlying population being sampled must not change during the exposure assessment period. Let's examine again our year's worth of 780 eight-hour shift exposures, but assume the process changed halfway through the year so that exposures doubled on average. Roughly half of our 10 random measurements would reflect exposures before the change and half would reflect exposures after the change. When we combined the samples for statistical analysis we would have neither an estimate of the exposure profile before the change nor an estimate of the exposure profile after the change. Instead we would have some combination of the two that would not accurately characterize the exposure profile of either the old or the new process. Furthermore, the distribution of exposures for the combined monitoring data would probably not be lognormal, and typical lognormal parametric statistics would give an inaccurate characterization of the exposure profile.

If the population changes significantly over the random sampling period, only calculations of simple descriptive statistics and decision making on the basis of professional judgment are recommended. Changes in process materials, process parameters, work practices, and performance of engineering controls are common examples of changes that can affect the population distribution of exposures. One simple procedure that can help subjectively check for population stability is to plot the monitoring data chronologically by time of monitoring. If any trends in the data are apparent, that is a sign the underlying process is not stationary.

Important to the exposure assessment strategy is a mechanism for following exposures that have been judged unacceptable with a system for prioritizing and implementing controls. Remedial actions might be required if the exposures are found unacceptable, and subsequent additional data gathering will be needed to determine whether the exposures are acceptable after such action has been taken. If changes have been made and the new data collected, they should be analyzed independently of the first set of data. Data pooled for analysis must represent a single SEG.

Example: Check for Stationary Population

Monitoring was performed in our hypothetical coil coating operation to evaluate 8-hour TWA octochlorostyrene exposures to the Helper during fluxing. The 8-hour TWA measurements are plotted to look for trends (see Figure 7.2). There are no apparent upward or downward trends in the magnitude of exposure.

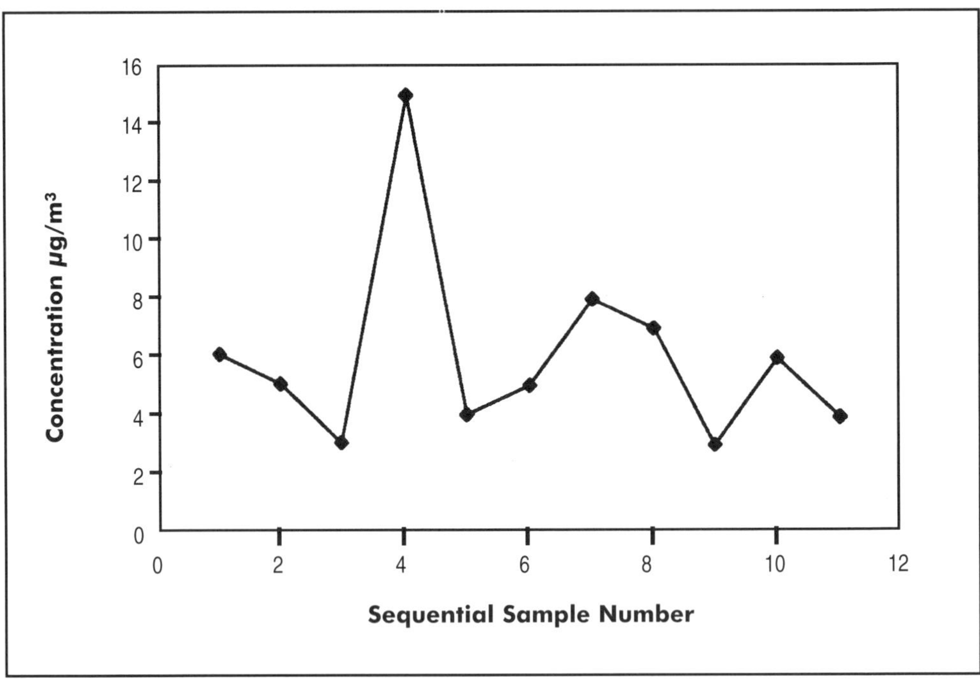

Figure 7.2 — Example sequential data plot.

Similar Exposure Interval

It has been suggested that the quality control concept of "lots" be applied to exposure assessment.[15] Each lot (or "similar exposure interval") would be defined as a period over which the distribution of an SEG's exposures would be expected to be stationary. The measurements needed to characterize the exposure profile would be taken randomly from within that similar exposure interval. This data set would then be used to describe the SEG's exposure profile for that specific interval. These similar exposure intervals would be set up using a combination of assessment tools, including statistical considerations, process knowledge, and past monitoring data.

Relationship of Averaging Times

Only data with similar averaging periods should be combined for statistical analysis. That is, combine full-shift data only with other full-shift data, and short-term data (e.g., STEL evaluations) only with other short-term data. It is inappropriate to average short-term data with full-shift data. Short-term data tends to be distributed differently than full-shift data (usually being more variable with a higher GSD). As pointed out previously, it is statistically inappropriate to combine data from different distributions into a single statistical analysis if we hope to get an unbiased picture of the exposure profile. In particular, mixing of data from different averaging times makes estimates of variance inaccurate and precludes use of most common statistical tools.[16]

Techniques are being developed to predict long-term exposure profiles based on a time-weighted combination of exposure profiles for the several short-term tasks making up the long-term exposure.[17,18] These techniques are computationally intensive and therefore beyond the scope of this book, but they hold great promise for providing more detailed characterizations of exposures and for optimizing sampling efficiency (i.e., getting the most accurate exposure profile for the least amount of effort and expense) using stratified random sampling of critical tasks.

Nondetectable Data

Monitoring results below the analytical limit of detection should not be discarded. They provide critical information about the exposure profile. Several techniques are available for including below detection limit data in statistical analysis. A simple approach is to use a fraction of the detection limit in the statistical analysis. A factor of 0.7 times the detection limit may be most appropriate for data with relatively low variability (GSD <3), while a factor of 0.5 times the detection limit may be best when the variability is high (GSD >3).[19] If more than 50% of data are below the detection limit then special techniques may be required.[20]

Probability plotting is another way to include data below the detection limit in the statistical analysis (see Appendix V). These plots allow extrapolation of the data above the detection limit to account for the data below the detection limit for determination of a reasonable estimate of the average and variability.[8]

Ultimately, the use of statistics for interpreting data must be done carefully, with considerable judgment. Practical problems with nonrandomized samples, nonstationary distributions, autocorrelation, and the difference between statistical significance and practical/toxicological significance reduces the reliance the assessor can have on the use of statistics alone.

Specific Statistical Techniques

There is no one ideal statistical technique for evaluating industrial hygiene monitoring data — all have advantages and disadvantages. Generally a good approach is to use a combination of tools to help form a statistical "picture" of the exposure profile. The assessor can then focus on the particular statistical tools that are most appropriate for the specific assessment, provide the most unbiased estimates, and are the appropriate type of statistics for the way that the data were collected. That information is then combined with the other knowledge gained during the exposure assessment's information gathering phase to form a judgment about the exposure profile and the risks it presents.

All measurements to be analyzed statistically should be valid in that 1) they were collected and analyzed using a reasonably accurate and reasonably unbiased sampling and analytical method, and 2) they adequately represent personal exposure.

Measurements should be representative in that 1) the production levels and level of environmental controls during sampling were not manipulated in any way, and 2) there was no known bias in the selection of either the employees or the days that were monitored.

Statistical tools are much easier to use (and misuse!) now that personal computers are readily available. All the basic statistical calculations discussed in this book can be entered onto a spreadsheet such as Microsoft Excel®, Corel Quattro Pro®, or Lotus 123®. Or an assessor can purchase "canned" statistical analysis programs. Some of these programs[(9,21)] have been designed specifically for statistical analysis of industrial hygiene data. A basic spreadsheet tool is supplied with this book (see Appendix XIII).

Descriptive Statistics

Start the exposure data analysis by making a sequential plot and calculating a sample arithmetic mean and standard deviation, sample median, range, maximum and minimum exposures, actual fraction of samples over the OEL, and sample size. These simple descriptive statistics provide summary information that can guide an experienced industrial hygienist through a subjective workplace exposure evaluation. They are discussed in more detail in Appendix IV.

Data representative of an SEG can be plotted on probability paper. The two types of paper most commonly used in industrial hygiene are logprobability paper and normal-probability paper. If the data plot as a straight line on either chart, that is strong evidence the data are adequately fit by a parametric distribution (lognormal or normal, respectively). If this is the case, the median (and geometric mean) and other percentiles (and percent exceedance levels) can be estimated directly from the plotted data — a real asset when one uses professional judgment on workplace exposures. More information on probability plotting and other methods for evaluating the underlying distribution for a sample data set are provided in Appendix V.

Inferential Statistics

Inferential statistics use characteristics of your sample to make inferences about the population from which it was drawn. They allow you to estimate various parameters of the population distribution (e.g., arithmetic mean, standard deviation, upper percentile) and quantify your confidence in the parameter estimates (e.g., confidence limits). Industrial hygienists have always "made inferences" about exposure profiles (e.g., exposure population of interest) based on a few monitoring results from that exposure profile (e.g., limited sample from the population). Industrial hygienists have even tempered their inferences with subjective judgments about how confident they were in their characterization of the exposure. Inferential statistical tools simply allow a more quantitative estimate of the exposure profile and better quantification of confidence in the exposure profile parameter estimates.

Two aspects of the distribution particularly useful to the industrial hygienist are the exposure distribution's arithmetic mean (AM) and upper tail. Emphasizing either one has advantages and disadvantages.[1,22] Focusing on the AM provides an average exposure estimate that is directly related to average dose and cumulative dose. Focusing on the distribution's upper tail provides insight to the upper extremes of exposure in the exposure profile and may be useful for evaluating agents with primarily acute effects and for evaluating the likelihood of noncompliance with OELs. Remember that if a decision must be made with a few measurements (e.g., 10), confidence is highest for the estimate of the mean, lower for the estimate of variance, and lowest for estimates of lower or upper percentiles.

When performing statistical analysis of industrial hygiene data, it is important to remember that OELs are established so that — with the highest certainty permitted by available data — most workers will not suffer health effects if exposed at the OEL day after day for a working lifetime. Implicit in that description is the possibility a small fraction might indeed experience health effects at or below the OEL. This is one reason why all exposures should be kept well below the OEL.

Focus on the Arithmetic Mean

For chronic-acting substances, the LTA exposure (exposure averaged over weeks or months, rather than for a single eight-hour work shift) is a relevant index of dose and, therefore, a useful parameter on which to focus for evaluating the health risk posed by such an exposure. This holds true for agents for which the dose or effect is cumulative, or for agents for which "body damping" of swings in exposure occurs to lessen the importance of variability and increase the mean exposure's importance.[1] Knowledge of occasional high exposures is not as critical because it is the arithmetic average that summarizes the total mass absorbed by a person.

Statistical tools are available for evaluating whether an arithmetic mean workplace exposure is less than an LTA–OEL.[23,24] In general, the OEL used for comparison should not be an OSHA PEL or an ACGIH threshold limit value (TLV®) but rather a specifically defined LTA–OEL.

If an 8-hour TWA–OEL is used for comparison with an arithmetic mean, a large fraction of exposures could still be above the OEL while the arithmetic mean exposure remains below the OEL. This is contrary to the interpretation of OSHA 8-hour TWA–PELs, which are enforced as though no 8-hour TWAs of exposure above the PEL are allowed.

One of the challenges facing the industrial hygiene profession is that OELs must be better defined in a manner that includes

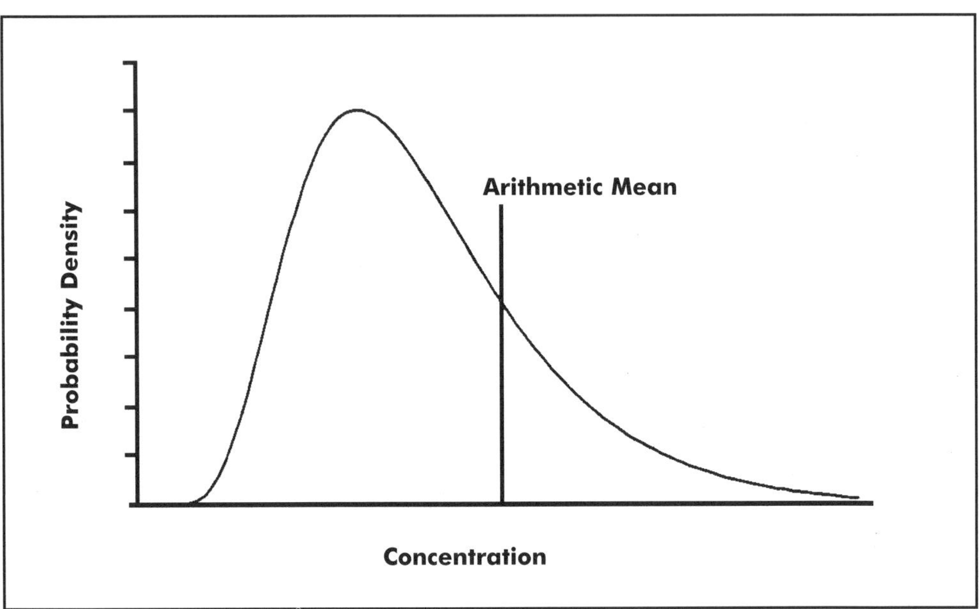

Figure 7.3 — Focus on the lognormal distribution's arithmetic mean.

definition of the appropriate statistical parameter.[5] This "statistically defined OEL" would be one in which an "acceptable" exposure profile was defined by the OEL's sponsoring organization. For example, it would be stated clearly whether the OEL was to be interpreted as a long-term average (i.e., arithmetic mean of the distribution of daily average exposures), a permissible exceedance of day-to-day exposures (e.g., 5%), or as a never-to-be-exceeded maximum daily average (e.g., 100% of the daily average exposures are less than the OEL). This acceptable exposure profile, where average and variability have been defined, would provide clear guidelines for consistent interpretation and serve as an achievable, practical goal for workplace exposures. To date, there are few statistically defined OELs.

Arithmetic Mean of a Lognormal Distribution of Exposures

It should be noted that the arithmetic mean of a lognormal exposure distribution, not the geometric mean, is the best descriptor of average exposure — and therefore of average and cumulative dose. In lognormally distributed data, the geometric mean is equal to the distribution median. Because the geometric mean is lower than the arithmetic mean in a lognormal distribution, using the geometric mean will underestimate the average exposure. The difference between the two grows as variance in the distribution increases. Thus, as the GSD gets larger, the geometric mean further underestimates the average exposure (see Figure 7.4).

Estimating the Arithmetic Mean of a Lognormal Distribution

There are several methods for estimating the arithmetic mean of a lognormal distribution based on a random statistical sample. The recommended method for all sample sizes and GSDs is the minimum variance unbiased estimate (MVUE).[25] It is preferred because it is unbiased and has minimum variance; however, if a programmable calculator or computer is not available, some might find the mechanics of the calculation complex. If so, the simple mean of the sample data is easy to calculate and works well for small sample sizes ($n < 20$) and small GSDs.[25,26]

The calculation and use of the MVUE, the simple arithmetic mean, and a third estimator — the maximum likelihood estimate (MLE) — are demonstrated in Appendix VI. The MLE is easy to calculate and is less variable than the simple mean for large data sets ($n > 50$) and high GSDs.[25,26]

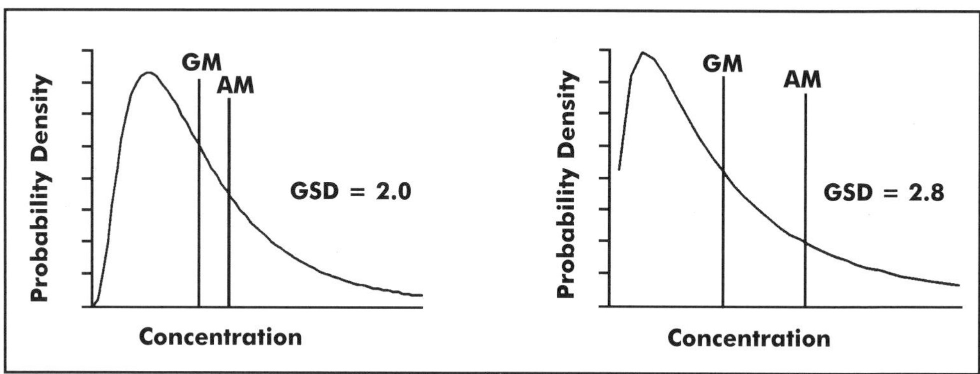

Figure 7.4 — Arithmetic and geometric means of lognormal distributions.

Confidence Limits Around the Arithmetic Mean of a Lognormal Distribution

A parameter point estimate (e.g., a mean, standard deviation, or percentile estimated from the statistical sample) hardly ever equals the population parameter's true value. Confidence limits are therefore calculated for the parameter point estimate in order to determine, with a specified degree of confidence, the range in which the true population parameter is likely to lie.

For example, one can calculate upper and lower confidence limits for an arithmetic mean exposure point estimate that will include the true exposure mean 90% of time (see Figure 7.5). These confidence limits allow one to gauge the uncertainty in

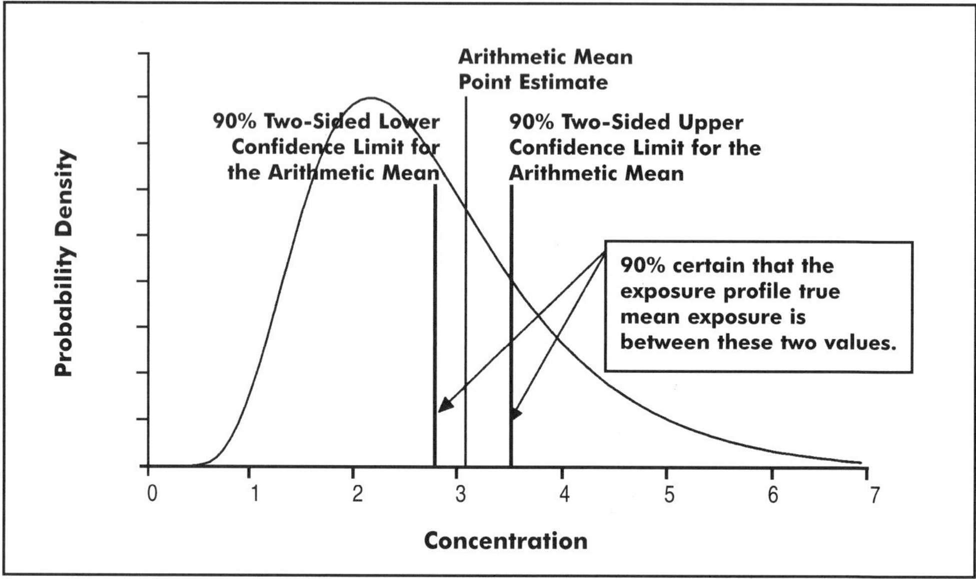

Figure 7.5 — Arithmetic mean estimate and its 90% upper and lower confidence intervals.

the parameter estimate — the wider the confidence limits, the less certain the point estimate. They can also be compared with a target or acceptable value (such as an LTA–OEL) to determine, with some known confidence, whether the target has been met or exceeded. Specific techniques for calculating and using confidence limits for arithmetic mean estimates, including Land's "exact" procedure, are discussed in Appendix VI.

Example: Arithmetic Mean

Monitoring was performed in our hypothetical coil coating operation to evaluate Helper 8-hour TWA exposures to octochlorostyrene during fluxing:

Date	µg/m³
January 6	6
January 25	5
February 17	3
February 18	15
April 24	4
April 28	5
May 3	8
May 12	7
May 13	3
May 14	6
June 1	4

The monitoring data were used to estimate the arithmetic mean of the SEG exposure profile for comparison with the new octochlorostyrene internal LTA–OEL, which was recently set by the Company at 10 µg/m³. Land's "exact" procedure was used to calculate the one-sided 95% upper confidence limit ($UCL_{1,95\%}$) for the arithmetic mean estimate.[25]

LOGNORMAL PARAMETRIC STATISTICS	
Estimated Arithmetic Mean – MVUE:	5.9 µg/m³
$UCL_{1,95\%}$ – Land's "Exact" Procedure:	8.2 µg/m³

Because the one-sided 95% upper confidence limit ($UCL_{1,95\%}$ = 8.2 µg/m³) is less than the internal LTA–OEL of 10 µg/m³, we are at least 95% confident that the true arithmetic mean exposure is less than the LTA–OEL and would probably rate this exposure as "acceptable." See Appendix VI for details on these calculation methods.

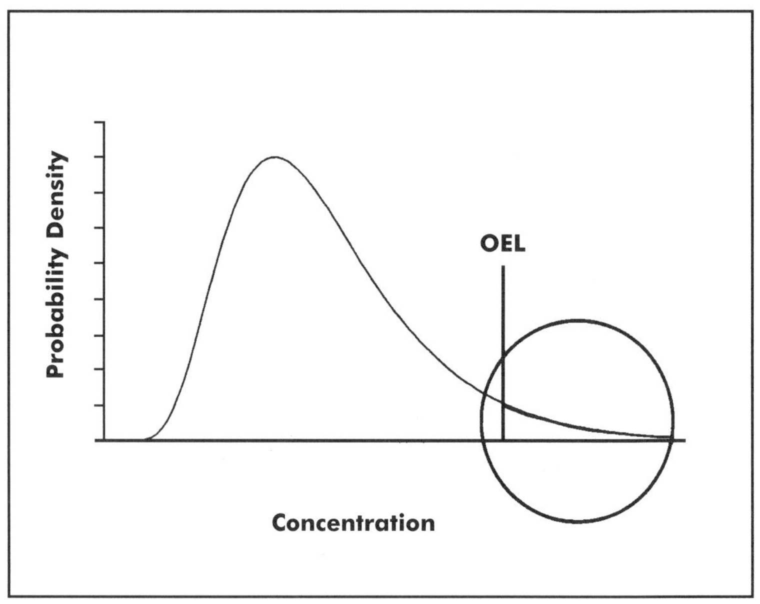

Figure 7.6 — Focus on the upper tail of a lognormal distribution.

Focus on the Upper Tail

Forming a "picture" of the exposure profile's upper tail is especially important when evaluating the health hazards of agents with acute health effects (such as hydrogen cyanide) or when evaluating the risk of noncompliance associated with exceeding an OEL (see Figure 7.6). In the case of an acute agent, the average exposure is not as important as understanding how high the exposure may get because those few high exposures might pose a more important risk to health than average exposures at lower levels. When evaluating the probability of exceeding an OEL, an examination of the exposure profile's upper tail will allow an estimate of the relative frequency with which the OEL may be exceeded.

Estimating Upper Percentiles

One way to form a picture of the upper tail is to estimate some appropriate upper percentile — usually the 95th percentile. This can be done through straightforward statistical techniques based on the underlying normal or lognormal distribution (see Appendix VII), or it can be done using linear- or logprobability plotting techniques (see Appendix V). Remember that when there is little monitoring data, your estimate of upper percentiles has low confidence. Calculating a tolerance limit enables you to quantify your confidence in the percentile estimate.

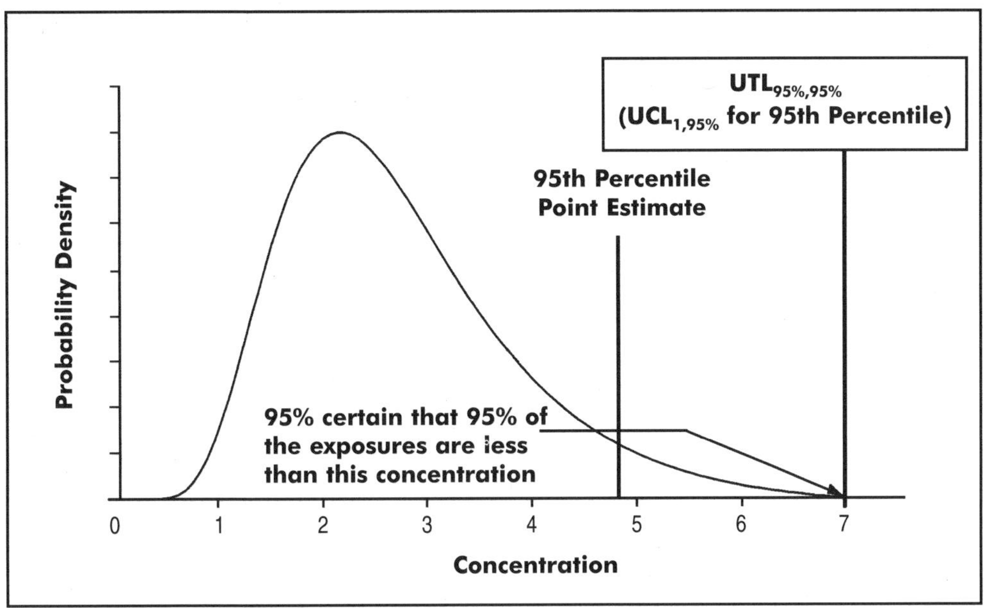

Figure 7.7 — 95th percentile point estimate and the upper tolerance limit.

Tolerance Limits

Because of the inherent variability of workplace concentrations, statistically guaranteeing that all exposures are below a guideline is usually impossible; however, demonstrating statistically that no more than a given percentage of exposures are greater than a standard with some confidence is possible. The most common procedure of this type is the tolerance limit approach.[26] This approach will permit the industrial hygienist to determine whether one can have, for example, 95% confidence that no more than 5% of the exposures exceed the standard. This is, in effect, an upper one-sided 95% confidence limit on the estimate of the 95% percentile (see Figure 7.7). An industrial hygienist can select whatever percentages are appropriate in light of an agent's toxic effects, warning properties, and general uncertainty of the population dose-response relationship.

Tolerance limits are helpful for defining the upper end of an exposure profile. A picture of relatively infrequent but extreme exposures can then be included in the assessment. This would be useful for evaluating whether an unacceptably high exposure to an agent with acute toxic effects is likely to occur.

The tolerance limit approach may also be appropriate for compliance testing. Keep in mind, however, that most regulatory standards are currently not written to allow any exposures in excess of the standard (a statistical impossibility given the inherent variability in workplace exposures). Regulatory noncompliance may be an important risk if exposures are above the OEL 5% of the time. The industrial hygienist will therefore have to spend time thinking about how much regulatory risk he or she is willing to take.

Unfortunately, tolerance limits are very sensitive to sample size and the distribution's standard deviation. With small sample sizes, this test has limited power to provide good confidence in an extreme percentile estimate, particularly for highly variable exposure profiles.(22) The method does not adequately evaluate the risk posed by primarily chronic toxicants. It makes no distinction between an exposure profile with a low mean but high variance and an exposure profile with a high mean and low variance.(22) Yet in the case of a chronic toxicant the risk posed by the latter would be much greater. In those instances, statistical techniques that focus on arithmetic mean exposures would be useful.

One should also not infer from this discussion that exposures above an OEL can be ignored when the 95th percentile exposure is less than the OEL. Good industrial hygiene practice dictates that all exposures above an OEL be investigated. A measured overexposure is a signal that the work environment for all members of the exposure group might be a problem or that there are individuals within the exposure group who routinely experience significantly greater exposures than the other employees — due to different work practices or effectiveness of controls.

There are both parametric and nonparametric versions of the tolerance limit approach (the nonparametric requires many more samples). The mechanics of using a parametric tolerance limit approach are described in Appendix VII. The use of nonparametric tolerance limits is discussed in Appendix VIII.

Example: Upper Tolerance Limit

Monitoring was performed in our hypothetical coil coating operation to evaluate short-term MIBK exposures to the Coil Feed Operator and Helper during cleanup.

Date	ppm
March 14	23
April 3	42
April 6	86
April 12	62
April 17	34
April 28	107
May 2	29
May 5	65
May 8	54
May 9	55

The monitoring data were used to estimate the 95th percentile of the SEG exposure profile and calculate a 95%,95% upper tolerance limit for comparison to the MIBK STEL of 75 ppm:

LOGNORMAL PARAMETRIC STATISTICS	
95th Percentile:	111 ppm
$UTL_{95\%,95\%}$:	204 ppm

Because the $UTL_{95\%,95\%}$ of 204 ppm is far above 75 ppm, we are not 95% confident that the true 95th percentile is less than the STEL OEL. We would probably rate this exposure as "unacceptable." See Appendix VII for details on these calculation methods.

Exceedance Fraction or "Probability of Noncompliance"

A twist on percentiles is the exceedance fraction or "probability of noncompliance" procedure.(28) This method calls for determining the point estimate of the percentile of the distribution that corresponds to the relevant OEL — the percentage of the distribution that lies above it equals the exceedance fraction. If, for example, the OEL happened to equal the 87th percentile of the distribution of day-to-day exposures, the best probability estimate that any given day's exposure would exceed the OEL would be 13%.

One must keep in mind when using this procedure, however, that confidence in estimates of a population's upper extremes is low when there are few measurements. These type of percentile estimates, therefore, have wide confidence limits for small sets of monitoring data.(29) Techniques for calculating exceedance fractions and their confidence limits are detailed in Appendix VII.

Example: Exceedance Fraction

In this example we will use the exceedance fraction technique to evaluate the same monitoring data collected in our previous example of Coil Feed Operator and Helper MIBK exposures during cleanup.

Date	ppm
March 14	23
April 3	42
April 6	86
April 12	62
April 17	34
April 28	107
May 2	29
May 5	65
May 8	54
May 9	55

The monitoring data will be used to estimate the percentage of the SEG exposure profile that exceeds the MIBK STEL of 75 ppm:

LOGNORMAL PARAMETRIC STATISTICS	
Percent exceeding OEL (% > OEL):	20%
$UCL_{1,95\%}$ (% > OEL):	42%

The exceedance fraction estimate is that 20% of the exposure profile is above the OEL. The one-sided 95% upper confidence limit ($UCL_{1,95\%}$) for that exceedance fraction tells us we are 95% confident that 42% or less of the exposure profile is above the OEL. Based on those results, we would probably conclude that it is too risky to have such a high proportion of the exposure profile above the STEL; we would rate the SEG as "unacceptable." For details on these calculation methods, see Appendix VII.

Which to Choose — The Mean or the Upper Tail?

Generally, given the ease with which parameters can be calculated using personal computers, it makes sense to routinely calculate estimates of the arithmetic mean and the upper percentiles, tolerance limits, and exceedance fractions. In that manner, characterization of the exposure profile should be more complete. As the industrial hygienist's understanding of the exposure profile develops, his or her judgment should focus more on one part of the overall picture than the other in making a final decision. That judgment will be based on an understanding of limitations of the statistical tests, the data on which they were based, the industrial hygienist's knowledge of the agent and its toxicity, the specific OEL, and many other qualitative factors typically included in the assessment.

In determining compliance with most regulatory and authoritative OELs that exist today, a focus on the upper tail would be most appropriate. In 1978, OSHA expressed in the preamble to its lead (Pb) PEL:[30]

> *OSHA recognizes that there will be day-to-day variability in airborne lead exposure experienced by a single employee. The permissible exposure limit is a maximum allowable value which is not to be exceeded: hence exposure must be controlled to an average value well below the permissible exposure limit in order to remain in compliance.*

More recently, in a guide to workplace exposure assessment, the Comité Européen de Normalisation (CEN) recommended that when the probability of exceeding the limit value is greater than 5%:[31]

> *The probability of exceeding the limit value is too high; appropriate actions have to be taken as soon as possible to reduce exposure.*

It is worth noting that each datum should also be reviewed individually. All measurements above the OEL should be investigated. Information collected along with the measurement should be examined to determine whether there was some reason (e.g., unusual process upset) that would cause exclusion of the datum from analysis with other SEG exposure data.

Analysis of Variance to Refine Critical SEGs

For some critical SEGs it is important to make sure no individual workers have exposures significantly higher than other workers in the SEG. Analysis of variance (ANOVA) is a statistical technique that can be used to compare the variability of individual workers' exposures with the exposure variability of the overall SEG. If a large difference is found, the industrial hygienist can further investigate the individual workers' exposures and determine whether there is a need to better refine the SEG.

In Chapter 4, two approaches to establishing SEGs were compared: the sampling approach and the observational approach. We suggested the observational approach generally be used to establish SEGs because of its advantages in prioritization and its ability to resolve many exposure judgments without monitoring. The sampling approach tends to be more objective and accurate, but there is a need to take many measurements. This approach can be used to check the homogeneity of the critical SEGs for which risk of individual misclassification is most severe and to reassign individuals as necessary.

ANOVA (described in Appendix IX) is a statistical tool that can be used in the sampling approach for determining whether SEGs have been defined appropriately. Several workers in the SEG are randomly chosen and air monitoring is performed to measure the exposures of each of the chosen workers several times. ANOVA is used to examine the exposure variability for each monitored individual (within worker variability) and compare it with the worker-to-worker variability in the SEG (between worker variability). If these differ substantially, that is evidence of worker misclassification in the SEG. That exposure group should then be examined more carefully, through additional monitoring or observation, to reclassify workers into appropriate SEGs.

Identifying Critical SEGs

As an exposure assessment system matures, the industrial hygienist will identify critical SEGs for which misclassification of workers presents the most risk. Generally, critical SEGs are those with exposure profiles near but below the OEL. If an individual worker assigned to those SEGs has an exposure that is significantly higher than the SEG exposure profile, he or she may be exposed to hazardous concentrations of the air contaminant. SEGs with exposure profiles above OELs can be excluded from further examination because resources should be directed at controlling those exposures rather than further refining them. SEGs with very low exposure profiles can be ruled out because exposure variability between workers would have to be extremely high for an individual's exposure to exceed the OEL (see Figure 7.8).

How low the SEG exposure profile must be before it can be excluded from the list of critical SEGs will depend on various factors. Exposure monitoring is suggested for all SEGs believed to have exposures above 10% of the OEL (see Figure 7.9). That initial exposure monitoring should consist of at least six to 10 measurements taken from workers and time periods that are chosen as randomly as possible. Nicas reviewed monitoring protocols for chronic toxicity agents (where the long-term average exposure is an appropriate focus for the judgment of acceptability) to determine when it would be critical to use additional monitoring and ANOVA to compare the within- and between-worker variability of SEGs.[32] He found that a reasonable cut-off would be to exclude exposure groups in which the initial monitoring found the SEG arithmetic mean exposure to be below 26% of the LTA–OEL with appropriate statistical confidence. For example, if the $UCL_{1,95\%}$ for the arithmetic mean of

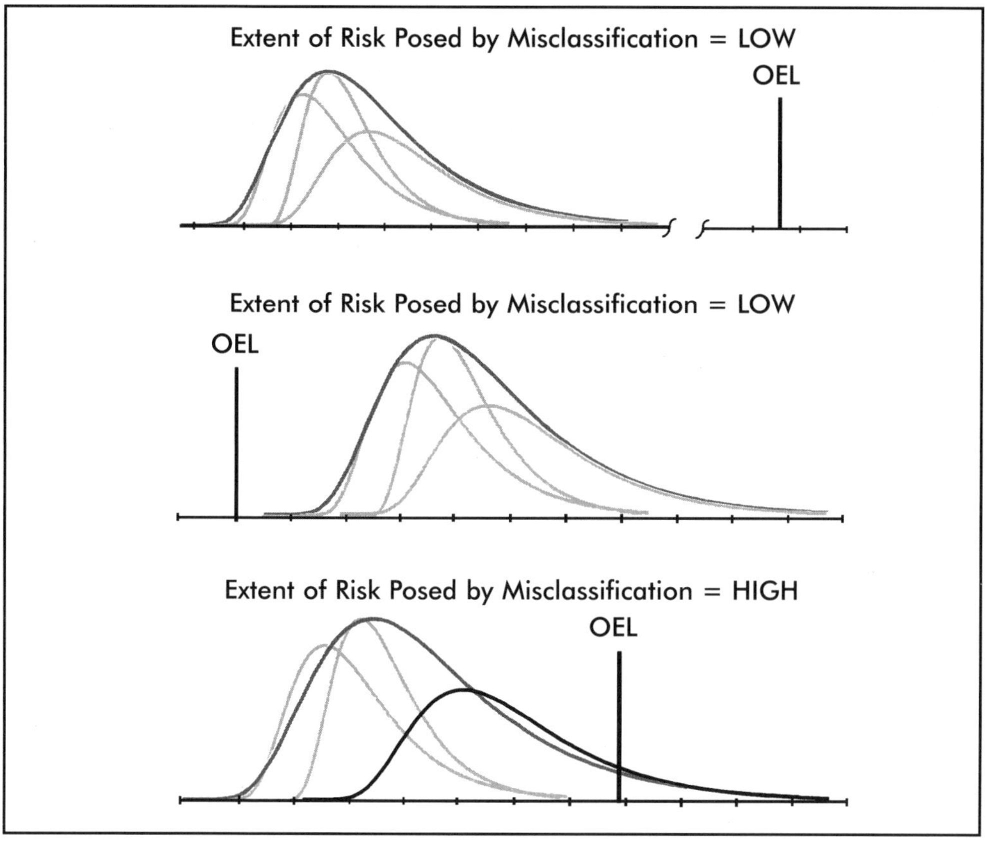

Extent of Risk Posed by Misclassification = LOW

OEL

Extent of Risk Posed by Misclassification = LOW

OEL

Extent of Risk Posed by Misclassification = HIGH

OEL

Figure 7.8 — Risk posed by misclassification of an individual worker's exposure.

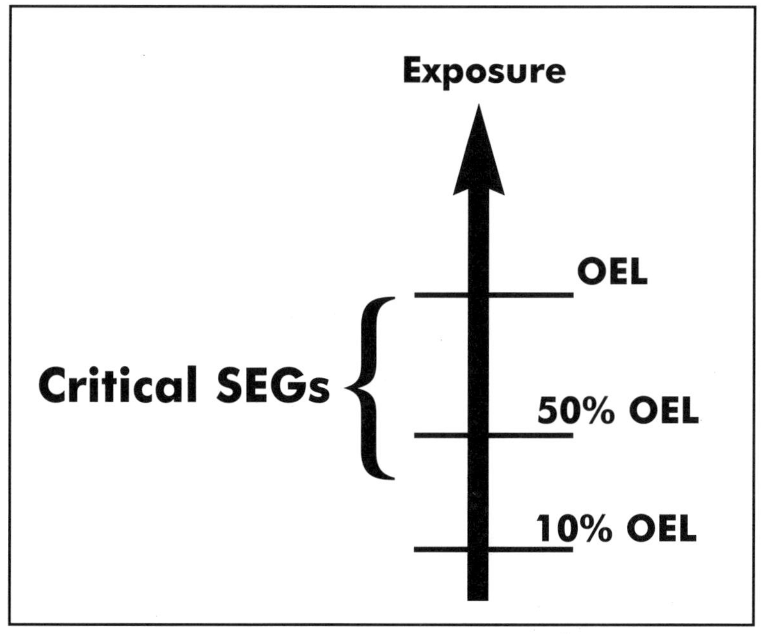

Figure 7.9 — Critical SEGs.

the SEG is below 0.26 × OEL, then one is 95% confident that the proportion of individuals with average exposures above the OEL is less than 5%. It is important to re-emphasize that this decision rule is limited to instances in which an LTA–OEL is appropriate.

By examining the list of critical SEGs, the industrial hygienist may be able to further prioritize them for extensive monitoring and ANOVA. This depends on:

- Higher priority if individual work practices are likely to influence exposures;
- Higher priority if the material is highly toxic;
- Higher priority if the material is a fast-acting toxicant; and
- Higher priority if unknown differences in process parameters, equipment emissions, or other workplace or environmental conditions are likely to influence exposures.

The use of ANOVA is discussed in more detail in Appendix IX.

Conclusion: Statistics to Aid the Judgment vs. Statistics to Make the Judgment

Statistical analysis of data that meets the strict conditions for use of parametric statistics undoubtedly can remove much subjectivity from a judgment on the exposure profile's acceptability. The method of random sampling and statistical analysis is the most accurate for defining SEGs. Statistical tests of the means or upper percentiles can give exact descriptions of the exposure profile for testing against some hypothesis of OEL exceedance.

Nonroutine Operations

Because during nonroutine operations it is difficult to collect sampling data that meet the data quality objectives for statistical analysis, overall reliance on statistics as a decision making tool is reduced. The macro level is where statistics can sometimes be used. Here, statistics can be used to describe the exposure of a population of workers involved in multiple, similar nonroutine operations. If, for example, multiple environmental restoration projects occur throughout an organization, the exposure data can be aggregated and analyzed to describe the exposure of this population of hazardous waste operation workers. This can be useful for health surveillance, regulatory compliance, and risk management. This perspective typically would be overlooked if each project were examined individually and not as part of the bigger picture.

Practically, however, it is difficult for industrial hygienists to meet the stiff requirements that must be met to rely on formal statistics alone. Lack of resources and trained personnel make it difficult to gather the large number of measurements needed to have high confidence in the parameter estimates, particularly of the variance and extreme percentiles. Practical problems get in the way of truly randomized sampling and in verifying that the population distribution is stationary and its shape known.

Even when all conditions are met to make precise estimates of the exposure profile parameters, there still might be a problem with what can be called "fuzzy" OELs. In other words, a precisely defined exposure profile can end up being compared with an imprecise OEL. We may be able to say with 95% confidence that the arithmetic mean of the exposure profile is below the LTA–OEL, but our knowledge of the LTA–OEL may still call for a judgment of unacceptable risk because the OEL contains inadequately characterized risk factors.

That is why this book focuses on statistical tools as aids to understanding exposure profiles for enhancing the industrial hygienist's professional judgment rather than as mechanisms for deciding an exposure's acceptability or unacceptability. A judgment must even be made about how much emphasis can be placed on the statistical analysis results. In cases in which the data fall far short of meeting the requirements of formal statistics (e.g., all measurements clustered into one or two days on an operation that changes systematically each season) the statistical analysis may play a very minor part. In cases in which measurements have been carefully randomized — and there are reasons to believe the exposure population is stationary and the underlying distribution is known — the statistical analysis may play a major role in the judgment.

It is, therefore, particularly important for industrial hygienists to understand statistics — not only the formulas but the conditions that underlie use of those tools.

As more data are generated, and as industrial hygienists gain a better understanding of exposures in the workplace through the exposure assessment process outlined in this book, critical SEGs will be identified. At that time, resources can be assigned to those high priority SEGs to gather data to refine the associated exposure profiles and judgments about their risks. It will then be possible to focus resources on gathering larger numbers of measurements and truly meeting the strict requirements involved in using statistical analysis to refine SEGs and their exposure profiles.

Summary: Steps for Analyzing Monitoring Data

Review the exposure assessment criteria for acceptability. Is, for example, the objective to ensure that the SEG's arithmetic mean exposure is below the LTA–OEL, or is it to ensure that less than 5% of the exposures in the SEG exceed the OEL. The following steps apply to baseline exposure assessments:

1. Design your sampling strategy. Consider the SEG and time interval being evaluated. Plan to gather at least six to 10 measurements to start. Randomize the measurements as much as possible. Try to avoid clustering of measurements into a single monitoring campaign covering successive periods.
2. Collect the measurements. Collect random samples as much as possible. Take care to record relevant information about the measurement and the process. If there is an unusual occurrence (e.g., spill, process shutdown) make a note of it. This information will help with data interpretation; however, be wary of excluding data — just because it is not "typical" does not mean it does not contribute to naturally occurring variability.
3. Plot the data in a time series as a subjective test for population stability. Trends in the data, as opposed to random variability, might indicate that the exposure distribution from which you are sampling is systematically changing over time. If systematic change is apparent, you must be extremely careful when pooling or omitting data for statistical analysis.
4. Calculate simple descriptive statistics (i.e., sample size, mean, median, minimum, maximum, standard deviation, GM, GSD, percent of actual data above OEL).
5. Plot the exposure data on logprobability paper. If the plot approximates a straight line, there is reason to believe the data are adequately described by a lognormal distribution. Try a normal-probability plot — the data may better fit a normal distribution. Review the sample data to look for outliers. Or consider that the SEG or similar exposure interval (SEI) was improperly defined. If the data fit a straight line on either the normal or lognormal paper, then the W-test can be used to quantitatively test the hypothesis that the data are parametric.
6. Use the eyeballed best-fit straight line through the points on the logprobability plot to estimate the GM (50% point) and the GSD (84% point divided by the 50% point). Examine

the plot to determine the 95th percentile to begin getting a picture of the upper extremes of the exposure profile.

7. Calculate the arithmetic mean estimate of the exposure profile and a confidence interval for that estimate.
8. Estimate the 95th percentile and the upper confidence interval (tolerance limit) for the percentile. Estimate the exceedance fraction and its upper confidence limits.
9. Review the available data, information, and statistical results for the SEG. Determine whether misclassification of individuals in the SEG is critical. If so, prioritize the SEG for further information gathering to better refine the SEG. If ANOVA will be used, randomly choose several employees from the SEG and monitor their exposures several times.
10. Judge the exposure to be acceptable or unacceptable in view of the exposure assessment objectives.

References

1. **Rappaport, S.M.:** Assessment of Long-Term Exposures to Toxic Substances in Air. *Ann. Occup. Hyg. J. 35(1):*61-121 (1991).
2. **Hawkins, N.C., M.A. Jayjock, and J. Lynch:** A Rationale and Framework for Establishing the Quality of Human Exposure Assessments. *Am. Ind. Hyg. Assoc. J. 53(1):*34-41 (1992).
3. **British Occupational Hygiene Society:** *Sampling Strategies for Airborne Contaminants in the Workplace* (Technical Guide No. 11). Leeds, United Kingdom: H & H Scientific Consultants Ltd., 1993.
4. **Leidel, N.A., K.A. Busch, and J.R. Lynch:** *Occupational Exposure Sampling Strategy Manual* (DHEW [NIOSH] Pub. No. 77–173). Cincinnati, Ohio: National Institute for Occupational Safety and Health, 1977. [National Technical Information Service (NTIS) Pub. No. PB274792.]
5. **Nicas, M., B.P. Simmons, and R.C. Spear:** Environmental Versus Analytical Variability in Exposure Measurements. *Am. Ind. Hyg. Assoc. J. 52(12):*553-557 (1991).
6. **Esmen, N.A., and Y.Y. Hammad:** Log-normality of Environmental Sampling Data. *J. Environ. Sci. Health A12(1&2):*29-41 (1977).
7. **Waters, M.A., S. Selvin, and S.M. Rappaport:** A Measure of Goodness-of-Fit for the Lognormal Model Applied to Occupational Exposures. *Am. Ind. Hyg. Assoc. J. 52(11):*493-502 (1991).

8. **Gilbert, R.O.:** *Statistical Methods for Environmental Pollution Monitoring.* New York: Van Nostrand Reinhold, 1987.
9. **Scheffers, T.M.L.:** "HYGINIST — A Computer Program for the Lognormal Evaluation of Air Exposure Data." Maastricht, The Netherlands: Scheffers IHPC, 1994. [Software.]
10. **Filliben, J.J.:** The Probability Plot Correlation Coefficient Test for Normality. *Technometrics 17:*111-117 (1975).
11. **Buringh, E., and R. Lanting:** Exposure Variability in the Workplace: Its Implications for the Assessment of Compliance. *Am. Ind. Hyg. Assoc. J. 52(1):*6-13 (1991).
12. **Francis, M., S. Selvin, R. Spear, and S. Rappaport:** The Effect of Autocorrelation on the Estimation of Workers' Daily Exposures. *Am. Ind. Hyg. Assoc. J. 50(1):*37-43 (1989).
13. **George, D.K., M.R. Flynn, and R.L. Harris:** Autocorrelation of Interday Exposures at an Automobile Assembly Plant. *Am. Ind. Hyg. Assoc. J. 56(12):*1187-1194 (1995).
14. **Symanski, E., and S.M. Rappaport:** An Investigation of the Dependence of Exposure Variability on the Interval Between Measurements. *Ann. Occup. Hyg. 38:*361-372 (1994).
15. **Manning, C.R.:** Considerations in the Design of a Sampling Strategy.
16. **Spear, R.C., S. Selvin, and M. Francis:** The Influence of Averaging Time on the Distribution of Exposures. *Am. Ind. Hyg. Assoc. J. 47(6):*365-368 (1986).
17. **Nicas, M., and R.C. Spear:** A Task-Based Statistical Model of a Worker's Exposure Distribution: Part I — Description of the Model. *Am. Ind. Hyg. Assoc. J. 54(5):*211-220 (1993).
18. **Nicas, M., and R.C. Spear:** A Task-Based Statistical Model of a Worker's Exposure Distribution: Part II — Application to Sampling Strategy. *Am. Ind. Hyg. Assoc. J 54(5):*221-227 (1993).
19. **Hornung, R.W., and L.D. Reed:** Estimation of Average Concentration in the Presence of Nondetectable Values. *Appl. Occup. Environ. Hyg. 5(1):*46-51 (1990).
20. **Cohen, A.C.:** Tables for Maximum Likelihood Estimates: Singly Truncated and Singly Censored Samples. *Technometrics 3:*535-541 (1961).
21. **Nelson, T.J., and S.W. Dixon:** "Management of Air Sampling Results." Paper presented at the American Industrial Hygiene Conference, Philadelphia, Pa., May 25, 1983.

22. **Selvin, S., S. Rappaport, R. Spear, J. Schulman, and M. Francis:** A Note on the Assessment of Exposure Using One-Sided Tolerance Limits. *Am. Ind. Hyg. Assoc. J. 48(2):*89-93 (1987).
23. **Evans, J.S., and N.C. Hawkins:** The Distribution of Student's t-Statistic for Small Samples from Lognormal Exposure Distributions. *Am. Ind. Hyg. Assoc. J. 49(10):*512-515 (1988).
24. **Rappaport, S.M., and S. Selvin:** A Method for Evaluating the Mean Exposure from a Lognormal Distribution. *Am. Ind. Hyg. Assoc. J. 48(4):*374-379 (1987).
25. **Attfield, M.D., and P. Hewett:** Exact Expressions for the Bias and Variance of Estimators of the Mean of a Lognormal Distribution. *Am. Ind. Hyg. Assoc. J. 53(7):*432-435 (1992).
26. **Selvin, S., and S.M. Rappaport:** A Note on the Estimation of the Mean Value from a Lognormal Distribution. *Am. Ind. Hyg. Assoc. J. 50(12):*627-630 (1989).
27. **Tuggle, R.M.:** Assessment of Occupational Exposure Using One-Sided Tolerance Limits. *Am. Ind. Hyg. Assoc. J. 43(5):*338-346 (1982).
28. **Leidel, N.A., K.A. Busch, and J.R. Lynch:** *Occupational Exposure Sampling Strategy Manual* (DHEW [NIOSH] Pub. No. 77–173). Cincinnati, Ohio: National Institute for Occupational Safety and Health, 1977. [National Technical Information Service (NTIS) Pub. No. PB274792.]
29. **Leidel, N.A., and K.A. Busch:** Statistical Design and Data Analysis Requirements. In *Patty's Industrial Hygiene and Toxicology,* Vol. 3A, 3rd Ed. (R.L. Harris, L.J. Cralley, and L.V. Cralley, editors). New York: John Wiley & Sons, 1994.
30. "Occupational Safety and Health Administration — Preamble to the Lead Standard," *Federal Register 43*: (14 November 1978). p. 52952.
31. **Comité Européen de Normalisation:** *Workplace Atmospheres — Guidance for the Assessment of Exposure by Inhalation to Chemical Agents for Comparison with Limit Values and Measurement Strategy* (EN 689). Brussels, Belgium: Comité Européen de Normalisation, 1995.
32. **Nicas, M.:** [Personal communication.] 1996.

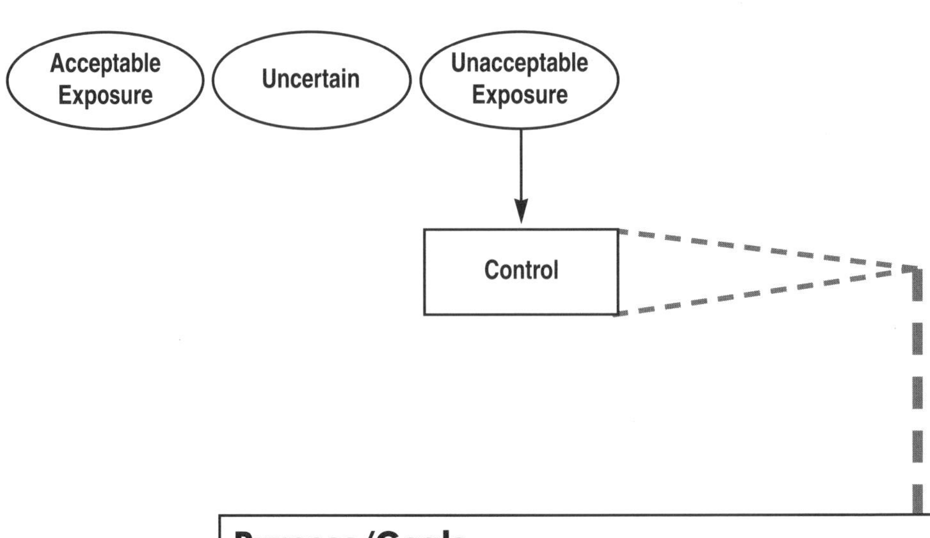

Purpose/Goals

- Prioritize exposure groups with unacceptable exposures for control.
- Develop strategy for control.
- Protect workers while long-term controls are put in place.

Tools

- Prioritization
  - Exposure rating
  - Toxicity rating
  - (Un)certainty rating
- Control options
  - Short term
    - PPE
    - Administrative
    - Work practices
  - Long term
    - Elimination
    - Substitution
    - Isolation
    - Enclosure
    - Ventilation

Outcome

1. Prioritized control plan
2. Control options: short term/long term
3. Exposures controlled

8 Health Hazard Control

Unacceptable exposures must be controlled — quickly and reliably! Control options include material elimination or substitution, engineering controls, work practice controls, administrative controls, and personal protective equipment. Implementing these measures, however, requires planning and resources. Designing and implementing long-term control solutions such as process modifications or local exhaust ventilation usually requires significant time and capital expenditures. Prioritizing the SEGs for control ensures that the limited resources are appropriated for those exposures that present the highest risks.

Once the SEGs are prioritized, the control strategy that is most effective should be determined for each SEG, while taking into account what industrial hygienists consider the fundamental "hierarchy of control." The control strategies for each of the prioritized unacceptable exposures can then be consolidated into a general health hazard control plan for the workplace. Following implementation of health hazard controls, the performance of these controls should be verified and workplace exposures to environmental agents should be reassessed.

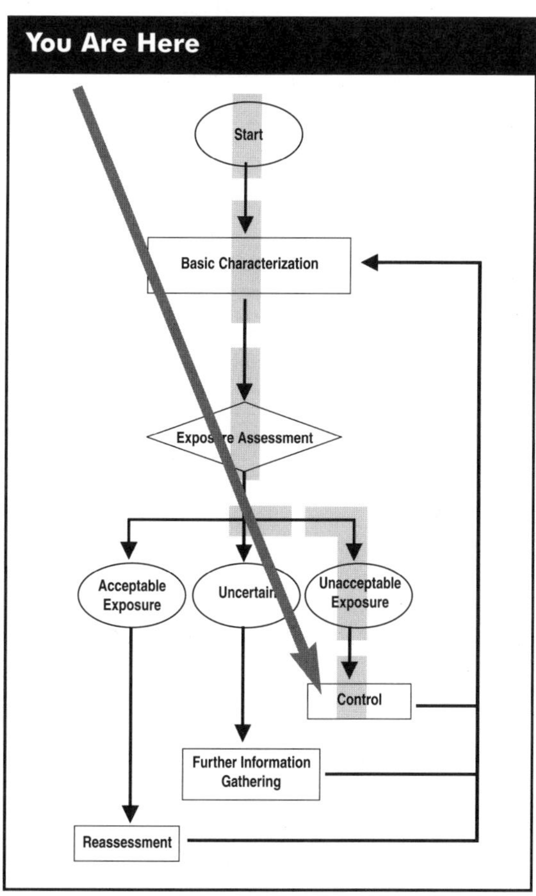

Prioritizing SEGs for Health Hazard Control

All unacceptable exposures must be controlled. These include those that present an unacceptably high health risk and those that present other unacceptable risks (such as risk of noncompliance with a government regulation). As discussed in Chapter 6, health risk increases with both exposure level and potential health effect. The higher the health risk, the higher the priority for action (see Figure 8.1).

Whether the action needed is control, information gathering, or a combination of the two depends on the extent of the potential health risk and the certainty of the exposure assessment (see Figure 8.2). If the assessment is highly certain, there is no need for additional information gathering — the industrial hygienist should move directly to defining control strategies for those SEGs that present a high health risk. If the assessment is uncertain, and the exposure has not been judged unacceptable, then information gathering will be the most appropriate action.

In Chapter 6, methods for prioritizing SEGs for more information gathering were discussed. Prioritization for control uses these same determinants, thereby making the two ranking and

Health Effect Rating				
4	4	8	12	16
3	3	6	9	12
2	2	4	6	8
1	1	2	3	4
	1	2	3	4
	Exposure Rating			

Figure 8.1 — Priority for action: health risk rating (health risk rating = health effect rating × exposure rating).

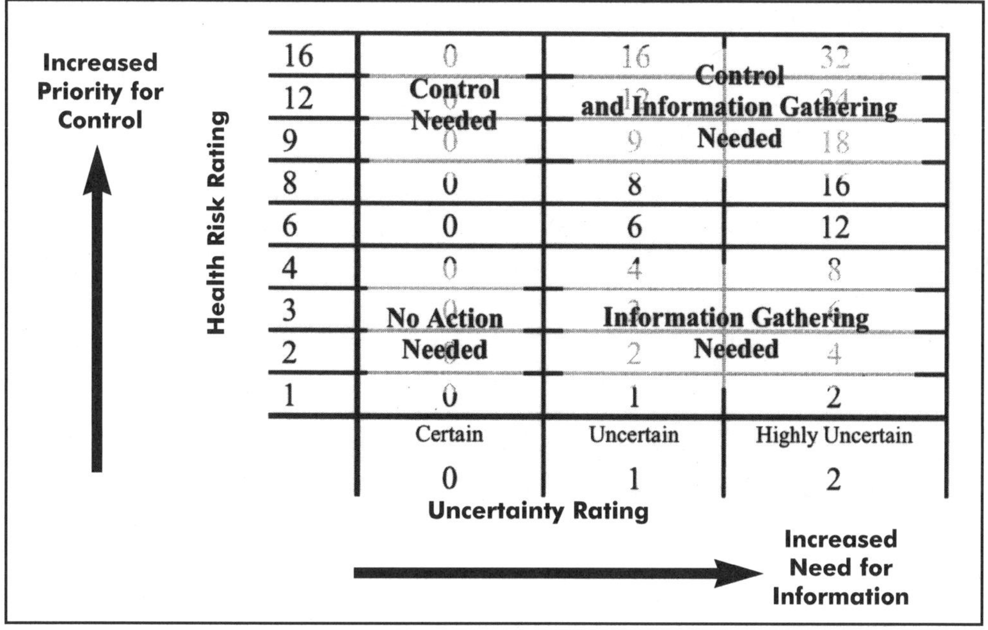

Figure 8.2 — Priority and action.

prioritization schemes compatible. As described in Chapter 6, SEGs assigned to a high health risk rating category with significant uncertainty should be given high priority for information gathering. If the potential health risk is severe enough, they may also be identified as deserving a quickly implemented short-term control (such as respirators) while additional information is generated. Depending on the potential health risk and the time it takes to implement long-term controls, there might also be times when temporary control measures are needed while the long-term control effort proceeds.

As is the case with prioritization for information gathering, the prioritization scheme provides only a rough ranking of risk. Prioritization schemes should not supplant the use of experience and judgment. The industrial hygienist is the most knowledgeable person to lead establishment of priorities and recommendations for controlling unacceptable exposures. In particular, all exposures potentially above the OEL (an exposure rating of 4 in this text) should be investigated and, if necessary, controlled.

After the SEGs are initially prioritized for control, the list of ranked SEGs should be reviewed to determine whether the result is consistent with the industrial hygienist's professional judgment in weighing all that is known about the SEG. The SEG priority rank may be raised or lowered based on the following data:

- Reliability of existing control methods;

- Number of workers exposed;
- Frequency of exposure;
- Concurrent exposures and the associated risk for additive or synergistic health effects; and
- Presence of workers whose personal health condition might put them at increased risk (e.g., pregnant workers, workers with respiratory disease, etc.).

The industrial hygienist may compare priority rankings for information gathering and control and judge simply to control the exposure rather than commit additional resources to further characterization. If, for example, an SEG has a high priority ranking for information gathering with an agent whose health effects are poorly characterized and the exposure occurs quite intermittently, it might be more effective to control the exposures than gather more information. This is especially true if an effective control strategy can be easily identified and deployed.

A major benefit of the control priority scheme is that it provides management with an easily understood framework around which judgments and decisions can be made. It also allows some standardization of response to health hazards in an organization. For example, respiratory protection could be immediately required for any SEG rated as having a "high" potential inhalation health risk with high uncertainty until exposure monitoring was completed to provide the needed additional information. More time might be given to gather information needed for further characterization of "low" potential health risk SEGs.

Example: Prioritization of SEGs for Health Hazard Control

Information for SEGs in our example coil coating operation is summarized in Table 8.1.

Priority for action depends to a great extent on the potential health risk. Whether the action needed is information gathering or control (or both) depends on the extent of the potential health risk and the degree of uncertainty. Arranging the SEGs according to the potential health risk rating (column 8) and uncertainty (column 7) allows prioritization for control and information gathering (see Figure 8.3).

As shown, SEG "N" has high priority for control with no need for further information gathering, and SEGs "R" and "G" have the highest priority for information gathering (column 9). SEGs "R" and "G" are also high on the list for control. Short-term controls such as the use of a respirator might be recommended while the needed information is gathered.

Table 8.1 — Manufacturing Plant Exposure Ratings

1	2	3	4	5	6	7	8	9
SEG ID	***Job***	***Task***	***Agent***	***Exposure Rating***	***Health Effect Rating***	***Uncertainty Rating***	***Pot. Health Risk Rating***	***Info. Gathering Priority Rating***
A	Coil Feed Operator	General	Noise–TWA	3	3	1	9	9
B	Coil Feed Operator	General	2-butoxyethanol	2	2	2	4	8
C	Coil Feed Operator	Cleanup	MIBK–STEL	3	2	1	6	6
D	Coil Feed Operator	Cleanup	Cyclohexanone–STEL	3	2	1	6	6
E	Discharge Operator	General	Noise–TWA	3	3	1	9	9
F	Discharge Operator	General	2-butoxyethanol	2	2	2	4	8
G	Discharge Operator	QC	MIBK–STEL	4	2	2	8	16
H	Discharge Operator	Cleanup	MIBK–STEL	3	2	1	6	6
I	Discharge Operator	Cleanup	Cyclohexanone–STEL	3	2	1	6	6
J	Helper	General	Noise–TWA	3	3	1	9	9
K	Helper	Cleanup	MIBK–STEL	3	2	1	6	6
L	Helper	Cleanup	Cyclohexanone–STEL	3	2	1	6	6
M	Helper	Lubricate	Packing grease 609	1	1	0	1	0
N	Helper	Fluxing	Heat	4	2	0	8	0
O	Helper	Fluxing	Hexachloroethane	1	2	1	2	2
P	Helper	Fluxing	Hydrogen chloride	4	1	0	4	0
Q	Helper	Fluxing	Hexachlorobenzene	3	4	1	12	12
R	Helper	Fluxing	Octochlorostyrene	3	4	2	12	24

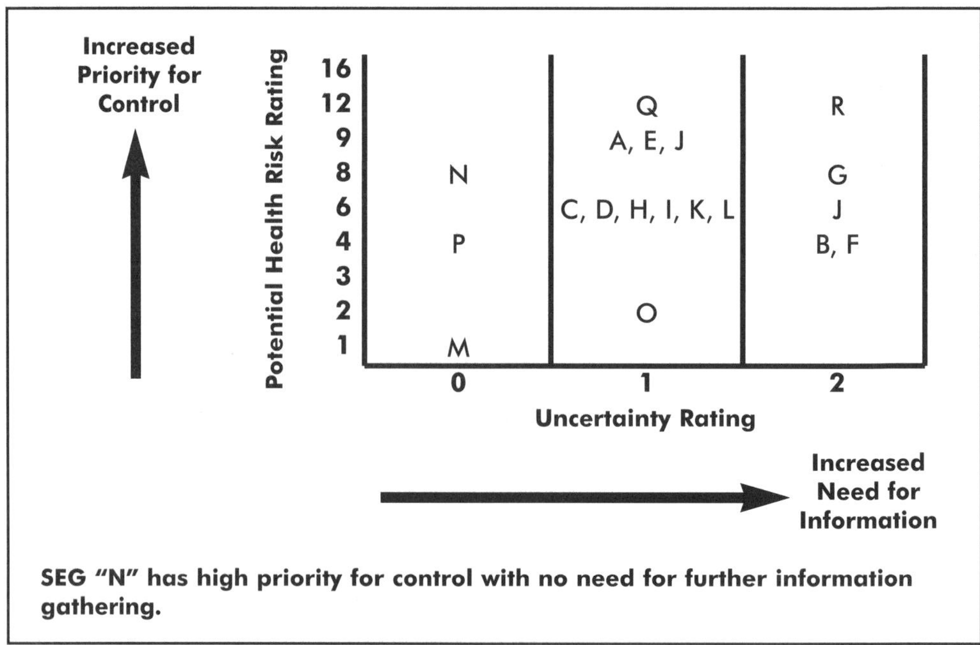

Figure 8.3 — Control/information gathering matrix.

SEG "Q" also received high priority for control. In this case, the industrial hygienist may choose to recommend short-term controls while more information is gathered, or he or she may decide to move directly toward implementation of permanent controls and save the time and money that would have been spent on additional information gathering (see Figure 8.3).

Hierarchy of Control

Industrial hygienists advocate use of a hierarchical strategy to select health hazard controls. Preference, of course, is given to the more reliable control methods. The following hierarchy should be applied when implementing permanent exposure control strategies for each SEG associated with unacceptable exposures:

- Elimination of the process, equipment, or materials giving rise to the exposure;
- Substitution with a less hazardous process, equipment, or material;
- Engineering controls (e.g., process modification, enclosure, exhaust ventilation, shielding, damping);
- Work practice controls and employee training;
- Administrative controls; and
- Proper selection, fitting, and use of personal protective equipment.

When occupational exposure assessments reveal unacceptable exposures, the exposures must be controlled expeditiously. It can take weeks, months, or longer to design and implement some of the more effective control strategies. In the interim, effective use of personal protective equipment will be necessary. Personal protective equipment is the last line of defense, and as such it is given the lowest rank in the industrial hygiene hierarchy of control.

Elimination or Substitution

Elimination, or substitution with a less hazardous agent, are generally the most effective and most preferred methods of control; however, although eliminating the source of the hazard may be the solution preferred by the industrial hygienist, it might be a sensitive subject for the process engineering and manufacturing staff. The industrial hygienist therefore should research the process thoroughly before suggesting changes. The chemical in question could be used for a specific reason and its elimination would be considered an impractical solution.

Another type of substitution that sometimes offers effective control is to change the form of process materials. A raw material supplied in a powder form might be replaced with a less dusty granular material, for example, or a spray coating operation might be replaced with dip coating.

In considering chemical substitutes, the safety and environmental implications should be reviewed to ensure that one hazard is not simply exchanged for another. A different chemical in the process might have a variety of impacts, including:

- Trigger environmental reporting;
- Change composition of waste streams;
- Cause emissions to be covered under the EPA Clean Air Act;
- Trigger coverage under the OSHA process safety management standard;
- Change requirements for sprinkler system coverage of storage areas; or
- Impact requirements on release of process water.

Similarly, when new processes are being designed — and when existing processes are being changed due to environmental, pollution prevention, or other initiatives — industrial hygiene and safety implications should be considered carefully.

Be wary of substituting an unknown hazard for a known hazard, particularly when replacing one material with another having similar chemical properties. The absence of toxicity warnings might be due to inadequate testing or lack of knowledge, so for that reason the industrial hygienist cannot simply assume one material is less hazardous than the one for which it is being substituted. It is more prudent to put programs in place to manage a known hazard than to risk mismanaging an unknown hazard.

Engineering Controls

Engineering controls generally are directed at modifying process equipment or at capturing emissions to maintain the environmental agent at an acceptable exposure level.

Isolation, which can be performed through physical barriers, time, or distance, is most readily implemented when emissions are diffuse or the operation is automated. General ventilation dilutes the concentration of the environmental agent and reduces exposures. It is used for low toxicity chemical agents and when there are indoor air quality issues. Local exhaust ventilation is based on capturing the agent at the point(s) of emission with a low volume, high velocity exhaust system. Local exhaust ventilation is typically more effective than general ventilation.

To avoid interference with normal operations and to allow for maintenance, the design of the engineering controls must consider how workers interface with the equipment. Maintenance worker exposure can easily be the most significant exposures associated with an operation. It is important to involve workers in the design and selection of engineering controls. After all, controls tend to be unused or bypassed when workers find them to be inconvenient.

Work Practice Controls

Work practice controls are prescribed work methods and procedures directed at controlling a health hazard (e.g., wetting down a surface to reduce the release of a particulate). Employee education and training is necessary for work practice controls to be implemented effectively, and because these controls depend on all employees following specific procedures, they will be only as good as the organization's ability to ensure adherence to prescribed (i.e., documented) procedures.

The effectiveness of newly adopted work practice controls should be verified through a reassessment of worker exposures or other techniques, such as job observations or inspections.

Administrative Controls

Administrative controls, which involve restrictions or redeployment of workers to reduce exposure time and safely spread the potential exposure over a group of many workers rather than among a few, have both strengths and weaknesses.

If the health effects associated with the environmental agent are well-characterized (i.e., little to no uncertainty in the health effects rating), it may be advantageous to devise an administrative control strategy that effectively manages worker exposures and health risks. A good example is application of administrative controls in hot environments. The health risks associated with heat stress are well-understood and there is little uncertainty about the potential health effects. During the hot season, for example, some organizations add employees to work crews to reduce the risk of heat-related illnesses. Overtime limitations are another form of administrative control.

On the other hand, if there is significant uncertainty about the potential health effects, administrative controls may not be a good strategy because more workers will potentially be exposed to an uncertain health risk. Administrative controls are normally not applied to managing carcinogen exposure when there is significant uncertainty about the dose-response relationship and the threshold of risk. Administrative controls would only serve to expose a larger number of workers to carcinogens. This concern is expressed in some OSHA standards, for instance where the agency does not permit administrative controls (e.g., OSHA's methylene chloride standard).[1]

Personal Protective Equipment

Personal protection for health hazard control includes respiratory protection, hearing protection, and use of equipment such as chemically protective clothing and gloves. Work area or task-specific personal protective equipment (PPE) rules should be established, and personal protective devices should be selected to reduce effective exposures below OELs.

It is essential that personal protective equipment is properly fitted, selected, and used — and effective PPE use depends greatly on worker acceptance and cooperation. Accordingly, employee education and training is necessary to ensure success in this area. Effective measures should also be considered to ensure that personal garments and protective equipment taken off site are not contaminated with environmental agents that pose a health risk to workers, their families, or the community.

Controlling Dermal Exposures

If a dermal exposure is judged unacceptable, the conditions of this exposure should be mitigated through material substitution, process changes, or engineering controls. Prescribed work practices and use of personal protective equipment should be fall-back protection when there is uncertainty about the reliability of controls.

A special emphasis on personal hygiene is advised when incidental or secondary skin contact is a concern. Employees should be encouraged to wash their hands and even their faces before eating, drinking, smoking, or applying cosmetics. Washing compounds should be carefully selected to ensure that the skin retains its ability to act as a natural contaminant barrier.(2) Food consumption and smoking are generally prohibited in the work area, and showering on exiting the work area is a recommended means to minimize skin absorption if there is a significant risk for contamination of work clothing.

Several factors (such as permeation, degradation, and penetration) can affect the protection provided by personal protective equipment and clothing. The industrial hygienist must consider the potential for permeation and degradation of the protective clothing being used. To do this, he or she must examine information such as the characteristics of the chemical (or formulation) that is in contact with the clothing, clothing construction and finish, garment design, and characteristics of the clothing material.

Laboratory glove permeation testing is commonly conducted to evaluate the permeation characteristics of a given contaminant–glove matrix, but other factors have to be considered, such as elevated temperature and the stressing and pressure applied to the glove during use. These factors have been found to significantly reduce the glove's effectiveness during actual use when compared with laboratory glove permeation data.(3) The effectiveness of protective clothing and equipment usually is influenced by the operation and work practices. For example, if a worker has to remove a glove to perform a task and replaces the glove without decontaminating his or her hands, the inside of the glove will likely become contaminated, thus contributing to dermal exposure.

A thorough determination of the effectiveness of protective clothing during actual use is quite complex, but it can be crucial. Use of engineering controls and other process controls to mitigate dermal exposures is recommended, of course, as the primary means of control.

Consistent Control Recommendations

Systematic and consistent exposure assessments allow consistent control recommendations. In Chapter 5, the Performance-Based Exposure Control Limit (PB–ECL) program used in the pharmaceutical industry(4) was described. In this program, chemical agents are managed in accordance with well-prescribed control strategies that address containment, general ventilation, local exhaust ventilation, surfaces, maintenance, cleaning, waste disposal, decontamination, personal protective equipment, monitoring, and medical surveillance. The choice of a particular control strategy is based on the containment levels defined by the PB–ECL. Ongoing monitoring and exposure assessment programs validate the ability of the various strategies to meet the control objectives. The unit operations control matrix used in this program is illustrated in Table 8.2.

Performance-based exposure control limits are also used in the American National Standard for the Safe Use of Lasers (ANSI Z136.1–1993). This standard defines hazard classifications for lasers; for each category, guidelines are provided for controlling exposure to laser radiation. The hazard classes and control recommendations are designed to ensure compliance with the underlying OELs for laser radiation expressed as maximum permissible exposure criteria.[5]

Control Plans

The control strategies or plans for each unacceptable exposure should be consolidated into a general health hazard control plan for the workplace. This plan should address health hazard abatement priorities and implementation schedules; it should be established and adopted by management.

Table 8.2 — Performance Based Exposure Control Limit (PB–ECL) Unit Operations Matrix – Solids: Charging/Transfers (Adapted from Naumann et al.[4])

PB–ECL Category	*1*	*2*	*3*	*4*	*5*
General corresponding numerical "exposure control limit" 8-hour TWA	In the range of 1–5 mg/m³	In the range of 0.1–1 mg/m³	In the range of 1–100 µg/m³	In the range of <1 µg/m³	In the range of 0.1 µg/m³
Containment level	Good manufacturing practices	Good manufacturing practices (with more stringent controls)	Essentially no open handling (closed systems should be used)	No open handling (closed systems must be used)	No manual operations, no human intervention
Vacuum conveyor (closed system)	yes	yes	yes	yes	yes
Half-suit isolator	yes	yes	yes	yes	yes
Glove box	yes	yes	yes	yes	yes
Iris valve	yes	yes	yes	yes	no
Open screw conveyor	yes	yes	yes	no	no
Open scooping (wet)	yes	yes	yes	no	no
Gravity (totes/drum dumping)	yes	yes	no	no	no
Dry open scooping with local exhaust ventilation	yes	yes	no	no	no

Reliability of Health Hazard Controls

The industrial hygienist's hierarchical strategy for health hazard controls can be used to rate control reliability. For example, exposure controls can be rated as follows:

7. Elimination of the process, equipment, or materials giving rise to the exposure.
6. Substitution with a less hazardous environmental agent.
5. Engineering controls with verification.
4. Work practice controls with verification.
3. Administrative controls with verification.
2. Personal protective equipment.
1. No controls.

Reliability is one element of the uncertainty associated with exposure assessment. As such, the reliability of existing exposure controls can be incorporated into prioritization schemes for further information gathering and health hazard control.

Hazard elimination, substitution, and engineering controls should be adopted to the greatest extent feasible. The following factors should be considered when assessing feasibility and ultimately selecting the most effective health hazard control strategy:

- Magnitude of health risk;
- Technical feasibility;
- Economic feasibility;
- Reliability of the control method;
- Worker acceptance;
- Consequences of control failure;
- Maintenance requirements;
- Associated safety hazards; and
- Associated environmental hazards.

A thorough analysis of the feasibility of implementing control options should make it easier to gain management support.

The industrial hygienist should consider calculating the costs and benefits for the various control options. Cost and benefits should be defined in terms of direct and indirect values. Personal protective equipment solutions to health hazards, although less expensive in the short term, often become more expensive than other more effective solutions in only a few years. Accordingly, the financial "net present values" associated with each control option should be considered for a multiple-year period.[6]

Continuous Monitoring Instrumentation

Use of continuous monitoring instrumentation and alarms should be considered in work areas where significant accidental exposures are possible due to toxic gases arising from combustion or chemical processes. For example, continuous monitoring instrumentation is advised in operations that use toxic compressed gases with poor warning properties (e.g., carbon monoxide).

SEG Exposure Assessment Update and Verification of Controls

If controls are modified in a manner that changes exposures, the affected SEGs' exposure profiles and judgments should be updated. The effectiveness of newly implemented controls should be verified through reassessment of worker exposures and other techniques. Initial and periodic testing of engineering controls is appropriate when the performance of controls can decline or fail (e.g., static pressure testing of local exhaust systems). ACGIH's *Industrial Ventilation — A Manual of Recommended Practice* provides procedures for performance testing of local exhaust systems.(7)

Summary

In most workplaces, problems compete for resources and it is frequently necessary to prioritize SEGs classified as having unacceptable exposures for health hazard control. The management of workplace exposures to chemical, physical, and biological agents is enhanced if prioritization for control is used in conjunction with prioritization for further information gathering. Most important, health hazard controls are selected in view of the commonly accepted "hierarchy of controls" where preference is given to the more reliable intervention strategies. Finally, exposures are reassessed following implementation of controls to verify that the occupational health risks have been reduced to acceptable levels.

References

1. **Occupational Safety and Health Administration:** *Methylene Chloride Standard.* Washington, D.C.: U.S. Government Printing Office.
2. **Packham, C.L.:** *Skin Care at Work: A Manual for the Prevention of Occupational Skin Disease,* 2nd Rev. Ed. Evesham, United Kingdom: Skin Care Services, 1994.

3. **Perkins, J.L.:** Chemical Protective Clothing: I. Selection and Use. *Appl. Ind. Hyg. 6:*222-230 (1987).
4. **Naumann, B.D., E.V. Sargent, B.S. Starkman, W.J. Fraser, G.T. Becker, and G.D. Kirk:** Performance-Based Exposure Control Limits for Pharmaceutical Active Ingredients. *Am. Ind. Hyg. Assoc. J. 57(1):*33-42 (1996).
5. **American National Standards Institute:** *American National Standard for the Safe Use of Lasers* (ANSI Z136–1993). New York: American National Standards Institute, 1993.
6. **Birkner, L.R., and L.S. Salzman:** Assessing Exposure Control Strategy Cost-Effectiveness. *Am. Ind. Hyg. Assoc. J. 47(1):*50-54 (1986).
7. **American Conference of Governmental Industrial Hygienists:** *Industrial Ventilation — A Manual of Recommended Practice,* 22nd Ed. Cincinnati, Ohio: American Conference of Governmental Industrial Hygienists, 1995.

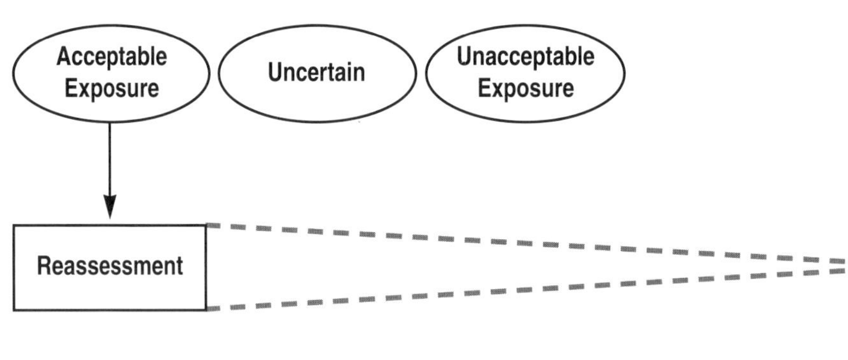

Purpose/Goals

- Periodically recharacterize and reassess exposures to:
  1. Update exposure groups and exposure profiles.
  2. Identify changes that may influence exposures.
  3. Identify unacceptable exposures for control.
  4. Identify uncertain exposures for further information gathering.

Tools

- Prioritization based on exposure, toxicity, and "instability" of the exposure (i.e., how likely the exposure is to change)
- Management of change process

Outcome

- Prioritized schedule for re-evaluation
- Updated basic workplace characterization
- Updated exposure groups and exposure profiles

9

Reassessment

Every workplace should be periodically reassessed to update SEGs, exposure profiles, exposure judgments, and information gathering and health hazard control priorities in view of significant changes in the workplace, work force, and environmental agents. Identification of new exposures and those exposures no longer present should be included in this reassessment process.

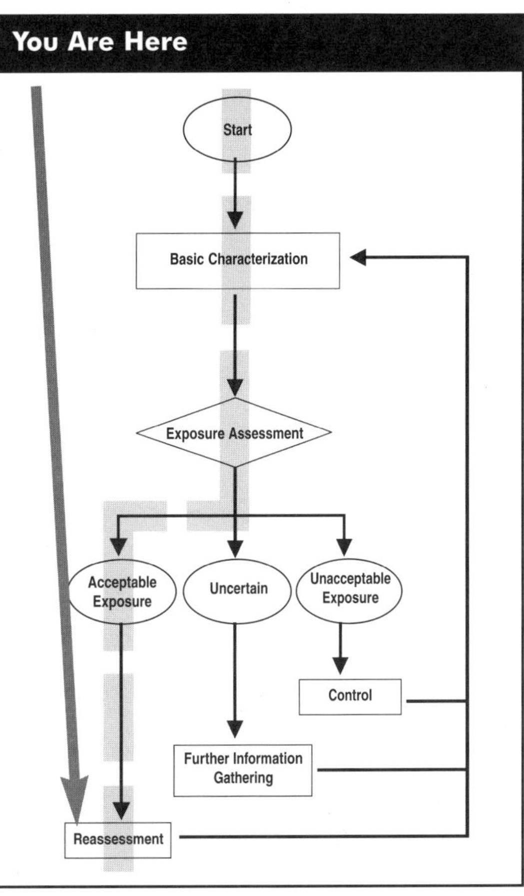

Reassessment Frequency

The written exposure assessment program should specify a frequency for periodic reassessment. A designated reassessment interval will help ensure identification of those changes in the workplace, work force, and environmental agents that might affect exposure assessments. Annual reassessments are performed in many workplaces, but the recommended frequency may depend on the nature of the work. The amount of change in the workplace is a good guideline. Certainly, those workplaces in which processes, job classifications, and use of environmental agents change rapidly should be reassessed more frequently.

A rigorous management-of-change process is needed to ensure

that the industrial hygienist is automatically appraised of significant changes between designated reassessment cycles. In this way the exposure assessments can be re-evaluated as needed. The industrial hygienist can keep abreast of significant changes by reviewing production, engineering, construction, or maintenance work orders. Some organizations, in fact, require formal health and safety reviews of new projects, process changes, or material substitutions.

A designated reassessment interval is important even if a good management-of-change procedure is in place. It helps ensure that a reassessment is performed to identify subtle but important changes that might not have been reported.

Reassessment Triggers

Significant changes in the workplace include changes in process and engineering controls that may affect exposure levels, such as a new filtration system in a chemical plant, a new welding system in an automotive operation, or an increase in production rate. Subtle changes in the workplace must be considered as well. Gradual wear and tear on critical equipment (e.g., fans, ducts, motors, gaskets, seals) can result in significant changes in exposure.

In reassessing exposures, significant work force changes should be considered. A reorganization of the work force may affect exposure assessments and the designation of SEGs. Work schedule changes also may affect exposure assessments. For example, a change from a conventional 8-hour-a-day work schedule to a 12-hour shift could lead the industrial hygienist to recommend a more conservative OEL, and the more conservative OEL may change the exposure assessment.

A work schedule change may also affect the exposure profile and thereby change the exposure assessment decision (i.e., acceptable or unacceptable). The exposure assessment may even be altered by significant changes in employment. For example, exposures for new hires may be significantly greater than exposures for more experienced workers in operations where exposure levels are largely affected by work practices.

Changes in the identity, quantity, and physical characteristics of the environmental agents used also may affect the exposure assessments, as may a significant change in the health effects information or the OEL. A change in the OEL, for example, could mean an exposure previously deemed acceptable is now unacceptable.

An exposure reassessment should be conducted if worker complaints are voiced or there is evidence of occupational illness or disease. It should go without saying that the industrial hygienist must work closely with the organization's medical staff, not only to provide the medical staff with insight into workplace exposures but also to learn in a timely and effective manner when there are worker complaints and concerns about exposure to chemical, physical, and biological agents.

Reassessment Scope

Reassessments should be complete. The industrial hygienist should start with information gathering to update the basic characterization and work through to assessment judgments, reprioritizations, and reports. Each significant change affecting the workplace, work force, or environmental agents should be reassessed using the cyclic exposure assessment process.

Each exposure reassessment should build on previous assessment information and results; therefore, typical reassessments should be less time-consuming than initial exposure assessments. Basic characterization data should be brought up to date, but there should be a base of documentation from the initial assessment from which to work. Past experience with the processes, tasks, materials, and workers should make reassessments proceed more smoothly. Often reassessments are simply a matter of confirming that exposures continue as before.

As in the initial exposure assessment, exposure monitoring is often not required to resolve exposure reassessments. When monitoring is required, however, care must be taken in comparing or combining new SEG monitoring data with previous monitoring data.

The concept of the similar exposure interval (SEI) was introduced in Chapter 7. Systematic reassessments will help the industrial hygienist identify when an SEI has ended and when a new SEI has begun. There may be a series of SEIs over the life of an SEG. Exposure histories can be derived for workers in the SEG if the beginning and ending dates of each SEI are documented.

Periodic Exposure Monitoring Strategies

Some organizations have established internal guidelines for periodic monitoring of workplace exposures.[1-3] If an organization's exposure assessment objectives include development of a historical database, the monitoring data acquired in conjunction with the reassessments can be applied toward building the database. In general, monitoring frequency and sample size are the variables for defining periodic monitoring. In some guidelines monitoring frequency is influenced by the exposure level and the environmental agent's health effects rating. The sample size may be influenced by the exposure variability and the number of employees in the SEG.

Random sampling is advised to minimize bias in the database, because collecting samples at the same time each year can result in a distorted database. If periodic surveillance samples are collected each summer, for example, the values may underestimate the long-term average exposure due to increased ventilation and lower exposure levels than may be present during the winter.

Statistical Techniques for Comparing Sampling Campaign Data Sets

To compare the newest exposure measurements with a reference exposure data set, several statistical methodologies are available. Specifically, methods that use the chi-square distribution and other statistics can test for a difference between parameters describing the periodic surveillance data and the previous exposure data. The Dutch Occupational Hygiene Society, for one, has developed a software program titled "HYGINIST" that contains various industrial hygiene statistical tools, including methodologies for comparing two data sets.(5)

If sufficient data are available to use statistical methodologies, graphical presentations of the data (such as logprobability and time series plots) should reveal any differences between the old and new data sets.(6)

A significant difference between the new and previous data sets means exposures have changed significantly and the assessment should be based exclusively on the new exposure data. If no significant difference is detected, the exposure should be reassessed using the periodic data pooled with the previous exposure data.

Statistical Control Charts

Once exposures are controlled to an acceptable level, some analysis of the trend of exposures over time may be appropriate. This time trend should be reviewed periodically not only to ensure that control is being maintained but to detect problems early.

Statistical control charts are excellent tools for analyzing exposure data and detecting trends over time. A mean chart plots the mean exposure values for each sampling campaign. Upper and lower control limits can be calculated. These means and confidence intervals can be plotted vs. monitoring dates. If the mean values of the campaigns remain within the control limits, exposure is stationary (i.e., not changing and in control). If exposures seem to be trending higher over time, more frequent monitoring campaigns might be needed. If trends are stable or exposure levels seem to be decreasing, less frequent monitoring usually is acceptable, which frees monitoring resources for higher priority SEGs. A "range chart" tracks variability over time.

Control chart methods plainly illustrate the need for meaningful sample numbers. Fifteen or more campaigns of 4–6 samples each may be needed. If fewer samples are collected, the data may seem out of control when, in fact, they are within the normal variability of the process. Control charting enforces the discipline involved in periodic reassessment of all exposure profiles.

In 1991, Hawkins and Landenberger wrote in *Applied Occupational and Environmental Hygiene* about the application of control chart methods in industrial hygiene.(7) The basic mechanics of control chart analysis are described in Appendix X.

Summary

Reassessment is an essential element of the exposure assessment and management process. No matter the size of the workplace, the industrial hygienist should conduct systematic reevaluations to identify any changes in the workplace, work force, and environmental agents that may lead to significant changes in the exposure profile, OEL, or exposure assessment decision. The reassessment process can be enhanced through use of periodic monitoring strategies, statistical analysis of monitoring campaign data sets, and control charts.

References

1. **Comité Européen de Normalisation:** *Workplace Atmospheres — Guidance for the Assessment of Exposure by Inhalation to Chemical Agents for Comparison with Limit Values and Measurement Strategy* (EN 689). Brussels, Belgium: Comité Européen de Normalisation, 1995.
2. **Nelson, T.J., and S.W. Dixon:** "Management of Air Sampling Results." Paper presented at the American Industrial Hygiene Conference, Philadelphia, Pa., May 25, 1983.
3. **Damiano, J.:** A Guideline for Managing the Industrial Hygiene Sampling Function. *Am. Ind. Hyg. Assoc. J. 50(7):*366-371 (1989).

4. **Harris, R.L.:** *Guideline for Collection of Industrial Hygiene Exposure Assessment Data for Epidemiologic Use.* Washington, D.C.: Chemical Manufacturers Association, 1993.
5. **Scheffers, T.M.L.:** "HYGINIST — A Computer Program for the Lognormal Evaluation of Air Exposure Data." Maastricht, The Netherlands: Scheffers IHPC, 1994. [Software.]
6. **George, D.K., M.R. Flynn, and R.L. Harris:** Autocorrelation of Interday Exposures at an Automobile Assembly Plant. *Am. Ind. Hyg. Assoc. J. 56(12):*1187-1194 (1995).
7. **Hawkins, N.C., and B.D. Landenberger:** Statistical Control Charts: A Technique for Analyzing Industrial Hygiene Data. *Appl. Occup. Environ. Hyg. 6(8):*689-695 (1991).

10 Communications and Record Keeping

Exposure assessment reports and records are critical elements of the exposure assessment and management process. Reports and records are needed to ensure effective communication of workplace findings and successful continuity of the industrial hygiene program. Each element in the assessment and management process should be documented: start (assessment goals and procedures); basic characterization; exposure judgments; information gathering needs; health hazard controls; and reassessment plans. As shown in our process flow diagram for assessing and managing occupational exposures (see Figure 1.2) a "communications and documentation" stage is not included. That is because communication of exposure assessment findings and maintenance of assessment data should be presumed throughout as essential features of an effective process.

All exposure assessment findings (i.e., the exposure profile and whether it is acceptable, unacceptable, or uncertain) should be documented, regardless of whether monitoring data were collected. Moreover, assessment findings should be communicated in a timely and effective manner to all workers in the SEG and those involved in worker health protection, such as management, labor representatives, and medical and engineering staff. If the assessment reveals unacceptable exposures, these determinations should be communicated rapidly along with recommendations for controlling the health hazard. When monitoring data are collected to support the exposure assessment, the monitoring data should be summarized and interpreted by the industrial hygienist.

Reporting Exposure Assessments

The exposure assessment report is essential for communicating assessment findings and health hazard control recommendations. For each report, include the following:

- *Summary:* This should describe the purpose of the exposure assessment, general observations, conclusions, and major recommendations.
- *Purpose:* The reason for performing the assessment must be stated clearly. Was it a baseline assessment, a reassessment, or was it in response to an employee complaint?
- *Exposure assessment strategy:* The report should make reference to the organization's written exposure assessment program and specify the assessment strategy (i.e., comprehensive or compliance).
- *Environmental agents:* For each environmental agent, the report should briefly identify the significant health effects and OEL(s) used in the assessment. The source of the OEL should be identified with reference to documentation describing the rationale for the OEL.
- *Exposure assessment data:* Assessment data should include assessment dates, name of the industrial hygienist performing the assessment, SEGs, exposure controls in place, exposure rating, health effects rating, uncertainty rating, and acceptability judgment (i.e., acceptable, uncertain, or unacceptable).
- *Monitoring data (if available for the SEGs being discussed):* Monitoring data should include sampling dates, SEGs, identity of workers who were monitored, measured exposure levels normalized to the integration period of the OELs (8 hours, 15 minutes, etc.), and use of relevant personal protective equipment.
- *Observations and conclusions:* Interpretive remarks should be provided. All assumptions and models should be identified or referenced. The report should conclude whether exposures were judged acceptable or unacceptable, or whether more data are needed to resolve the assessment. A diagnostic exposure assessment report should provide observations and conclusions about the sources of exposure and the effectiveness of controls (e.g., engineering, work practices, etc.).
- *Recommendations:* As appropriate, specific recommendations should be provided (e.g., engineering controls, process changes, work practice controls, personal protective equipment). A re-evaluation frequency may be recommended.

Graphical tools and performance measures can be used in written reports and oral presentations. If available, monitoring results can be summarized graphically or through the use of tabulated statistics. Assessment findings can be used to prepare charts reporting:

- A list of unacceptable exposure SEGs, thus serving to help focus health hazard control efforts.
- Total number of workers incurring unacceptable exposures, excluding the use of personal protective equipment. This metric serves as a measure of health hazard control. (The report should appropriately acknowledge the use of personal protective equipment.)
- A list of SEGs for which the exposure profile exceeds medical surveillance triggers.
- For hazard communication, a list of exposure agents for each SEG.
- Chronological charts to illustrate upward or downward trends in a SEG's exposure levels.

The organization's assessment results can be summarized graphically.[1] This may be a simple pie chart of general assessment results (see Figure 10.1) or a matrix designed to communicate the relative health risks identified by the assessment (see Figure 10.2).

Occupational Exposure Database

The data documentation and management efforts required by a comprehensive exposure assessment approach in medium- and large-sized organizations will be difficult to manage without a computerized system.[2] An exposure database is especially important if the organization commits to maintaining worker

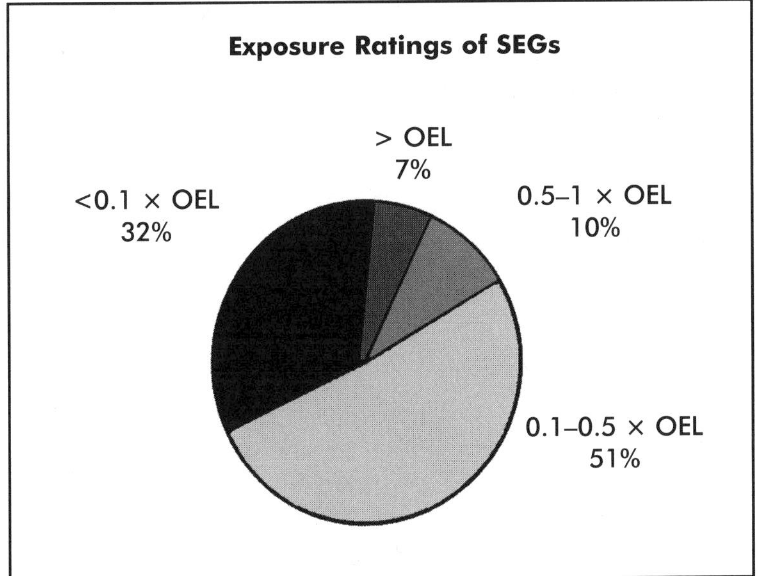

Figure 10.1 — Exposure ratings of SEGs.

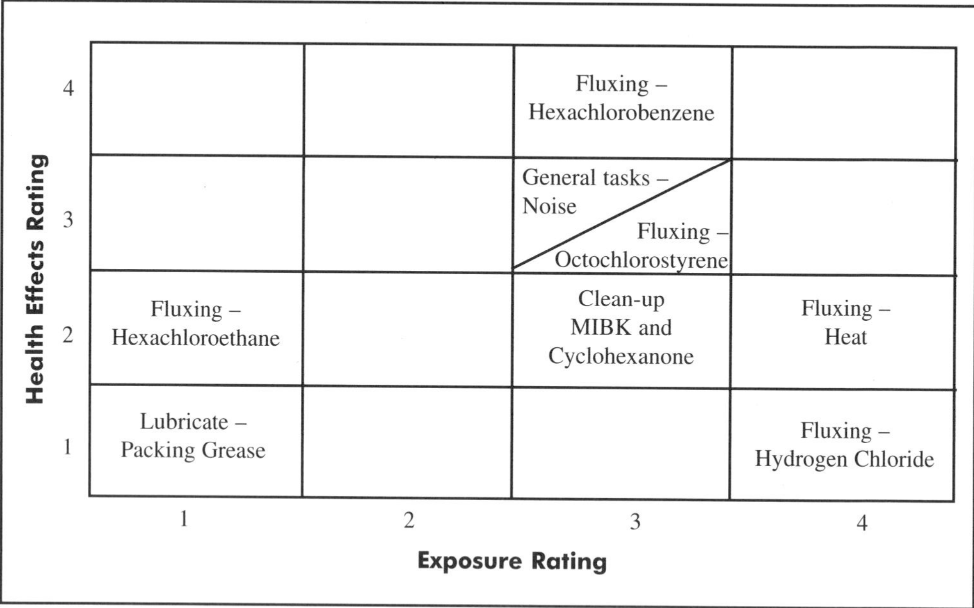

Figure 10.2 — SEG matrix (helper in casting and coil coating processes — task and environmental agent).

exposure histories.[3-7] Another driving force is the need to document OEL compliance; however, it may be possible to accomplish this simply with exposure assessment reports.

In compiling an occupational exposure database, the industrial hygienist should carefully consider how exposure data will be used. Records should be established and maintained so that pertinent questions can be answered accurately and within a reasonable period of time. The industrial hygienist should recognize that other disciplines may have an interest in exposure data, such as the work force, management, medical, engineering, and legal personnel, and even governmental agencies and industry associations. Exposure records are also a critical component of future epidemiological studies.[8,9]

The industrial hygienist should focus on which questions are likely to be asked and what information is needed to adequately answer these questions. Here are some frequently asked questions:

- What environmental agents are associated with a particular work area or SEG?
- Who belongs to the SEG?
- What is the magnitude and variation in exposure for each SEG?
- What processes or tasks were associated with the exposure?
- How long did the exposure last?
- How frequent was the exposure?

- What are the acceptable and unacceptable exposures in the workplace?
- Who qualifies for medical surveillance?
- Is there evidence of upward or downward trends in exposure levels?
- What is a worker's occupational exposure history?

Occupational exposure histories can be maintained through a database that captures information on the workplace, work force, environmental agents, SEGs, monitoring data, and exposure assessment findings. A good reference for designing a database is a recent article in *Applied Occupational and Environmental Hygiene* titled "Data Elements for Occupational Exposure Databases: Guidelines and Recommendations for Airborne Hazards and Noise."(6) Some important data elements are identified below.

Workplace Data

A workplace file can be established where the workplace is described in words, process flow diagrams, maps, and floor plans with noted points of interest (e.g., sources of noise, ventilation hoods).

The site can be described by the following data elements:

- Organization (e.g., Company); or
- Facility name.

The work area can be described by:

- Department;
- Building/zone;
- Room/area; or
- Production unit or center.

The operation can be described by:

- Process (including frequency and duration);
- Task (including frequency and duration);
- Equipment; or
- Health hazard controls (e.g., engineering, work practice, administrative, personal protective equipment).

Environmental Agent Data

An inventory of chemical, physical, and biological agents is necessary for any industrial hygiene program. The environmental agent database can be organized around mixtures and specific agents.

Mixtures

Information listed in the database may include:

- Trade name;

- Manufacturer;
- Chemical components (e.g., percentage of component);
- Quantities in use;
- OEL for mixture, if appropriate;
- Begin date of use;
- End date of use;
- Application (i.e., how used?);
- Link to material safety data sheet (MSDS);
- Physical form (e.g., solid, powder, liquid, gas); and
- Degradation products.

Specific Agents

The following may be included:

- Name;
- Unique code (e.g., CAS number);
- Health effects rating (see Tables 6.1 and 6.2 in Chapter 6);
- Occupational exposure limits;
- Physical form (e.g., dust, mist, fume, gas, noise, radiation, heat, vibration, ergonomic);
- Other properties (e.g., vapor pressure); and
- Sampling and analytical method.

SEG Data

The following data elements provide a good historical record of each SEG:

- SEG identifier(s): Name of group, basis for group, and/or data elements describing the group (e.g., process, job, task, environmental agent); and
- Work schedule (e.g., 8, 10, or 12 hours per day).

Written descriptions of the processes, jobs, and tasks are important to ensure an accurate understanding of the SEG by those who will access the database in the future.

Worker Data

Workers should be linked to exposure assessment findings and monitoring data through the SEGs. To create a historically accurate record of exposures, the following data should be collected and maintained for each worker:

- Employee name;
- Unique identifying code;
- Work crew (e.g., day shift, night shift); and
- Links to participation in each SEG, with begin dates and end dates.

Monitoring Data

The data elements for each measurement should include:

- Unique identification number;
- Date collected/measured;
- Collected by (i.e., industrial hygiene technician);
- Date of analysis;
- Sample duration: begin and end measurement times;
- Plant site and location;
- SEG (e.g., process, job, task, environmental agent);
- Monitored worker and his or her unique identification number;
- Work schedule and shift length;
- Sample type (e.g., personal, biological, positional/area);
- OEL averaging time (e.g., instantaneous for a ceiling limit assessment; 15 minutes for a STEL; 8, 10, or 12 hours for a full-shift TWA);
- Sampling strategy or reason for monitoring: baseline (random), compliance (worst-case), or diagnostic. [NOTE: For worst-case monitoring, document the worst-case scenario.];
- TWA assumptions: exposure during unsampled time;
- Measured exposure level and unit of measure;
- TWA exposure level and unit of measure;
- Conditions during measurement (e.g., typical, upset, etc.) and explanation; and
- Observations and comments, including information describing where the measurement was collected (e.g., building, production line), work practices, and observations on the potential for exposure via skin contact or inadvertent ingestion. Such information must be recorded since it might affect interpretation of the monitoring data or recommendations for control. Observations and comments are important aspects of professional judgment, and exposure assessments cannot be made without professional judgment.

The monitoring and analytical methods are critical when the measured result may differ depending on the monitoring and analytical method. For example, noise dosimeter samples collected in accordance with a 5-decibel (dB) doubling rate should not be mixed with samples collected with a 3-dB doubling rate. Monitoring and analytical information should be linked to monitoring data. These data elements should include:

- Monitoring method;
- Monitoring media;
- Monitoring device;
- Noise dosimeter settings (e.g., integration threshold, doubling rate);

Nonroutine Operations

Direct-reading, area, or diagnostic monitoring data can be misleading when it is not properly described and qualified. When examined historically, one may mistakenly believe these data represent typical exposures or something other than what they truly represent. Nonroutine operation logbooks are full of handwritten observational data and notes. Industrial hygienists are obligated to describe accurately what their exposure data represent because these logbooks may be examined by others in the future as part of a retrospective exposure assessment study.

- Flow rate;
- Calibration documentation;
- Analytical method; and
- Analytical laboratory.

Personal protective equipment information should be linked to monitoring data. These data elements should include:

- Hearing protection: Worn? Type?
- Respirator: Worn? Type?
- Gloves: Worn? Type?
- Protective clothing: Worn? Type?
- Eye/face protection: Worn? Type?

Exposure Assessment Data

The following data should be collected and maintained for each exposure assessment:

- SEG identifier (includes environmental agent);
- SEI begin and end dates;
- Name of industrial hygienist who performed the assessment;
- Date of exposure assessment;
- Route(s) of exposure (e.g., air, skin, whole body);
- Exposure rating (see Tables 5.1 and 5.2 in Chapter 5);
- Uncertainty rating (see Table 6.4 in Chapter 6);
- Decision: acceptable, unacceptable, or uncertain; and
- Significant concomitant exposures (i.e., risk for additive or synergistic effects associated with concomitant exposures).

Some organizations have developed algorithms for processing exposure assessment data. These algorithms have been integrated into "expert" software systems.(10) Also, to improve and leverage the use of models in exposure assessment, it may be valuable to collect and document various determinants of exposure conditions relevant to modeling, such as ventilation and generation rates.(11)

Summary

Communications are the vital link between the industrial hygienist's efforts and employee health protection. Workers and management must understand the health risk present in the workplace since their support and participation is vital to implementation of health hazard controls. Industrial hygiene communications must be timely and effective. Exposure assessment findings must be shared with all similarly exposed workers and those in the organizations who support employee health protection. Exposure assessment findings may be communicated through both written reports and oral presentations. Graphical tools and statistical parameters can be used to enhance communication of exposure assessment findings and health risks.

A carefully designed and well-maintained exposure assessment database can support resolution of future questions regarding past exposures, which undoubtedly will surface in many organizations. Exposure histories can be derived from exposure data, maintained in six relational databases.

References

1. **Bonorden, J.:** "Exposure Assessment Strategies Implementation: Hurdling the Barriers." Roundtable presented at American Industrial Hygiene Conference & Exposition, Washington, D.C., May 22, 1996.
2. **Holzner, C.L., R.B. Hirsh, and J.B. Perper:** Managing Workplace Exposure Information. *Am. Ind. Hyg. Assoc. J. 54(1):*15-21 (1993).
3. **Ott, M.G., S.K. Norwood, and R.R. Cook:** The Collection and Management of Occupational Exposure Data. *Am. Statist. 39:*432-436 (1985).
4. **Gómez, M.R., and G. Rawls:** Conference on Occupational Exposure Databases: A Report and Look at the Future. *Appl. Occup. Environ. Hyg. 10:*238-243 (1995).
5. **Damiano, J.:** Quantitative Exposure Assessment Strategies and Data in the Aluminum Company of America. *Appl. Occup. Environ. Hyg. 10(4):*289-298 (1995).
6. **Joint ACGIH–AIHA Task Group on Occupational Exposure Databases:** Data Elements for Occupational Exposure Databases: Guidelines and Recommendations for Airborne Hazards and Noise. *Appl. Occup. Envir. Hyg. 11:*1294-1311 (1996).
7. **Rajan, B., R. Alesbury, B. Carton, M. Gérin, H. Litske, H. Marquart, E. Olsen, T. Scheffers, R. Stamm, and**

T. Woldbaek: European Proposal for Core Information for the Storage and Exchange of Workplace Exposure Measurements on Chemical Agents. *Appl. Occup. Environ. Hyg. 12(1):*31-39 (1997).

8. **Harris, R.L.:** *Guideline for Collection of Industrial Hygiene Exposure Assessment Data for Epidemiologic Use.* Washington, D.C.: Chemical Manufacturers Association, 1993.
9. **Stewart, P.A., A. Blair, M. Dosemeci, and M. Gómez:** Collection of Exposure Data for Retrospective Occupational Epidemiologic Studies. *Appl. Occup. Environ. Hyg. 6(4):*280-289 (1991).
10. **Tait, K.:** The Workplace Exposure Assessment Expert System (WORKSPERT). *Am. Ind. Hyg. Assoc. J. 53(2):*84-98 (1992).
11. **Jayjock, M.A., and N.C. Hawkins:** A Proposal for Improving the Role of Exposure Modeling in Risk Assessment. *Am. Ind. Hyg. Assoc. J. 54(12):*733-741 (1993).

11 Conclusion: Exposures Occur Whether We're There or Not

The industrial hygienist's view of exposures in the workplace can be either narrow or broad. If your focus tends to be narrow, we suggest you step back from your subject and, in a manner of speaking, begin using a wide-angle lens — you will quickly notice there is so much more to see. While doing this, keep the following in mind:

- Your field of view should address the exposures for all workers, not just those present when you visit the workplace.
- Your field of view should address the exposures for all workers on all days. Steer away from focusing exclusively on the conditions at the time of your visit.
- Your field of view should address the exposures for all workers on all days for all environmental agents. Steer away from focusing exclusively on environmental agents with formally established OELs (such as OSHA PELs or ACGIH TLVs).

When it is time to meet the challenge of managing exposures for all workers on all days for all environmental agents, we will probably find our clarity reduced: this is not the same as being able to focus only on a relatively small number of workers, over a few days, for a limited number of environmental agents. A trade-off results, and unfortunately when we choose to use the comprehensive approach in the assessment process, we are also incorporating a great deal of uncertainty.

The picture, of course, will be "fuzzy." To include all workers in the exposure assessment process, we will need to engage in the inexact exercise of establishing SEGs. It is disconcerting to address day-to-day variability in exposure levels, but we must do so to address exposures across time. Moreover, it can be disconcerting — and sometimes painful — to examine the OELs and discover that the health effects data are weak or, worse yet, no OEL is available.

Keep in mind that in this book we have dissected the underlying criteria and hallmarks of professional judgment — the industrial hygienist's primary tool for managing the uncertainty associated with occupational exposure assessments. We can choose to manage the uncertainty and deal with it effectively, or we can revert to our narrow practice of industrial hygiene and enjoy a higher level of confidence in our exposure assessments. Again, we suggest you choose the comprehensive approach because exposures occur regardless of whether or not they are being managed.

According to NIOSH, "improved exposure assessment methods will lead to better identification of at-risk workers, better identification of the most cost-effective control and intervention strategies, better understanding of exposure-response relationships, and improved baseline data for standards-setting and risk assessment, all of which are central to improving occupational health and safety."[1]

Some of the other advantages of comprehensive exposure assessment detailed and illustrated in this book are:

- Comprehensive understanding of exposures: Because the approach is systematic and comprehensive, users can be confident the resulting description of exposures is thorough and accurate.
- Prioritized exposure management efforts: Comprehensive exposure assessment allows the industrial hygienist to focus his or her efforts on the exposures that present the highest risks. Management can be sure that resources are being spent effectively on those issues that most ensure compliance with regulations and protection of employees and the organization.
- Improved industrial hygiene programs: A detailed and complete understanding of exposures allows the industrial hygienist to establish programs that are thorough and focused.
- Documented exposure judgments: Comprehensive exposure assessment provides a mechanism for documenting each exposure judgment, regardless of whether the judgment was made for a low exposure or high exposure situation. This helps ensure that judgments and their rationales are not forgotten and enables continuity in the industrial hygiene program over time. It ensures that exposure judgments will be available for future use when employee

questions need to be answered. It also helps address legal issues involving employee exposures, provides exposure information for future epidemiology, and allows management to understand and focus on possible changes in environmental agent toxicology.

- Efficient ongoing exposure assessment and management: Well-documented basic characterizations and exposure profiles mean the industrial hygienist can confidently leverage monitoring data from one process to similar processes. Likewise, an understanding of exposures in one process can be used to assess more efficiently exposures in similar processes or processes further up or down the production chain.
- Employee confidence and comfort: As a result of their participation in the comprehensive exposure assessment process, employees can be more confident that harmful exposures are being identified and managed. This increased confidence and comfort usually results in better employee satisfaction and helps ensure good productivity and product quality.
- Increased process understanding: A comprehensive exposure assessment increases understanding of the process and the materials being used. The material ingredients, their physical and hazardous properties, the amounts being used, and the ways they are used are all better understood. This increased understanding can trigger investigations and activities that can improve the process in several areas, from industrial hygiene to safety, environmental, quality, or productivity concerns.

In this book, we advocate a comprehensive approach to exposure assessment and management for all workers on all days for all environmental agents. We trust we have convinced you of these and numerous other benefits, and have given you ideas for incorporating the strategy into your industrial hygiene program. Now is the time to get started. After all, the exposures occur whether we're there or not!

References

1. **National Institute for Occupational Safety and Health:** "National Occupational Research Agenda" (April 1996).

Appendix I

Estimating Airborne Exposure with Physical–Chemical Models

Introduction

Personal air monitoring of an individual quantifies the concentration of the agent of interest in the person's breathing zone. The interface of this airborne concentration with the person defines the exposure.[1] One can also estimate this airborne concentration with physical–chemical models. This appendix provides some of the currently used techniques for modeling, but it is not exhaustive in its treatment. Please consult the references for more detailed information.

Inhalation exposure models are not generally well developed or validated. The reasons for this are presented elsewhere;[1,2] however, suffice it to say that current models represent relatively crude estimators of exposure. Given their rather coarse state of development, there is a fairly large degree of uncertainty associated with model use. To guard against underestimation of exposure, risk assessors typically use models that overestimate exposure potential. This tendency is directly proportional to the amount of uncertainty (i.e., lack of data or information) in the analysis. In situations where there are very little data on which to base the model, the overestimation can be high.

We usually start with relatively simple models that have overestimating assumptions. Depending on the conclusions of the predicted level of exposure to the OEL, we may need to use more sophisticated modeling tools. Unfortunately, as mentioned above, the total modeling resource at hand is relatively weak, and we sometimes run out of modeling resources before we reach a definitive answer. In these cases one needs either to develop a better model or perform representative air monitoring. The second solution is almost invariably chosen because it is relatively inexpensive and answers the question at hand expeditiously. This, however, has delayed development of improved physical–chemical models, leaving us without improved theoretical resources.

The fact that our current models are underdeveloped does not mean they are not useful or valuable industrial hygiene tools. Indeed, models are invaluable in the preliminary assessment process to determine the need for further studies and for supplying critical insights about the nature of the exposure. As an example, consider a material with a molecular weight of 100, a room temperature vapor pressure of 0.1 Torr (or mmHg), and an OEL of 300 ppm v/v (1230 mg/m^3). As you will see below, application of a relatively simple, overestimating saturation model will render an estimate of 132 ppm v/v (538 mg/m^3). Thus, this simple model shows that overexposure to vapors at room temperature is essentially impossible. On the other hand, if the OEL happened to be 100 ppm in this example, the model would not have allowed this conclusion of relative safety and we would be forced to use a more sophisticated model or perform representative air monitoring.

Other potential uses of exposure models include:

- Evaluation of an existing operation for different emission activity scenarios;
- Exposure control selection and design;
- Preliminary assessment of material substitutions;
- Retrospective exposure evaluations; and
- Evaluation of potential exposure during new product development.

It is the authors' hope that the future will bring exposure model development that provides industrial hygienists with better, more cost-effective means of estimating exposure than are available today. This investigative work will also provide a foundation for a growing and evolving science of human exposure assessment.(2) Until then, the tools presented here represent the current state of the science for the practicing industrial hygienist.

Background

Exposure models attempt to use a mathematical construction to quantitatively estimate exposure. Classical modeling techniques define a source term for the contaminant and describe transport and fate of the contaminant in time and space to predict airborne concentrations. Receptors (humans who encounter this airborne concentration) are then integrated into the predicted contaminant field and their time-weighted average exposure estimated.

There is a broad range of model sophistication;[1,3] this appendix will cover only the following types as the most useful for the practicing industrial hygienist:

- Saturation model;
- Box model;
- Back pressure box model; and
- Dispersion model.

They are presented in order of increasing sophistication and level of information needed to use them successfully.

The estimation of vapor pressure is critical when estimating airborne exposure to vapors in the workplace; there will be further discussion on this elsewhere in this appendix. The connection between modeling and monitoring becomes particularly important when one has some monitoring data to add to the estimates. A brief discussion is presented on linking monitoring data into the models.

Saturation Model

The saturation model is to be used for gases and vapors emitted without mist formation when no information on ventilation or details of use are available.

A basic but conservative approach to inhalation exposure assessment is to calculate the maximum possible concentration of vapor (i.e., saturation) in air. For any liquid, saturation will eventually occur in the air above a liquid surface when no ventilation is present and the evaporation rate ultimately overwhelms any removal mechanism such as absorption, adsorption, or chemical transformation.

The equilibrium saturation concentration (C_{sat}) in volume parts of contaminant per million volume parts of air (ppm v/v) will be:

$$C_{sat} = \frac{(10^6)(\text{vapor pressure})}{(\text{atmospheric pressure})} \quad (1)$$

Vapor pressure at any ambient temperature is an experimentally determined quantity; however, it can also be estimated for any class of liquids from boiling point data either at atmospheric pressure or under vacuum.[4] The vapor pressure of components within mixtures can also be estimated using established procedures.[5] A brief discussion of the estimation of vapor pressure of an organic compound mixture is presented below. A discussion of vapor pressure as a function of temperature is presented at the end of this appendix.

This saturation model is usually conservative for the prediction of workroom air concentrations. It has been the authors' experience that it overestimates workroom air concentrations of vapor (i.e., nonparticulate) in all but worst-case scenarios (such as large spills indoors with very poor ventilation) by a factor ranging from 1 to 4 orders of magnitude (10–10,000×). This observation is the result of comparing scores of measured concentrations of organic air contaminants in occupational settings with their saturation concentrations calculated from vapor pressure or boiling point data. Worst-case scenarios include those in which significant aerosol is released or there is a relatively large area (greater than a few square meters) of evaporating liquid.

This model's value lies in its simplicity as a screen with only a few basic physicochemical properties required as input. As a conservative estimate it represents a good "first step" in a tiered risk assessment. If exposure levels determined by the model are below the compound's OEL, it is likely that actual vapor concentrations do not pose an unacceptable risk to worker health via inhalation exposure. Of course, other types of exposure (such as dermal or oral) and aerosol generation are not considered in this method.

Box Model

The box model is used with data on source rate and ventilation for gases and vapors emitted without mist formation.

Equilibrium Model

The box model considers the conservation of air contaminant mass in a volume of workroom air. Airborne concentrations are derived using the following general equation:

$$C = \frac{(A_{in} - A_{out})}{\text{volume of the box}} \tag{2}$$

where:

C = concentration after some finite time t_i (assume $C = 0$ at $t_0 = 0$) in units of mass/volume

A_{in} = mass of contaminant that went into the box during time interval $t_i - t_0$

A_{out} = mass of contaminant that has left the box during time interval $t_i - t_0$

A more specific differential equation can be used to describe this situation:

$$VdC = Gdt - QCdt - kCdt \quad (3)$$

where:

- V = volume of the box
- C = concentration of air contaminant (mass/unit volume)
- G = generation rate of contaminant (mass/time)
- k = nonventilatory removal coefficient (volume/time)
- Q = ventilation rate (mixing volume of air/unit time)

The term kCdt describes the loss of contaminant from the air in the box from the combined effects of absorption and adsorption onto environmental surfaces (including walls, floors, machinery, clothes, and skin) and chemical transformation. The assumption is that the rate of contaminant loss from these mechanisms is proportional to the concentration of the contaminant in the workroom air. One can choose to ignore this factor and solve the equation without any consideration of these nonventilatory losses within the box. Although convenient, this approach can lead to dramatically conservative overestimates of inhalation exposure potential. This is especially true of contaminants that are highly reactive or have high molecular weight or a high boiling point, and thus a tendency to adhere to environmental surfaces. *A priori* estimates of k or any other term describing these types of losses are virtually impossible. Some early work has been done,[6] but we need significantly more experimental activity to explain the nature of this factor and to use and predict the level of its effect.

The term QCdt describes the removal of contaminant from the air in the box by general ventilation with mixing volumes of clean air. It assumes perfect and instantaneous mixing of the entire volume of air in the box with the incoming air. Since almost all modelers have recognized that perfect mixing does not exist in the real world, this term is often modified to render a lower effective ventilation rate. Thus Q in Equation (3) becomes Q´, which is defined as:

$$Q' = Q(m) \quad (4)$$

where:

- Q´ = effective ventilation (air volume/time) into and out of the box
- m = mixing factor, with a possible range of 0–1.0 (dimensionless)

An experimental study using a tracer gas technique to determine mixing factors found m values in the range of 0.3–0.7 in small rooms without fans.[7] The proper assignment of values for Q and m in any particular scenario is problematic and depends greatly on the workroom air box size, which in turn is determined by factors affecting diffusion of the contaminant within that volume. This sizing of the box of air around any contaminant source is covered in detail elsewhere[8] with a discussion of "affected volume." The conclusion of this analysis is that a convenient and appropriately conservative affected volume is approximately 230 m^3 (8000 ft^3) cube with a mixing factor (m) of 0.15.

Conceptually this volume would represent the workroom section of greatest concern because it would contain by far the highest concentrations of toxicant. A significantly larger volume would require mixing factors (m) that will diminish rapidly to much less than 0.1. A much smaller volume could overestimate concentrations near the source because the dilution ventilation rate is proportional to the affected volume. More important, ascribing a small affected volume also suggests that there is relatively little exposure potential beyond its boundaries. Depending on the level of eddy diffusion and the ratio of Q′ to G, this may not be true.

In practice, the person doing the modeling must determine or estimate the number of mixing air changes per hour and the resulting ventilation rate (Q) in this conceptual affected volume (a 20-foot cube around the source). Combining this ventilation rate and mixing or safety factor (m = 0.15) will allow one to render a worst-case estimate of the average concentration in this box of workroom air after he or she also estimates the generation rate (G).

The term Gdt describes the total input of contaminant into the air volume of the box (i.e., emission rate). The contaminant can enter the air through direct injection or evaporation. In some instances toxicants may exist as both thoroughly mixed gas molecules (either gas or vapor) and as suspended particulate (aerosols). Examples of direct injection include spraying or displacement of contaminated air, such as from the head-space of a drum during its filling. Evaporation will occur from any liquid at an air–liquid interface in which the air is not saturated with that liquid's vapor.

The determination of G in many operations involving direct injection is relatively straightforward, using material balance determinations (in the case of spraying) and verifiable assumptions about displacement of contaminated air (as in charging operations). For example, as a worst case, assume that the headspace volume of a receiving vessel is displaced into the work room air and that this volume contains saturated vapors (C_{sat}) of the material(s) being transferred. The following equation would describe the generation rate:

$$G = (\text{volume of receiving vessel})(C_{sat})(\text{number of vessels filled per hour}) \quad (5)$$

The determination of G from vaporization is more complicated and requires input of the contaminant's vapor pressure, the surface area of the air–liquid interface, and some determination of the diffusion mass transfer coefficient for the molecules going from liquid to vapor state. Methods to estimate G from evaporation have been put forward in the last two editions of the *EPA Manual for the Preparation of Engineering Assessments.*[9,10]

Other methods for estimating G from evaporation that involve more input variables and more complicated calculation have been summarized.[11-15] It remains for experimental verification to determine which method or combination of methods will ultimately be the most effective in predicting contaminant evaporation rates into occupational settings when criteria of accuracy, practicality, and ease of use are taken into account.

Solving the combination of Equations (3) and (4) under the following conditions:

1. C_{eq} is at steady-state equilibrium (i.e., $dC/dt = 0$).
2. G, Q, k, and m are all constant.

yields the relatively simple relationship:

$$C_{eq} = G/(Qm + k) \quad (6)$$

Assuming a state of ignorance regarding the removal rate kC, we are forced to be conservative (i.e., overestimating) and assign k a value of zero resulting in the simple relationship of:

$$C_{eq} = \frac{G}{(Q)(m)} \quad (7)$$

Thus, knowledge of the effective general ventilation rate and contaminant source rate allows the estimation of the equilibrium contaminant air concentration in any affected volume or box of workroom air. This model typically assumes that there is no concentration of air contaminant in the outdoor or recirculated air that makes up the incoming ventilation. These can be accounted for in the model when they are significant. For example, modeling of a carbon dioxide source indoors would require accounting for the ambient concentration of about 300 ppm v/v of carbon dioxide that always comes in with outdoor or recirculated air. The details and examples of this expanded modeling are available elsewhere.[16]

Nonequilibrium or Time–Course Model

Equations (6) and (7) are independent of volume (V) and the only thing required about time t is that it is "long enough" to have attained steady-state. The model shown in Equations (6) and (7) is thus appropriately applied only to situations that have come to equilibrium. That is, an equilibrium model will render an equilibrium concentration, but it does not tell you about the time course of the exposure.

One might ask:

1. How long must a typical operation run before equilibrium is established?
2. How can we estimate an exposure that occurs before equilibrium is established from a source that starts at t = 0?
3. How can we estimate exposure that occurs after equilibrium is established from a source that is then turned off?

Since theoretical steady-state is approached but rarely achieved, a practical solution to the problem of gauging the time scale of concentration buildup is to calculate the time required to achieve some percentage of equilibrium. Combining Equations (3) and (4) and solving the resulting differential equation for time (with C = 0 at $t_0 = 0$) yields:

$$t = \frac{-V}{(Qm + k)} \ln [(G - (Qm + k)(C))/G] \tag{8}$$

at 90% of equilibrium

$$C = \frac{0.90\ (G)}{(Qm + k)} \tag{9}$$

Combining Equations (6) and (7) gives:

$$t\ (\text{at } 90\% \text{ of equilibrium}) = 2.303\ V/(Qm + k) \tag{10}$$

Equation 10 means that large volumes with low ventilation rates and poor mixing take a relatively long time to reach a substantial portion of equilibrium. The practical lesson: if one is modeling essentially batch processes where C = 0 at t = 0 and the length of time for the exposure is of relatively short duration (less than two hours), then one needs to consider the time-weighted average concentration the worker may be exposed to under non-steady-state conditions.

In the converse situation, there is a workroom where the air volume contains a concentration of toxicant in which the source has been turned off or removed. Under the same conditions (i.e., large volume, low ventilation rate, poor mixing) it will take a relatively long time to clear this concentration. This scenario is examined and presented below in more detail.

The above analysis and equations of the time variation of airborne concentration assume that the initial concentration is nil (i.e., C = 0 at t = 0), which is the common situation; however, in many industrial situations the initial concentration should not be neglected. For example, if you are modeling worker exposure in the morning and afternoon, and the source is turned off at lunch time, then it might be important for the afternoon estimate to include an initial concentration term based on the decay calculated for the lunch period.

With the source turned off (G = 0):

$$C = C_0 e^{-\frac{(Q)(m)(t)}{V}} \qquad (11)$$

where:

C_0 = concentration just before lunch and just before source was turned off
C = concentration immediately after the lunch period
t = elapsed time for lunch period

After lunch one may need to model the situation as the source is again turned on. This is done by combining Equations (3) and (4), setting k to 0 (unless you have some data on k) and solving the resulting algorithm:

$$C = \frac{G}{(Q)(m)} + C_0 - \frac{G}{(Q)(m)} e^{-\frac{(Q)(m)(t)}{V}} \qquad (12)$$

In this situation, set C_0 in Equation (12) to be equal to the C from Equation (11): that is, the final airborne concentration after the lunch break becomes the initial concentration for the beginning of the afternoon work session.

To understand the time course of exposure for increasing concentrations from C = 0 at t = 0, one needs to doubly integrate

Equation (3) to solve for average concentration C over time (t) with the assumption of constant contaminant release that begins at t = 0. This yields:

$$C_{avg} = \left(\frac{G}{(Qm+k)}\right) - \left(\frac{GV}{t(Qm+k)^2}\right)(1 - e^{(-t(Qm+k)/V)}) \qquad (13)$$

where:

C_{avg} = average concentration
t = elapsed time
e = natural log base number (2.7182...)

Average concentrations calculated for "long" time intervals — such as large values of the quantity t(Qm+k)/V — approach the equilibrium concentration presented in Equations (6) and (7). However, short time intervals, low ventilation rates, large volumes, and poor mixing will substantially decrease the actual integrated exposure (relative to the airborne steady-state equilibrium concentration-exposure) for any person exposed during a batch operation.

It may appear strange at first that low ventilation rates can decrease exposure potential. It becomes easier to understand, however, when one realizes and calculates that the low ventilation rates retard the establishment of steady-state equilibrium concentration within any volume. Thus, those exposed during the time of concentration buildup will have less exposure relative to a similar time of exposure to the equilibrium concentration. For example, consider a batch job lasting one hour in a cubic room 6.1 m (20 ft) to a side with poor mixing (m = 0.1) and 14,160 L/min (500 cfm) general ventilation. The TWA exposure or dose is less than 20% of that calculated by using Ceq for the one-hour period. This is not to say that high ventilation rates cause high exposures; they merely cause less relative difference in the total exposure potential of batch vs. steady-state exposures. Thus, the potential to overestimate exposure using a steady-state model (Equation [6] or [7]) is higher in situations with low general ventilation rates. Of course, the converse case is also important (i.e., clearing a concentration from workroom air under these conditions can take a relatively long time). Assuming quick or an instantaneously purged air concentration following source removal could result in an underestimation of exposure.

Note that when modeling a scenario in *steady state* (i.e., one at *equilibrium* relative to airborne concentration of contaminant) you do not have to account for or keep track of initial concentrations. In these cases, Equations (6) and (7) should be used.

The question of whether you should use an equilibrium or nonequilibrium model is probably best answered by looking at the scenario of interest and using a reasonable worst-case approach. The product of $(C_{eq})(t)$ will always render the highest estimate of exposure for any reasonably constant source. If, however, this typically overestimated value is not satisfactory for the evaluation of exposure, one may need to do the more sophisticated analysis of integrating nonequilibrium conditions. Relatively long exposure times and a steady source rate will render essentially the same estimates of exposure regardless of whether one uses an equilibrium or nonequilibrium model.

Instances in which the validity of all the above models may be compromised is in workroom scenarios where contaminant release occurs close to the worker's breathing zone or the ratio of G to Q′ is high enough to cause displacement of clean ambient air by essentially saturated vapor. In these cases, the appropriate affected volume will have to be sized considerably smaller to render an accurate estimation of breathing zone concentrations.

Back Pressure Box Model

This model deals exclusively with evaporating sources with relatively large surface areas. The rate of evaporation from any source (G) is driven by the gradient in concentration between the source and the receiving volume. Just as water evaporates fastest on a day that has low relative humidity, the evaporation rate of any compound is maximized when there is little or no partial pressure of that compound in the air above it. As the amount of compound in the air increases toward its saturation level (C_{sat}) the evaporation (generation) rate (G) decreases until it is zero when the air is saturated. Thus, the evaporation rate (G) is inversely proportional to the airborne concentration in the room over the source. We term this effect "back pressure."[17] This factor is ignored in the standard box model; however, modeling large evaporating sources indoors requires the inclusion of back pressure. Equation (12) describes the time–course of exposure build up from a steady source.

A two-film theory of volatilization has been developed by Liss and Slater.[18] Subsequent to the development of this theory, a physical–chemical model to estimate the source strength of a volatilizing liquid has been presented by Thibodeaux:[19]

$$G = (10^3)\,\frac{(K_t)(MW)(AREA)(VPP - VPB)}{(R)(TL)} \qquad (14)$$

where:

G = generation rate (mg/min)
K_t = mass transfer rate (m/min)
MW = molecular weight (g/mole)
AREA = volatilizing surface area (m^2)
VPP = equilibrium or Henry's law vapor pressure exerted by the compound under equilibrium or closed conditions (atm)
VPB = time-dependent actual vapor pressure exerted by the compound under local conditions of ventilation (i.e., back pressure [atm])
R = gas constant (8.205×10^{-5} atm-m^3/((mole)(°K)))
TL = temperature of the volatilizing liquid (°K)

For any particular volatilizing species at constant temperature, the constant terms can be collected into the following simplified relationship:

$$G = K\,(VPP - VPB) \tag{15}$$

Note: $K = \text{a constant} = (10^3)\,\dfrac{(K_t)(MW)(AREA)}{(R)(TL)}$

Thus, given a relatively large and constant evaporating surface we have the following sequence of events. When evaporation begins (t = 0) the airborne concentration (C) equals zero. At this point the evaporation rate (i.e., generation rate) is at its maximum because there is no concentration in the air and the concentration gradient is at a maximum. After any time elapses there is contaminant in the air, resulting in some finite reduction of the gradient. Some back pressure is now acting to slow down the evaporation rate (G). Ultimately, the system reaches equilibrium at an evaporation rate lower than the maximum rate that occurred at time zero. In situations in which the equilibrium concentration is very close to the saturation concentration (e.g., when you find large surface areas of evaporation in rooms with poor ventilation) the evaporation rate will be lowered to near zero.

The ideal gas law can be used to convert airborne concentration in units of mg/m^3 to partial pressure (i.e., back pressure) using the following relationship:

$$VPB = \frac{(C)(T_{air})(8.2 \times 10^{-8})}{MW} \tag{16}$$

where:

C = airborne concentration (mg/m^3)
T_{air} = air temperature (°K)
MW = g/mole

The constant, 8.2×10^{-8} combines the universal gas constant R and units of conversion [atm-m^3/((mole)(°K))]. Note: For our purposes, we set T_{air} = TL the temperature of the volatilizing liquid (°K).

Our approach to modeling this scenario is to use a personal computer to do stepwise solutions in the following sequence:

- Step 1: At t = 0 minutes, set concentration (C) = C_0 = 0 and VPB = 0.
- Step 2: Calculate the airborne concentration (C) using Equation (12) for the time interval from t = 0 to t = 1 (i.e., t = 1 minute).
- Step 3: Calculate the back pressure (VPB) using Equation (15).
- Step 4: Calculate G using Equation (14).
- Step 5: Calculate the airborne concentration (C) using Equation (12) by setting C_0 equal to the C that was calculated in Step 2 and the slightly reduced G calculated in Step 4. Again, the time interval is 1 minute (i.e., the period for the second interval is between t = 1 and 2 minutes).

Repeat Steps 3 through 5 repeatedly for subsequent 1-minute periods (i.e., t = 2 to 3 minutes, t = 3 to 4 minutes, ... t = n to n + 1 minutes) until the airborne concentration does not change (i.e, it reaches equilibrium).

A standard form mathematical solution for airborne concentration at any point in time for this specific model has been determined:[20]

$$C = \frac{(10^3)(MW)(K_t)(AREA)(VPP)}{(TL)(R)((K_t)(AREA) + Q')}\left(1 - e^{-((K_t)(AREA)+Q')(t)/V}\right) \qquad (17)$$

The agreement between the stepwise model and the exact solution is good for fine time increments of a minute or less. An advantage to using the stepwise approach is its versatility in allowing the simple substitution and use of other expressions for the generation rate which may be experimentally derived. Also, the stepwise model can be expanded to account for a time-dependent VPP (from a time-dependent change in concentration for a binary solution) or an increasing (growing puddle) or decreasing (shrinking) evaporating source without resorting to calculus.

Dispersion Models

Dispersion models can describe contaminant concentration patterns created by emission sources. Mass balance models based on the diffusion of a contaminant mass into a specified volume have been applied with some success to outdoor sources and, more recently, to indoor ones. Dispersion models have a notable advantage over the previously described mass balance models. That is, for a specific set of conditions, they describe how concentration increases as the distance to a source decreases.

Diffusion theory is based on the random motions of molecules that result in a net movement from an area of high concentration into areas of low concentration.[(8)] The relation between mass migration or flux of the molecules and the rate of change in concentration is known as Fick's law. The dimension of the flux from the source is (mass per time) per area. The dimension of the concentration gradient is (mass per volume) per length. The ratio of the two is a proportionality constant called the molecular diffusivity and has the dimension of area per time.

Diffusion in workroom air occurs principally because of the air's turbulent motion.[(21)] In most industrial environments, molecular diffusion is not significant between the emission source and the worker's breathing zone. Instead, there is an eddy-like motion that has the effect of hastening the mixing of the contaminant mass with the workroom air. Applications of diffusion models in industrial environments must use experimentally determined diffusion coefficients called eddy or effective diffusivities.

The eddy diffusivity term can be based on experimental measurements at the site being modeled. (Some eddy diffusivity values are also available in the literature.[(22-24)]) Measurements of D in indoor industrial environments have ranged from 0.05 to 11.5 m^2/minute, with 0.2 m^2/minute being a typical value.

An example is the eddy diffusion model for a point source. The model describes the workspace as having a hemispherical or spherical concentration gradient within several meters around a point source.

If the point source emits all of the contaminant instantaneously, the model assumes the following conditions:

- Contaminant mass emitted instantly without significant momentum;
- No concentration gradient remains around the source from a previous emission event;
- Random air movement, no directional movement of workroom air;

- Eddy diffusivity is constant throughout the space; and
- No surface deposition.

In the case of a spherical region (i.e., emission from an elevated source), a solution of the diffusion equation for an instantaneous contaminant release is:[(25)]

$$C = \frac{M}{8(D\pi t)^{1.5}} \, e^{\left(\frac{-r^2}{4tD}\right)} \qquad (18)$$

If the point source emits the contaminant continuously, the model assumes the following conditions:

- Contaminant emitted continuously without significant momentum;
- Steady-state emission rate during the time period;
- Random air movement, no directional movement of workroom air;
- Eddy diffusivity is constant throughout the space; and
- No surface deposition.

The equation for a continuous point source is found by integrating Equation (18) for the concentration at position r and time t.

$$C = \left(\frac{G}{4\pi Dr}\right)\left[1 - \text{erf}\left(\frac{r}{\sqrt{4tD}}\right)\right] \qquad (19)$$

where:

"erf" = error function
C = concentration, mass/volume (mg/m^3)
G = steady-state emission rate, mass/time (mg/minute)
M = mass of vapor emitted at time t (minute)
r = radius of hemisphere, length (meter)
D = effective or eddy diffusivity, area/time (m^2/minute)
t = elapsed time (minute)

Plotting the calculated C at one position, r, for many values of time, t, gives a time/concentration curve that approaches a steady-state concentration. The average concentration at this position can be calculated by integrating Equation (19) with time and dividing by the averaging time.

An approximating algorithm (Equation [19a]) can be used by people unfamiliar with the error function to estimate the concentration calculated in Equation (19) to within a few percent:

$$C = \frac{G}{4\pi Dr}\left[1 - \sqrt{1 - e^{-\frac{r^2}{\pi tD}}}\right] \qquad (19a)$$

At equilibrium, Equation (19) simplifies to:

$$C = \frac{G}{4\pi Dr} \qquad (20)$$

Equation (19) is an estimator of the maximum concentration at position r for a continuous source. It shows that contaminant concentration varies inversely with distance from the source, not the square of the distance.(21)

Equations (18), (19) [or (19a)], and (20) work for a spherical dispersion pattern. If the source is close to a flat surface such as a floor, a hemispherical pattern may be more appropriate. In this case, multiplying their results by 2 can appropriately modify the equations.

Equations (18), (19) [or (19a)], and (20) can be solved with a calculator. The calculations can be repeated for several values of distance r. Estimates of exposure can be made based on the workers' positions in these concentration gradients. At some point the predicted concentration will be close in magnitude to the background concentration of the workroom. The background concentration can be estimated by the box model. The distance from the source to the background concentration is the zone where the concentration gradient around the source is important. This distance is usually within several meters of a source.(18)

Molecular diffusion theory applies strictly to vapors and gases; however, particulate matter with aerodynamic diameters of less than 10 μm follow random workroom air currents in a similar manner. Using the eddy diffusion models to describe the concentration gradients of inhalable dusts and fumes as well as gases and vapors is a reasonable approach if the assumptions of the models are satisfied.

The above model is for completely random dispersion. In any situation where there is a steady direction to the indoor air movement one should use a Gaussian plume dispersion model:

$$C = \frac{G}{4\pi Dr} e^{\left[\frac{-U}{2D}(r - X)\right]} \qquad (21)$$

This is a simplification of the general air dispersion Gaussian plume model and assumes an unvarying wind direction and speed. It also assumes that the eddy diffusivity (D) is the same in all directions and there is no plume rise.

where:

C = airborne concentration (mg/m^3)
D = eddy diffusivity (m^2/minute)
r = sample distance from the source (meters).
X = downwind distance from the source along the centerline of the plume (meters). [If r is on the center line, then r - X = 0.]
G = emission rate, mg/minute
U = velocity in meters/minute

Another derivation of the Gaussian plume model has been suggested for use indoors for exposures within 3 meters of a source:(12)

$$C = 7353 \left(\frac{G/60{,}000}{X^{1.84} - U/60} \right) \qquad (22)$$

For downwind distances from 3 to 100 meters the following equation is suggested:(26)

$$C = 3012 \left(\frac{G/60{,}000}{X^{1.81} - U/60} \right) \qquad (22)$$

Estimation of Vapor Pressure from Mixtures

When estimating the vapor pressure of the individual components of a mixture, one is faced with a number of choices; you must use your best judgment. The simplest method is to use Raoult's law:

$$VPM_x = (VPP_x)(MF_x) \qquad (24)$$

where:

VPM_x = vapor pressure of compound x over the solution
VPP_x = vapor pressure of pure compound x
MF_x = molefraction of compound x in the solution

$$MF_x = \frac{\text{moles of compound x}}{\text{total moles of all compounds in the solution}} \qquad (25)$$

Thus, the vapor pressure of the pure compound x is essentially attenuated by the fact that it is in solution and is expressed proportionately to its molefraction in the solution. Raoult's law assumes there is negligible interaction between the components. It can be considered to be reasonably accurate for compound mixtures in which all the components are of the same homologous series or close structural analog (e.g., a mixture of methylene dichloride and dichloroethane or a solution of benzene and toluene).

Mixtures of dissimilar materials can result in severe deviations from Raoult's law. For example, an organic compound in water will have a vapor pressure above the solution and typically will not follow this relationship. Given liquids in a nonideal mixture, one can apply a variable correction factor (commonly known as the activity coefficient):[(5)]

$$VPM = (\gamma)(VPP_x)(MF_x) \qquad (26)$$

A common technique used to estimate g is the UNIFAC method, which uses compound structural activity and group contribution. The basic idea behind this method is that, while there are many thousands of organic compounds, the number of functional groups that constitute these compounds is much smaller.[(5)] The methodology — although somewhat simple in concept — is quite arduous in its mathematical execution. This difficulty has been somewhat alleviated by the modern PC and available software.[(27)]

In the case of nonideal solutions, the concept of Henry's law will be more accurate and useful than Raoult's law without the activity coefficient correction. For our purposes, Henry's law can be considered a generalization of Raoult's law:

$$VPM_x = (\text{a constant})(MF_x) \qquad (27)$$

Another way of expressing this is that the ratio of vapor concentration of compound x in the head space to its concentration in the bulk liquid is a constant. If we designate these concentrations in the same unit of measure (e.g., mg/m^3) their ratio will be dimensionless. This is the definition of the dimensionless Henry's law constant (HLC):

$$HLC = \frac{[\text{HEAD SPACE}]}{[\text{BULK SOLUTION}]} \qquad (28)$$

Note: HEAD SPACE and BULK SOLUTION concentrations have the same units of weight per unit volume.

One practical means of determining HLC for mixtures of organic compounds is by analytical determination of the head space and bulk concentrations. If elevated temperatures are involved in the application, it would be worthwhile to determine this at 25°C and some appropriately elevated temperature such as 35°C or 40°C. Once one has an HLC and information about the bulk concentration, it is simple to estimate the vapor pressure from the head-space concentration calculated by the use of Equation (28).

The most accurate source for an HLC of an organic compound in an aqueous solution is an experimentally derived value; however, the database of experimentally determined HLC values is extremely small in comparison to the thousands of organic compounds of potential interest. A structural activity relationship (SAR) method for estimating HLC of organic compounds in water, developed by Hine and Mookerjee,[28] has become a preferred structural activity method for HLC estimation, in situations lacking reliable water solubility and vapor pressure data. This method relies on bond contribution or chemical group contribution values to estimate the HLC for a particular compound. The bond contribution method is able to estimate HLCs for most types of organic structures and is relatively accurate when applied to hydrocarbons, monofunctional compounds, and many multifunctional compounds contained in an aqueous solution. As chemical structures become more complex, however, the bond contribution method is more likely to be inaccurate.

This methodology has been codified into a personal computer program developed by the Syracuse Research Corporation. The program will rapidly calculate HLCs for most organic compounds[29] using bond contribution values derived by Syracuse Research Corporation from a data set of 345 chemicals having either reliable experimental Henry's law constants or reliable vapor pressure and water solubility data. A coefficient of determination (R^2) of 0.96 was derived for the validation set of the known Henry's law constants and those Henry's law constants estimated by the bond contribution method.[30]

In summary, the four methods described herein for evaluating the vapor pressure of a component in mixture are:

- Raoult's law for organic compounds that are close structural analogs;
- Raoult's law corrected with an estimated activity coefficient (γ);
- Henry's law estimation using bond contribution for organic compounds in water; and

- Analytical determination of the head space and bulk concentrations.

Relationship of Vapor Pressure and Temperature

The vapor pressure of a material is a measure of that substance's tendency to volatilize. The saturation model (Equation [1]) requires only the vapor pressure to estimate the airborne concentration at equilibrium. A substance's vapor pressure rises with temperature and equals the surrounding or atmospheric pressure at its boiling point. Thus, the vapor pressure of any pure substance is equal to 760 mmHg at the normal boiling point of the material. If the substance is put under a partial vacuum it will boil at a lower temperature because the vapor pressure equals the pressure in the partial vacuum. Thus, when a compound boils at 50°C under a partial vacuum of 5 mmHg, the vapor pressure of this compound at 50°C is 5 mmHg.

The relationship between temperature and vapor pressure is described by the classic Clausius-Clapeyron equation:(31)

$$\log\left(\frac{P_{nb}}{P_{ob}}\right) = \frac{\Delta H_{vap}}{2.303R}\left(\frac{T_{nb} - T_{ob}}{T_{ob}T_{nb}}\right) \qquad (29)$$

where:

all temperatures are in Kelvin; all pressures in Torr or mmHg

$T_{nb}P_{nb}$ =normal boiling point and normal boiling pressure (i.e., 760 mmHg)

$T_{ob}P_{ob}$ =observed temperature and vacuum pressure for boiling under vacuum

ΔH_{vap} = molal heat of vaporization in units of J/moles

R = Universal Gas Constant (8.3145 Pa m^3/(°K moles))

This relationship has been rearranged and presented elsewhere.(4)

$$\Delta T = \frac{(273.1 + T)(2.8808 - \log p)}{\Phi + 0.15\,(2.8808 - \log p)} \qquad (30)$$

where:

$\Delta T = T - T_b$

T = ambient temperature in °C

T_b = normal boiling point temperature in °C

$\Phi = \Delta H_{vap}/(2.303RT_b)$
$p =$ vapor pressure in mmHg

Another way of expressing this relationship is:

$$p = 10^{\left(\frac{(-\Phi)(\Delta T)}{(T + 273.1 - 0.15\Delta T)}\right) + 2.8808} \qquad (31)$$

You can therefore calculate the vapor pressure if you have the boiling point at two pressures (i.e., normal and under vacuum) or an estimated boiling point and the heat of vaporization.

Linking Modeling and Monitoring Data

One can estimate (or refine purely model-estimated) exposures for an agent by combining the information from monitoring with the theoretical construct of the model.

A relatively simple example is to run a model on a chemical mixture that then predicts an exposure to a number of components of that mixture. If we happen to have monitoring data on one of the components in the modeled scenario, we can check and refine the estimates. That is, we can not only determine how well the model performed but, more important, we can use the monitoring data on the substance to predict the airborne levels of the other components. This is done by using the ratios predicted by the model and multiplying the monitored data by these ratios in order to predict the concentrations of the other components.

As a concrete illustration of this let us assume we have exposure data on substance X, (X_{ppm}) but need to estimate the exposure for substance Y (Y_{ppm}). Both are components of the same mixture in a process stream. We know their percentage in the stream (%x and %y) and their vapor pressures (VPx and VPy). Assuming their molecular weights are similar, we can use the percentage concentration in place of their mole fractions.

$$Y_{ppm} = \left(\frac{\%_y}{\%_x}\right)\left(\frac{VP_y}{VP_x}\right)X_{ppm} \qquad (32)$$

Of course, this assumes the mixture acts as an ideal solution.

The main reason for this linking is that modeled ratios combined with monitored data can give more refined estimates of exposure for monitored species.

References

1. **National Research Council:** *National Research Council Committee on Advances in Assessing Human Exposure to Airborne Pollutants: Human Exposure Assessment for Airborne Pollutants — Advances and Opportunities.* Washington, D.C.: National Research Council/National Academy of Sciences, Board on Environmental Studies and Toxicology/Commission on Geoscience, Environment, and Resources, 1991. p. 12.
2. **Jayjock, M.A., and N.C. Hawkins:** A Proposal for Improving the Role of Exposure Modeling in Risk Assessment. *Am. Ind. Hyg. Assoc. J. 54(12):*733-741 (1993).
3. **Hawkins, N.C., M.A. Jayjock, and J. Lynch:** A Rationale and Framework for Establishing the Quality of Human Exposure Assessments. *Am. Ind. Hyg. Assoc. J. 53(1):*34-41 (1992).
4. **Haas, H.B., and R.F. Newton:** Correction of Boiling Points to Standard Pressure. In *CRC Handbook of Chemistry and Physics,* 59th Ed. Boca Raton, Fla.: CRC Press, 1978. p. D-228.
5. **Lyman, W.J., W.F. Reehll, and D.H. Rosenblat:** Chapters 11, 14, and 15. In *Handbook of Chemical Property Estimation Methods.* New York: McGraw-Hill, 1982.
6. **Sparks, L.E.:** Modeling Indoor Concentrations and Exposure. *Ann. N.Y. Acad. Sci. 641:*102-111 (1992).
7. **Drivas, P.J., P.G. Simmonds, and F.H. Shair:** Experimental Characterization of Ventilation Systems in Buildings. *Environ. Sci. Technol. 6:*609-614 (1972).
8. **Jayjock, M.A.:** Assessment of Inhalation Exposure Potential from Vapors in the Workplace. *Am. Ind. Hyg. Assoc. J. 49(8):*380-385 (1988).
9. **U.S. Environmental Protection Agency:** Appendix F. In *A Manual for the Preparation of Engineering Assessment.* Washington, D.C.: U.S. Environmental Protection Agency/Office of Toxic Substances, Chemical Engineering Branch, Economics and Technology Division, 1984. [Unpublished draft.]
10. **U.S. Environmental Protection Agency:** Chapter 4. In *Preparation of Engineering Assessment, Vol 1: CEB Engineering Manual.* Washington, D.C.: U.S. Environmental Protection Agency/Office of Toxic Substances, Chemical Engineering Branch, 1991.

11. **Schroy, J.M., and J.M. Wu:** Emission from Spills. In *Proceedings on Control of Specific Toxic Pollutants.* Gainesville, Fla.: APCA/Florida Section, 1979.
12. **Chemical Manufacturers Association:** *PAVE – Program to Assess Volatile Emissions, Version 2.0.* Washington, D.C.: Chemical Manufacturers Association, 1992. [Software.]
13. **U.S. Environmental Protection Agency:** *Evaporation Rate of Volatile Liquids* (PACE Laboratories Inc. Project 890501.315 [EPA/744–R–92–001]) by K.O. Braun and K.J. Caplan. Washington, D.C.: U.S. Environmental Protection Agency/Office of Pollution Prevention and Toxics, 1989. [National Technical Information Service (NTIS) Pub. No. PB92–232305.]
14. **Hummel, A.A., K.O. Braun, and M.C. Fehrenbacher:** Evaporation of a Liquid in a Flowing Airstream. *Am. Ind. Hyg. Assoc. J. 57(6):*519-525 (1996).
15. **Fehrenbacher, M.C., and A.A. Hummel:** Evaluation of the Mass Balance Model Used by the Environmental Protection Agency for Estimating Inhalation Exposure to New Chemical Substances. *Am. Ind. Hyg. Assoc. J. 57(6):*526-536 (1996).
16. **Wadden, R.A., and P.A. Scheff:** *Indoor Air Pollution, Characterization, Prediction, and Control.* New York: John Wiley & Sons, 1983. p. 105.
17. **Jayjock, M.A.:** Back Pressure Modeling of Indoor Air Concentrations from Volatilizing Sources. *Am. Ind. Hyg. Assoc. J. 55(3):*230-235 (1994).
18. **Liss, P.S., and P.G. Slater:** Flux of Gases Across the Air-Sea Interface. *Nature 247:*181-184 (1974).
19. **Thibodeaux, L.J.:** Exchange Rates Between Air and Water. In *Chemodynamics.* New York: Wiley-Interscience, 1979.
20. **Tuggle, R.M.:** "Standard Mathematical Form Solution for Back Pressure Model." Oct. 26, 1990. [Personal correspondence to M.A. Jayjock, AIHA Exposure Assessment Strategies Committee.]
21. **Roach, S.A.:** On the Role of Turbulent Diffusion in Ventilation. *Ann. Occup. Hyg. 24:*105-132 (1981).
22. **Wadden, R.A., P.A. Scheff, and J.E. Franke:** Emission Factors of Trichloroethylene Vapor Degreasers. *Am. Ind. Hyg. Assoc. J. 50:(9)*496-500 (1989).
23. **Wadden, R.A., J.L. Hawkins, P.A. Scheff, and J.E. Franke:** Characterization of Emission Factors Related to Source Activity for Trichloroethylene Degreasing and

Chrome Plating Processes. *Am. Ind. Hyg. Assoc. J. 52(9):*349-356 (1991).

24. **Scheff, P.A., R.L. Friedman, J.E. Franke, L.M. Conroy, and R.A. Wadden:** Source Activity Modeling of Freon Emissions from Open-Top Vapor Degreasers. *Appl. Occup. Environ. Hyg. 7:*127-134 (1992).
25. **Carslaw, H.S., and J.C. Jaeger:** *Conduction of Head in Solids,* 2nd Ed. London: Oxford University Press, 1959. pp. 260-261.
26. **Lipton, S., and J. Lynch:** *Handbook of Health Hazard Control in the Chemical Process Industry.* New York: John Wiley & Sons, 1994.
27. **BRI Software Inc.:** "UNIFAC." Atlanta, Ga.: BRI Software Inc., 1993. [Software.]
28. **Hine, J., and P.K. Mookerjee:** The Intrinsic Hydrophilic Character of Organic Compounds — Correlation in Terms of Structural Contributions. *J. Org. Chem. 40:*292-298 (1975).
29. **Syracuse Research Corporation:** "Henry's Law Constant." Syracuse, N.Y.: Syracuse Research Corporation, Chemical Hazard Assessment Division, Environmental Chemistry Center, 1991. [Software.]
30. **Meylan, W.M., and P.H. Howard:** Bond Contribution Method for Estimating Henry's Law Constants. *Environ. Toxicol. Chem. 10:*1283-1293 (1991).
31. **Thibodeaux, L.J.:** *Chemodynamics.* New York: Wiley-Interscience, 1979. p. 44.

Appendix II

Dermal Exposure Assessments

Historically, more attention has been given to airborne exposures than dermal exposures. In many scenarios, in fact, it is the airborne exposure potential that dominates the overall picture, but there are numerous situations in which dermal exposure is important and sometimes critical. A good example is phenol. The principal route of exposure for phenol (in the absence of a mist) is skin contact and absorption. For some chemical agents, both inhalation and skin absorption may be significant routes of exposure (hexachlorobenzene, for example). The importance of dermal exposure is recognized by ACGIH, AIHA, and other organizations responsible for publishing exposure limits. Specific compounds that can be absorbed through the skin are designated with what is known as a "skin" notation.[1]

The industrial hygienist should begin to assess dermal exposures to chemical agents when the basic characterization reveals tasks and work practices in which skin contact may occur directly or through secondary contact with contaminated tools, work surfaces, or personal protective equipment. Of course, the presence of skin contact alone is not enough to create a health risk. A review of available information on the toxicology of the chemical agent and its chemical and physical characteristics should quickly indicate whether dermal exposure presents a health risk. Information on the toxicity of the environmental agent and its chemical (e.g., lipophilicity) and physical (e.g., pH) characteristics — including dermal absorption characteristics — should provide some insight into the target organs that might be affected.

Skin contact may be the principal route of exposure for high molecular weight compounds exhibiting low volatility. Another factor that enhances the dermal absorption of a chemical agent is a relatively high degree of lipophilicity for the compound.

That is, compounds that are more soluble in oil than water tend to go through the skin more readily.

External and Internal Target Organs

In proceeding with the dermal exposure assessment, there is some practical value in differentiating between chemical agents whose target organ is the skin and other chemicals that are absorbed through the skin and whose target organs are internal. Some chemical agents, of course, might affect both the skin and internal organs.

The skin is the principal target organ for acids, alkalies, and other chemicals exhibiting irritating or corrosive effects on the skin or eyes. Some chemical agents principally target the skin but have a toxicity less acute than acids or alkalies. Epoxy resins are a good example, where repeated skin contact might lead to skin sensitization and dermatitis.

When the skin is the principal target organ, the industrial hygienist should carefully identify the tasks and work practices in which routine or accidental skin exposure to the chemical agent could occur and control the exposures. In the case of dermal sensitizers, careful consideration should be given to the control of incidental and relatively minor skin exposure occurring through contact with contaminated work surfaces, tools, and personal protective equipment. The industrial hygienist must judge exposures and the associated health risks to be either acceptable, unacceptable, or uncertain.

When skin contact is a significant route of exposure, and the principal target organs are internal, many industrial hygienists choose the same approach toward managing exposures. That is, they identify the tasks and work practices in which routine or accidental skin exposure to the chemical agent can occur and control the exposures. This simple approach, however, might not be an effective strategy when the health risk is proportional to the internal dose. If so, it is useful to apply the same exposure assessment methodology that underlies exposure assessments in which inhalation is the principal route of exposure. The industrial hygienist can use either biological monitoring or skin exposure assessments.

Biological Monitoring

Biological monitoring is an attractive method of assessing exposure when skin absorption is a major route of exposure. A good example is the use of p-aminophenol in urine to assess exposure to aniline. A good source for more information on biological monitoring strategies is the ACGIH monograph *Topics in Biological Monitoring*.[2]

Some of the uncertainty associated with air monitoring can be a lesser concern with biological monitoring. For example, since many biomarkers reflect the integrated effect of exposures over time, there is less uncertainty about the effect of day-to-day variability in exposure levels. Also, the uncertainty associated with the inferential use of air monitoring data collected on some members of a similar exposure group (and applied to all members of the SEG) is a lesser concern with biological monitoring since biological specimens are normally collected from all exposed workers. This helps to reduce the exposure assessment problem associated with between-worker variability in exposures due to differences in work practices.

Unfortunately, biological monitoring is often not an option. Both a validated biological monitoring method and an occupational exposure limit (such as ACGIH's biological exposure indices [BEIs]) must be available to biologically assess exposure to chemical agents. Relatively few BEIs, or similar limits, have been established by ACGIH and other organizations. Also, the personal and invasive nature of biological monitoring tends to limit its use in occupational exposure assessments.

Skin Exposure Assessments

"Skin exposure assessment" is the other approach that can be applied when skin contact is a significant route of exposure and the principal target organ is internal. This methodology is described below; however, prior to discussing skin exposure assessments, keep in mind there are scenarios in which the target organs are both internal and external (skin). One example is hydrofluoric acid, which is corrosive to the skin and also absorbed through the skin, thereby endangering internal organs. Another example is dermal exposure to coal tar pitch. Coal tar pitch absorbed into the epidermis can cause transient photosensitization. Moreover, coal tar pitch is also absorbed through the skin and may contribute to an increased risk for bladder cancer. The industrial hygienist may need to use a combination of methodologies for assessing and controlling dermal exposures when the target organs are both external and internal.

As mentioned previously in this book, the evaluation of exposure is only meaningful in the context of our knowledge and understanding of the health risks associated with the exposure levels. Thus, we rely on the OEL to help differentiate acceptable from unacceptable exposures; however, nearly all OELs for chemical agents are presented in units of airborne concentration in the breathing zone of workers. The development of dermal exposure limits is under investigation. Dermal limits could be based on: 1) workplace surface contamination levels; 2) skin or clothing contamination levels; and 3) biological measures of exposure or internal dose.[3]

When dermal exposure limits are absent, one could convert OELs expressed in units of airborne concentration to meaningful metrics of dermal exposure to determine whether additional control measures to reduce skin contact are needed. Although a worker's respiration rate varies with activity, workers generally breathe about 10 m^3 of air in a workday. Thus, one can convert an inhalation exposure limit expressed in mg/m^3 to an equivalent total body dose in units of mg/day using the following relationship:

$$\text{Exposure (mg/day)} = \text{OEL}(\text{mg/m}^3) \times \text{inhaled air volume}(10\ \text{m}^3/\text{day}) \qquad (1)$$

One can then estimate the potential dermal dose in mg/day and compare it with the converted limit. A few publications recently proposed strategies for addressing the contribution of dermal exposure.[4,5]

Note that this approach is valid only for compounds that exert their toxicity as a systemic effect. It is not appropriate to use this methodology for agents for which the primary health effect is local tissue response (e.g., hydrochloric acid). In this case, a dermal exposure limit would have to be determined by other means and would most likely be expressed as an allowable amount per skin area per day. Good industrial hygiene practice would limit dermal contact with these types of agents, and work force surveillance coupled with an appropriate skin care program should help minimize the incidence of occupational skin disease.[6,7]

Dermal exposure assessment is often based on limited information on the magnitude of the skin exposure and dynamics of dermal absorption. This generally leads to conservative (i.e., overestimating) assessments of dermal exposure because overestimation of risk is preferred to underestimation.

Determining the amount of skin contact generally is performed using an approach whereby the surface area of the skin potentially exposed to the environmental agent (in units of cm^2), and the amount of environmental agent transferred to the skin during the exposure event (in units of mg/cm^2/event) are determined. It usually is not possible to determine the actual amount transferred to the skin during the activity, meaning the amount transferred to the skin (or a surrogate skin such as a glove) is determined at completion of the activity. This amount is influenced by the transfer to, from, and through the skin. Multiplying the skin surface area and the amount of the agent transferred to the skin with the number of exposure events per day provides an estimate of the amount of skin contact per day. The estimated amount absorbed through the skin is then combined with the amount of skin contact to predict the daily potential dermal dose.

The following equation can be used as a screening level estimate of the daily dermal dose rate in units of mg/day, assuming deposition on the skin followed by absorption. Once the predicted dermal absorbed dose rate has been determined, it can be easily compared with an OEL expressed in units of mg/day.

$$DA = (S)(Q)(FQ)(ABS)(WF) \tag{2}$$

where:

DA = dermal absorbed dose rate, mg/day
S = surface area of skin available for contact, cm^2
Q = quantity deposited on the skin per event, mg/cm^2 – event
FQ = number of events per day
ABS = fraction of applied dose absorbed through the skin during the event
WF = weight fraction of the substance in the mixture, unitless

Some environmental agents will be absorbed through the skin during the exposure event, some will be absorbed after the event (if not removed before the next event), and some will be removed before absorption occurs. It is reasonable to use a conservative approach by assuming a fraction absorbed through the skin during a reasonable time frame (e.g., 4 hours). It also is reasonable to assume that the agent remaining on the skin after four hours will not be absorbed, but will be removed.(8)

To determine the surface area of the potentially exposed skin, the industrial hygienist will need to gather information on the activities and tasks performed by the worker, and the types, number of skin surfaces (e.g., one hand, two hands, etc.) potentially exposed during the activities. Fortunately, the mean skin surface areas for various parts of the body have been measured for adults and children by several researchers, allowing development of statistical descriptors for skin surface area.(9) Table II.1 presents measured skin surface area values commonly used by the EPA as

Table II.1 — Surface Area by Region of the Body for Adults 5th to 95th Percentile

Region of the Body	*Men* *Mean, cm^2*	*Min.–Max., cm^2**	*n*	*Women* *Mean, cm^2*	*Min.–Max., cm^2**	*n*
Head	1180	900–1610	29	1100	953–1270	54
Trunk	5690	3060–8930	20	5420	4370–8670	54
Arms	2280	1090–2920	32	2100	1930–2350	13
Upper Arms	1430	1220–1560	6	—	—	—
Forearms	1140	945–1360	6	—	—	—
Hands	840	596–1130	32	746	639–824	12
Legs	6360	2830–8680	32	4880	4230–5850	13
Thighs	1980	1280–4030	32	2580	2580–3600	13
Lower Legs	2070	930–2960	32	1940	1650–2290	13
Feet	1120	611–1560	32	975	834–1150	13
Total	**19,400**	**16,600–22,800***	**48**	**16,900**	**14,500–20,900***	**58**

* 5th percentile to 95th percentile, respectively
Source: U.S. Environmental Protection Agency[11]

default input values in predicting dermal dose. Note that various parts of the human body have differing rates of absorption.[10]

In using the deposition approach for predicting dermal dose, care must be taken in interpreting the number of exposure events occurring per day. The vast majority of the dermal deposition data has been collected for a single exposure event. The relationship between the amount of agent deposited on the skin and the amount absorbed over time has not been characterized. It is reasonable to presume that the amount of the agent retained on the skin will increase linearly over time to a level at which the skin's affinity to retain the substance reaches its maximum level, and the amount retained will increase nonlinearly thereafter to the point of equilibrium[12].

Although determining the skin surface area potentially exposed during the various tasks is fairly straightforward, determining the amount of the environmental agent deposited on the skin can be challenging. In the absence of dermal exposure monitoring data, the default values for the amount retained on the skin per event as presented in Table II.2 can be used to develop screening level estimates of potential dermal dose. It should be noted that the default values are based on the limited amount of data available to the present, and are fairly uncertain. The data were collected using a variety of measurement methods, and much of the data were collected over a single exposure event; the relationship to total dermal dose when multiple events are performed per day is unknown.

The data generally represent exposure received by workers wearing no personal protective equipment, and many of the samples were collected on surrogate skin (e.g., gloves), which may result in biased estimates of the actual exposure. Furthermore, the amount of agent retained on the skin may vary over several orders of magnitude and depends on specific activities performed by the worker.[6,7,13-15] Several studies have demonstrated that the hands generally receive the highest exposure, but other parts of the body may also receive significant exposures.[16] Generally, theoretical and empirical considerations advise that cotton as a surrogate skin collection device leads to overestimation of exposure levels.[8]

Because of the limited amount of data and information available with which to estimate workplace-related dermal exposure, assumptions are generally made when developing estimates. Some common assumptions are 1) the amount of the agent measured on the absorbent pad is uniformly deposited within a specific area of the body, and 2) the retention rate on absorbent pads or surrogate skin is equivalent to that of the skin. The exposure assessment should also consider the impact of the varying measurement methodologies used by investigators, and extrapolation from pesticides mixing and loading data (in agricultural pesticide application operations) to various industrial mixing and loading operations.[16] Nevertheless, the data can be useful in developing screening level estimates of the potential for dermal exposure during some activities. An EPA evaluation of the available literature and field data determined that the screening level estimates developed using deposition modeling of dermal exposure for occupational exposures appear to be reasonable, but they might overestimate exposures for some activities.[16]

In addition to estimating the surface area of the exposed skin and the quantity of the environmental agent transferred to the skin, the industrial hygienist should also consider the exposure time (e.g., minutes/event) and the dermal penetration properties. Frequently, little is known about dermal penetration. Consider a chemical with unknown dermal penetration properties. The conservative default assumption would be to consider any material in contact with the skin to be instantly (time of absorption = 0) and completely (percentage adsorbed = 100) absorbed. This, of course, could lead to a dramatic overestimation of exposure. Without proper data, however, it might be the only choice available.

Although few surface contamination limits have been established for chemical agents, it can be instructive to collect surface wipe samples on work surfaces, equipment, inside protective clothing, and in nonprocessing areas for use in training workers regarding procedures to minimize contamination. Colorimetric wipe test kits have been developed for aromatic

Table II.2 — Amount of Contaminant Retained on the Skin per Event

Activity	*Description*	*Exposure to hands, range, (mg/event)*[A]	*Quantity transferred to the skin per event (Q), (mg/cm²/event)*[B]	*Source*
Manual weighing and dumping of powder	Scooping; weighing; cutting bags; dumping powder; mixing dry powder, flakes and granules into liquid.	100–4200	0.06–2.1	Lansink et al.[C] PHED[D]
Handling bags of powder	Manually moving bags of powder from storage to the production area, and disposing of empty bags.	50–1100	0.03–0.55	Lansink et al.[C]
Monitoring the process in the chemical industry (liquids)	Monitoring the production process; collect process samples; preparing equipment for maintenance; filling waste drums; unloading raw material. Limited direct contact with liquids in the chemical industry.	0.002–2.4	<0.001–0.033	Anonymous[E]
Maintenance in the chemical industry (liquids)	Instrument/electrical maintenance; mechanical maintenance in the production area; repairing and replacing pumps in the production area.	0.0009–505	<0.001–6.89	Anonymous[E]
Handling wet or dried material in a filtration and drying process (powder, slurry)	Removing filter cake; loading wet or dry product onto filter tray; unloading dry material from plate and frame filter press.	—	0.005–0.63	EPA[F]
Handling of liquids without immersion of hands into liquid (suspensions, solutions, pure liquids)	Opening containers; pouring into mixer; mixing; handling wet rags; spill cleanup.	—	<0.3–2.1	PHED[D], Versar[G]
Immersion of hand into a liquid	Immersion of hand into a liquid, followed by a partial wipe of the skin with a clean cloth.	—	1.3–10.3	Versar[G]

Table II.2 — Amount of Contaminant Retained on the Skin per Event (continued)

[A] The amounts were originally determined as total amounts for one or two hands (in some cases including part of the forearm). Amounts in mg/cm^2 were calculated assuming a specific surface area exposed. The actual surface area exposed was not determined in most studies and will probably have been smaller than the assumed area, leading to an *underestimate* of the adherence in mg/cm^2. At least the same area exposed should be used as was assumed for calculating the adherence when calculating total exposure from adherence and surface area exposed in an assessment. The adherence for immersion into a liquid is based on an experiment with fully exposed surface area. When assessing exposure due to adherence, the real surface area exposed in the assessed situation should be used in the calculation.

[B] Data for adherence are calculated from total amounts on the skin of one or two hands (in some cases including part of the forearm). Only in experiments by Versar was full exposure of the exposed surface area established.(18) In the other studies the exposed surface area is assumed, based on either the area of the glove monitors used or on standard assumptions of the area of a hand.

[C] The sampling strategy for this study included collecting skin exposure measurements from two workers in 10 different paint factories, although this was not achieved for all samples taken. Blank and spike samples were collected and analyzed, and other quality control procedures were followed. The number of samples collected per task ranged from 6 to 19. Workers wore cotton gloves (with 28-cm sleeve length) which were analyzed and measured for calcium carbonate using atomic absorption spectrometry (AAS). It is believed that the cotton gloves (surrogate skin) retained a larger amount of calcium carbonate than the hands would have, and thus this data is believed to be conservative (i.e., overestimates exposure.) The study did not evaluate the effect of multiple contacts. The study measured the total amount transferred to the gloves covering two hands and part of the forearms. For use with Equation (1), the data has been converted to mg/cm^2/event by dividing the total amount transferred by 1980 cm^2, the skin surface area for two hands and part of the forearm, based on Table II.1. This assumes that the amount transferred to the glove is equally distributed across the glove, which is a simplifying assumption.(13)

[D] Measurements from the mixing and loading files of the Pesticide Handlers Exposure Database (PHED) have been normalized by time and adapted to present estimates of the gross amount transferred to the skin for the entire formulation (measurements in PHED are for the active ingredient AI). The 90th percentile estimated gross transfer rate has been time-normalized for a 4-hour exposure period. The two highest grades of PHED data have been used in this analysis.(14)

[E] Blank and spike samples were collected and analyzed, and other quality control procedures were followed. Workers wore nitrile gloves with an average surface area of 1258 cm^2 for Size 10 gloves, and 1106 cm^2 for Size 9 gloves. Gloves served as surrogate skin and were changed every two hours. The nitrile gloves were analyzed using gas chromatography with electron capture detector, following a typical work day. For use with Equation (1), the data has been converted to mg/cm^2/event by dividing the total amount transferred by the surface area of the nitrile gloves as an average of 73.312 cm^2, as reported in the study. This assumes that the amount transferred to the glove is equally distributed across the glove, which is a simplifying assumption. Measurements of cotton gloves worn under the nitrile gloves were also taken to document skin exposure while wearing gloves (e.g., skin exposure while protected). The measurements for process operators ranged from 0.0032–0.0074 mg/day, and for maintenance mechanics from 0.0024–0.200 mg/day. The processing operation is a closed system, and the facility has a strong commitment to procedures and use of personal protective equipment. Process operators worked a 12-hour shift during the study. Maintenance workers worked an 8-hour shift during the study.(15)

[F] Four to eight measurements were collected from rinsing of hands after the operation. Measurements reflect exposures to the hands and part of the forearms.(17)

[G] The liquids (mineral oil, cooking oil, and bath oil) were applied to the hands from a saturated cloth, or for immersion, by placing the hand in a jar of the liquid. The amount of liquid retained on the skin was determined by the weight differential of the cloth (or for immersion, the jar of liquid) before and after contact. Four to six replicates per subject–liquid–application/removal technique from four subjects were collected and analyzed.(18)

amines and isocyanates, thereby providing an opportunity to immediately recognize surface contamination.[7]

Dermal Exposure Monitoring

The amount of an environmental agent deposited on the skin has been shown to vary by activity, but the factors that influence the adherence of particles to the skin, and the mechanisms for absorption through the skin for liquids, have not been well-characterized.[19,20] A variety of methods are used for quantifying dermal exposure, and many summaries have been prepared.[21-23] There also are numerous methods for measuring dermal exposure or the source of the exposure: absorbent pad and clothing sampling, glove and hand wash sampling, surface wipe sampling, fluorescent tracer, and other techniques. The most common methods are described in this section.

Wipe sampling is a fairly common technique used by occupational health professionals to estimate the amount of contamination on a surface. The interpretation of wipe sampling data can be difficult, and standardization of the sampling technique is critical. Often, moistened cotton gauze pads are used to sample a standardized area of contamination. The number of times a surface is wiped has not been standardized, and a weight may be added to the sampling pad to exert a uniform pressure on the sampling device. Fenske recommends that the goal of wipe sampling should be to estimate the potential transfer of surface residue to the skin, with an estimated dermal transfer coefficient estimated for specific activities.[22]

Absorbent pad and clothing sampling are probably the most frequently used method overall for dermal exposure assessment. This technique involves attaching gauze pads, treated cloth, or alpha-cellulose pads to various sites on the worker's outer clothing or skin to capture the contaminant that would have been deposited on the skin. An estimate of the potential dermal exposure can then be developed by multiplying the amount of contaminant deposited on a unit area of the absorbent pad by the surface area of the body area for which the pad is positioned to represent. The assumption is that the contaminant deposited on the pad is uniformly distributed and that the deposit of contaminant on a given skin surface area is represented by that deposited on the absorbent pad. This technique is generally used for sampling nonvolatile contaminants or those with very low vapor pressure, although charcoal-impregnated cloth has been evaluated for sampling of volatile compounds.

There are advantages and limitations associated with the use of absorbent pad sampling and interpretation of the data can be quite challenging. One of the most prominent uncertainties is extrapolating the amount of contaminant captured on a small area covered by the pad to the particular section of the skin surface area. For this reason, "whole body" exposure assessment methods (e.g., using an entire garment as the absorbent pad) is considered to be superior to sampling using pads. Removal of the patches and handling of patches is a critical aspect of the procedure and care should be taken not to contaminate the patches or to inadvertently cause loss of contaminant from the patch.

Glove and hand wash sampling are also fairly common methods for evaluating dermal hand exposure, although interpretation of the results can be quite difficult. Sections of lightweight absorbent gloves may be analyzed. The hands may be swabbed or rinsed with appropriate liquids, using various techniques. It has been demonstrated that use of standard hand washing techniques for removal of pesticides are not likely to be representative of actual exposures because of uncertainty associated with the removal efficiency.(24) Other authors note that bag rinsing, particularly with solvents, is of questionable value and can be quite dangerous.(22) Standardization of the hand rinse procedure is important since the removal efficiency can vary with the chemical loading on the skin, the time between exposure and washing, and the type of wash solution used.(24)

Example: Dermal Exposure Assessment

An industrial hygienist was contacted to investigate an incidence of skin disease among maintenance workers responsible for repairing water service lines for the facility. The initial basic characterization and information gathering revealed that workers reported some "tingling" sensation in their hands, but the primary symptom was dryness and "peeling" of the skin of the hands. Acrylamide grouting compounds were used by the workers, and the potential for dermal exposure had been minimized as much as possible; however, glove use was still required for portions of the grouting task.

The ACGIH TLV for acrylamide (0.03 mg/m^3 as a TWA) was selected as the OEL to be used in judging whether exposures were acceptable, and exposure during the grouting operation was believed to occur primarily through skin contact. Acrylamide is an animal carcinogen as defined by ACGIH and has been identified as a suspected human carcinogen.(1) The TLV carries a skin notation that cautions that air sampling alone may be insufficient to adequately quantify exposure and that taking preventive actions to mitigate skin absorption might be needed.[1] There is no dermal exposure limit for acrylamide, and ACGIH has not established a BEI.

The industrial hygienist determined that a qualitative rating of 2 (incidental contact with the grout) was appropriate, but though the exposure was very uncertain the health hazard was significant, resulting in an "unacceptable" initial judgment. The exposure was rated among those needing additional information gathering. The industrial hygienist proceeded to use modeling to try to resolve the exposure judgment. Converting the airborne inhalation OEL to total body dose using Equation (1) provided an equivalent total body dose of 0.3 mg/day:

$$(0.03 \text{ mg/m}^3) \times (10 \text{ m}^3\text{/day}) = 0.3 \text{ mg/day total body dose}$$

Since no dermal monitoring data were available, a screening level estimate of potential dermal dose was developed, using Equation (2), and default values from Tables II.1 and II.2. Specific activities include mixing the two-part acrylamide product (acrylamide as powder with activator and other materials), evaluating the consistency of the acrylamide gel (manually pouring a small amount of liquid mixture from one cup to another), assembling the grouting equipment, and using the equipment to fill the leak in the water line.

Using Equation (2) on page 215:

$$DA = (S)(Q)(FQ)(ABS)(WF)$$

where:

DA = dermal absorbed dose rate per day, mg/day
S = surface area of skin available for contact, cm^2
Q = quantity deposited on the skin per event, mg/cm^2 – event
FQ = number of events per day
ABS = fraction of applied dose absorbed through the skin during the event
WF = weight fraction of the substance in the mixture, unitless

The potential dermal absorbed dose estimates depicted in Table II.3 were developed.

The skin permeation for acrylamide has been determined to be 25%, based on laboratory studies conducted by several researchers.[25] When compared with the OEL in units of

Table II.3 — Screening Level Estimates of Acrylamide Dermal-Absorbed Dose During Grouting Activities

Activity	*S, cm²*	*Q, mg/cm² – event*	*WF, weight percent*	*FQ events/day*	*ABS percent*[A]	*DA mg/day*[B]
Pour acrylamide into mixing tank	840 (two hands)	0.06–2.1[C] (dump bags of powder)	1	1	0.25	13–440
Manually test for consistency	420 (one hand)	0.002–2.4[D] (monitoring the process)	0.05	1	0.25	0.01–13
Assemble equipment	420 (one hand)	0.002–2.4[E] (monitoring the process)	0.05	1	0.25	0.01–13
Perform grouting	840 (two hands)	<0.3–2.1[F] (assume level of contact is similar to that of handling a rag)	0.05	2	0.25	3–44

[A] Adapted from Reference # 2.
[B] Estimates are developed assuming no use of gloves or other control measures are in place (e.g., unprotected exposures).
[C] Adapted from Reference # 13.
[D] Adapted from Reference # 14.
[E] Adapted from Reference # 1.
[F] Adapted from Reference # 18.

mg/day, the screening level estimates (column DA in Table II.3) identified a potentially unacceptable exposure, even though it was acknowledged that the screening level estimates were believed to overestimate the true dose.

The industrial hygienist took immediate action to reduce dermal exposures by instituting improvements in the glove practices, housekeeping, and prescribed work practices controls. Skin exposure monitoring also was performed to confirm that the work practices and protective equipment were effective. Also, the bags of powder acrylamide were replaced with a liquid form of acrylamide, further reducing the potential contribution of exposure due to inhalation.

Following the implementation of health hazard controls, the measured dermal exposure range was 17–90 μg/day, with a surface contamination measurement range of 6.2–234 μg/100 cm² on top of the acrylamide mixing tank. The major sources of exposure were contact with contaminated work surfaces, equipment, and tools. Comparison with the OEL in units of mg/day (by adjusting for percent absorbed) revealed that exposures could be effectively controlled (i.e., 0.004–0.02 mg/day for the measured dermal exposures), although the surface contamination measurements indicated that exposures could be reduced further. The industrial hygienist sought other means of further reducing dermal exposures, such as evaluating possible substitutes for acrylamide grout.

References

1. **American Conference of Governmental Industrial Hygienists:** *1996 Threshold Limit Values (TLVs®) for Chemical Substances and Physical Agents and Biological Exposure Indices (BEIs®).* Cincinnati, Ohio: American Conference of Governmental Industrial Hygienists, 1996.
2. **American Conference of Governmental Industrial Hygienists:** *Topics in Biological Monitoring.* Cincinnati, Ohio: American Conference of Governmental Industrial Hygienists, 1996.
3. **Fenske, R.A., and J.J. van Hemmen:** Occupational Skin Exposure to Chemical Substances: Setting Limits. *Ann. Occup. Hyg. 38(4):*333-336 (1994).
4. **Fiserova-Bergerova, V., J.T. Pierce, and P.O. Droz:** Dermal Absorption Potential of Industrial Chemicals: Criteria for Skin Notation. *Am. J. Ind. Medicine 17:*617-635 (1990).
5. **DeCock, J., D. Heedrik, H. Kromhout, and J.S.M. Boleij:** Strategy for Assigning a "Skin Notation": A Comment. *Ann. Occup. Hyg. 40:*611-614. (1996).
6. **Packham, C.L.:** *Skin Care at Work — A Manual for the Prevention of Occupational Skin Disease,* 2nd Rev. Ed. Evesham, United Kingdom: Skin Care Services, 1994.
7. **Colormetric Laboratories, Inc.:** "Implementation of a Dermal Exposure Protection Program." Des Plaines, Ill.: Colormetric Laboratories, Inc., 1995. [Brochure.]
8. **Marquart, J.H.:** Jan. 20, 1997. [Personal correspondence to Cathy Fehrenbacher, AIHA Exposure Assessment Strategies Committee.]
9. **U.S. Environmental Protection Agency:** *Exposure Factors Handbook* (EPA 600/8–89–043). Washington, D.C.: U.S. Environmental Protection Agency/Office of Health and Environmental Assessments, Exposure Assessment Group, 1989.
10. **VanRooij, J.G.M., J.G.C. de Roos, M.M. Bodelier-Bade, and F.J. Jongeneelen:** Absorption of Polycyclic Aromatic Hydrocarbons through the Human Skin: Differences Between Anatomical Sites and Individuals. *J. Toxicol. Environ. Health 38:*355-368 (1993).

11. **U.S. Environmental Protection Agency:** *Development of Statistical Distributions or Ranges of Standard Factors Used in Exposure Assessments* (EPA 600/8–85/010). Washington, D.C.: U.S. Environmental Protection Agency/Office of Health and Environmental Assessments, 1985.
12. **Marquart, J.H.:** Jan. 20, 1997. [Personal correspondence to Cathy Fehrenbacher, AIHA Exposure Assessment Strategies Committee.]
13. **Lansink, C.J.M., M.S.C. Beelen, J. Marquart, and J.J. van Hemmen:** *Skin Exposure to Calcium Carbonate in the Paint Industry. Preliminary Modeling of Skin Exposure Levels to Powders Based on Field Data* (TNO Report V 96.064). Rijswijk, The Netherlands: TNO Nutrition and Food Research Institute, 1996.
14. **Health and Welfare Canada, U.S. Environmental Protection Agency, and National Agricultural Chemicals Association:** "Pesticide Handler's Exposure Database (PHED, Version 1.1 update)." February 1992. [Software.]
15. **Anonymous:** "Worker Dermal Exposure to Trichloroketone — Laboratory Final Report." [Data submitted to U.S. Environmental Protection Agency for the Premanufacture Notification Program.] Washington, D.C.: U.S. Environmental Protection Agency/Office of Pollution Prevention and Toxics, 1996.
16. **U.S. Environmental Protection Agency:** *Occupational Dermal Exposure Assessment — A Review of Methodologies and Field Data. Final Report* (Contract No. 68–D2–0157, WA No. 2–50). Washington, D.C.: U.S. Environmental Protection Agency/Office of Pollution Prevention and Toxics, 1996.
17. **U.S. Environmental Protection Agency:** *Exposure and Release Estimations for Filter Press and Tray Dryer Operations Based on Pilot Plant Data* (EPA 600/R–92/039). Washington, D.C.: U.S. Environmental Protection Agency/Risk Reduction Engineering Laboratory, 1992.
18. **U.S. Environmental Protection Agency:** *Exposure Assessment for Retention of Chemical Liquids on Hands* by Versar, Inc. (Contract No. 68–01–6271). Washington, D.C.: U.S. Environmental Protection Agency/Exposure Evaluation Division, 1992.
19. **Kissel, J.C., K.Y. Richter, and R.A. Fenske:** Field Measurement of Dermal Soil Loading Attributable to

Various Activities: Implications for Exposure Assessment. *Risk Analysis 16(1):*115-125 (1996).

20. **U.S. Environmental Protection Agency**: *Dermal Exposure Assessment: Principles and Applications* (EPA/600/8–9–91). Washington, D.C.: U.S. Environmental Protection Agency/Office of Research and Development, 1992.
21. **McArthur, B.:** Dermal Measurement and Wipe Sampling Methods: A Review. *Appl. Occup. Environ. Hyg. 7(9):*599-606 (1992).
22. **Fenske, R.A.:** Dermal Exposure Assessment Techniques. *Ann. Occup. Hyg. 37(6):*687-706 (1993).
23. **Ness, S.A.:** *Surface and Dermal Monitoring for Toxic Exposures.* New York: Van Nostrand Reinhold, 1994.
24. **Fenske, R.A., and C. Lu:** Determination of Handwash Removal Efficiency: Incomplete Removal of the Pesticide Chlorpyrifos from Skin by Standard Handwash Techniques. *Am. Ind. Hyg. Assoc. J. 55(5):*425-432 (1994).
25. **Ramsey, J., J. Young, and S. Gorzinski:** "Acrylamide: Toxicodynamics in Rats." 1984. [Unpublished Dow Chemical Company Report.] In *Assessment of Health Risks from Exposure to Acrylamide.* Washington, D.C.: U.S. Environmental Protection Agency/Office of Toxic Substances, 1990.

Appendix III

Uncertainty Analysis

The purpose of this appendix is to impress you with the importance of uncertainty analysis and to provide a quick overview of some of the more common techniques. Those wishing to learn more should consult references 1 through 6.

The respected scientist Jacob Bronowski once remarked that any time we are absolutely certain of a fact, we are almost surely wrong.[7] Indeed, we cannot measure any physical quantity without error. Also, any activity that aspires to gain and transmit knowledge — including the industrial hygiene practice of risk assessment — is, to quote Dr. Bronowski, "personal and responsible . . . [and] at the edge of uncertainty."[7] Thus, the understanding and communication of uncertainty is of central importance to our science.

When examining the scientific uncertainty of worker exposure determinants, it is useful to consider them as resulting from two sources or types. Type # 1 is the natural variability of these predictors in any particular scenario of interest; type # 2 is our lack of knowledge of the basic nature of these variables (i.e., our fundamental ignorance of the reality and relationships within that reality that cause the exposure to occur).

Given data, we can describe type # 1 uncertainty using sampling statistics. These in turn describe a tolerance of knowledge around the measurement or estimate.

The second source of uncertainty (type # 2 signifying our lack of basic knowledge) is typically much more immense and troublesome; as such, this source tends to dominate. It presents us with the humbling fact that to a significant extent "we don't know what we don't know." It is therefore vital to understand and describe this lack of basic knowledge in as much detail as possible so that those who use our work are able to comprehend and appreciate its strengths and limitations and make informed decisions.

Two classes of uncertainty analysis are presented in this appendix. The first and more conventional method is to look at predictions based on reasonable worst cases and the impact or sensitivity of the uncertainty for individual variables. The second method uses more recent computer simulation techniques and software — such as Crystal Ball[8] and @Risk[9] — to estimate a range of outcomes and the sensitivity associated with predictor variables.

The example for this appendix is a simple indoor air model with three variables:

$$C = \frac{G}{Q} \qquad (1)$$

where:

C = equilibrium airborne concentration of a toxicant (mg/m^3)
G = steady generation rate (mg/hour)
Q = steady ventilation rate (m^3/hour)

Reasonable Worst Case

A traditional way to address or describe uncertainty in risk assessments is to assign "reasonable" worst-case conditions for evaluations or models. In this case we would typically pick the worst case (highest G and lowest Q) to estimate a worst case for C. This then could be combined with "best-case" estimates (lowest G and highest Q) to provide a range for C. Finally, the impact or sensitivity of G or Q on either best- or worst-case scenarios could be determined by calculating the results of varying these predictors, from maximum to minimum individually.

The practical truth of this approach is that when a single or "bright-line" prediction for exposure potential is required, often only the worst-case estimate is reported and used. This single worst-case value is the compounding of all the worst-case uncertainty in all of the predictors. Our example has only two variables; in cases with many predictors the estimate of exposure often becomes compounded to a much higher order. Historically, mention of the "average case" or "best case" is often omitted. Doing so essentially hides valuable information about the uncertainty since those viewing the results have no knowledge — and thus no sense — of the relative width of the error band around the prediction.

Given our example, let us assume we have data on the source rate (G) that indicate it is normally distributed with a mean of 50 mg/hour and a standard deviation of 5 mg/hour for the particular source of interest. (This is an example of uncertainty type # 1 above — a known and measured quantity with natural variability.) We might interpret a worst-case estimate of G as the mean plus 3 standard deviations. This is 50 + 15, or 65 mg/hour, which is a value greater than 99.8% of the values in this predicted set of values. Best case would be the mean minus 3 standard deviations, or 35 mg/hour.

The result is: 1) reasonable worst case G = 65 mg/hour; 2) average case G = 50 mg/hour; and 3) reasonable best case G = 35 mg/hour.

For the ventilation rate (Q) in this case, however, we have much less certain information or knowledge. (This is an example of uncertainty type # 2 — uncertainty from ignorance or lack of knowledge.) We know that this particular source will be used in large and small industrial settings almost invariably without benefit of local exhaust. From our understanding of the literature we are reasonably confident that the general ventilation rate likely will not be less than 0.2 mixing air changes per hour and will most likely not be higher than 30 air changes per hour. (Note that Q = [air change per hour][room volume]). Given our knowledge base in this hypothetical example we have no positive sense of what the average or "most likely" level of ventilation might be. We could guess that it is halfway between 0.2 and 30, but if we have no knowledge or confidence that this is true it would be unwise to do so.

So we have: 1) worst case air change per hour = 0.2; and 2) best case air change per hour = 30. Using the old "reasonable worst case" approach we can simply take a worst-case estimate of G (the mean plus 3 standard deviations = 50 + 3[5] = 65) and use the worst-case estimate of ventilation as 0.2 air changes per hour. Given a relatively small room of 3 m × 3 m × 2 m (note that we could have used a variable room size in this analysis, but in the interest of keeping this example simple we did not), this renders an estimated worst-case equilibrium concentration of:

$$C = \frac{65 \text{ mg/hour}}{(0.2\text{/hour})(18 \text{ m}^3)} = 18.1 \text{ mg/m}^3$$

The best case would be:

$$C = \frac{35 \text{ mg/hour}}{(30\text{/hour})(18 \text{ m}^3)} = 0.065 \text{ mg/m}^3$$

There is no average case since we do not have enough confidence in our estimate of an average ventilation rate to use one.

The prediction of exposure in this treatment varies 278-fold from best to worst case.

Obviously, the ventilation rate is the most sensitive predictor because it varies more than 150-fold from 0.2 to 30 while the generation rate varied less than a factor of 2 from 35 to 65.

Monte Carlo Computer Simulation

Computer-aided stochastic (i.e., random, involving chance) probability analysis as typified by the Monte Carlo technique[1,2] allows one to present more readily and completely information about the exposure predictions and the uncertainty associated with these predictions. In essence, the predictor variables — in this case G and Q — are described as "distributions" rather than point estimates of best, worst, or average.

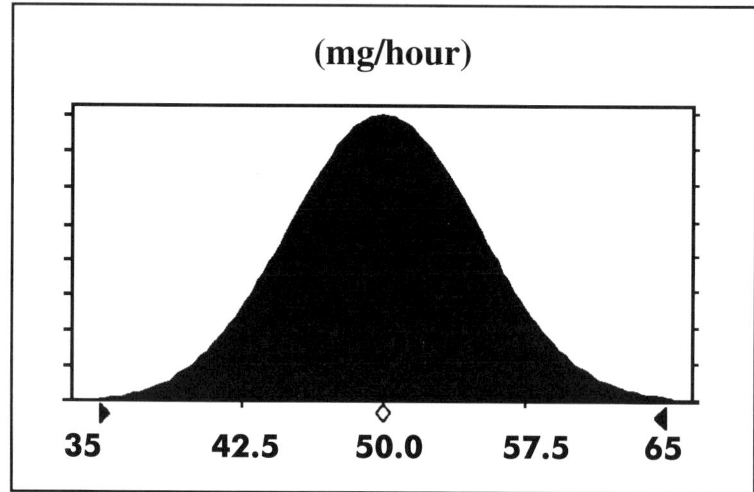

Figure III.1 — Normally distributed generation rate.

In this example, G has a normal or Gaussian distribution, the mean equals 50, the standard deviation equals 5.0 (see Figure III.1), Q equals a uniform (i.e., totally random) distribution from 0.2 to 30 air changes per hour (i.e., a distribution in which there is an equal probability of any values occurring within this range and a zero probability of any value occurring outside the range; see Figure III.2). In a room sized 3 m × 3 m × 2 m, this is a uniform distribution range of 3.6–540 m^3/hour.

Note that the distribution chosen for the air changes per hour is a direct result of our lack of knowledge about it. It is important to consider that this distribution is not reality but is a best

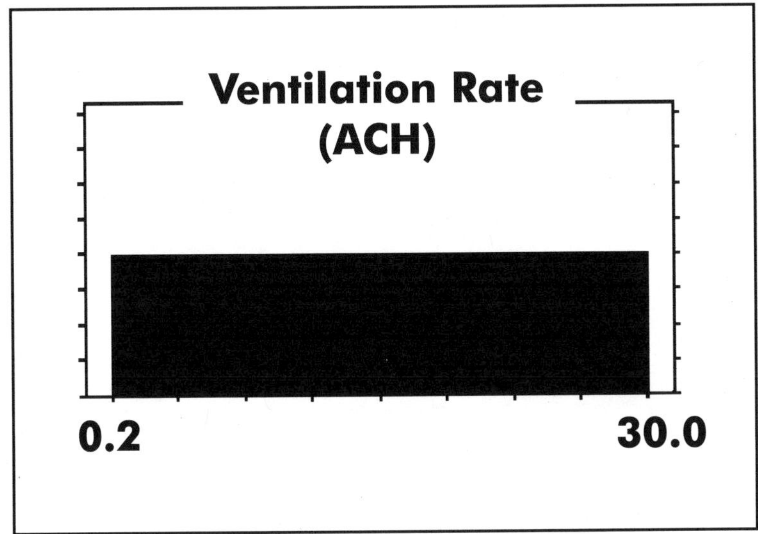

Figure III.2 — Uniformly distributed ventilation rate.

subjective description of our knowledge of reality. There is most likely some finite probability of air change rates being below 0.2 or above 30, and there is certainly some central tendency to this universe of values; however, this distribution represents the quantification of our best knowledge and professional judgment for this situation. If we had access to better data, we could use the information to refine this estimating distribution to be closer to reality.

This analysis therefore allows for a "distribution" (more accurately termed a "probability distribution function" or PDF) of values to be used for these two input variables (G and Q). These PDFs reflect the quality of our understanding and data. Using a personal computer and readily available software (e.g., Crystal Ball[(8)]) a large number (usually 10,000 or more) of independent "samples" consisting of sets of values for each of the input variables are obtained and the corresponding distribution of predicted airborne concentration is calculated. This is done by repeated computer runs through the concentration estimation algorithm using PDF-selected values for the input parameters. These values are constrained by the known or inferred ranges, means, and probability distributions of the individual input parameters. The resulting output is displayed as a forecast chart that shows the entire range of possible outcomes and the likelihood of achieving any of them. This includes a mean concentration and the probability for any concentration above and below the mean. It also provides the upper and lower limits as a measure of dispersion (see Figure III.3).

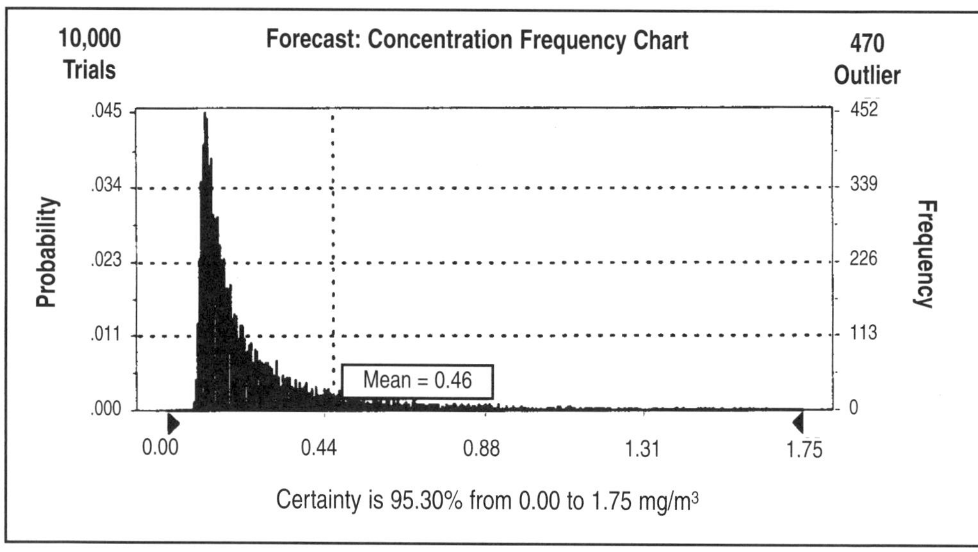

Figure III.3 — Forecast: concentration frequency chart.

In this example, the median equals 0.19 mg/m^3; the mean equals 0.46 mg/m^3; the 5th percentile equals 0.09 mg/m^3; and the 95th percentile equals 1.7 mg/m^3.

Interestingly, our worst-case estimate of 18.1 mg/m^3 was not reached in the 10,000-run simulation; the highest prediction in this run (i.e., the 100th percentile) was 14.5 mg/m^3. Likewise, the lowest value (i.e., the 0 percentile) was 0.07 mg/m^3, which is relatively close to the 0.065 mg/m^3 value as our absolute best case.

An added benefit of Monte Carlo analysis is that a common byproduct of this computerized examination is a sensitivity analysis that shows how much each predictor variable contributed to the uncertainty or variability of the predictions. This in turn tells the risk assessor and risk manager alike which portion of the variability is from natural fluctuation as opposed to how much is caused by lack of knowledge. Given this informa-

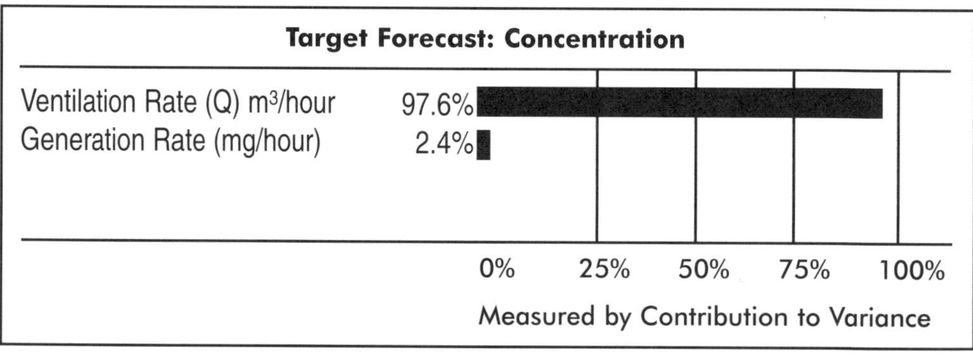

Figure III.4 — Sensitivity chart.

tion, decisions can be made about where the most cost-effective allocation of resources may occur to refine the estimate of exposure and risk. In our example, the sensitivity analysis shows the distribution of variance for the model as depicted in Figure III.4.

In Figure III.4, estimates of G contributed 2.4% and estimates of Q contributed 97.6% of the variance of the predictions.

Clearly — and not surprisingly — our lack of knowledge of the ventilation (Q) in this scenario added most of the uncertainty to this analysis. More important, it made our estimate of the 95th percentile concentration significantly higher than it would have been with a more accurate description of the ventilation rates in these scenarios.

Validation

This brings us to the final topic of this appendix: validation. In some instances, one may have actual exposure data for the scenario of interest. As mentioned earlier, the distribution for a Type # 2 uncertainty might not be reality, though it should still represent our best estimate of the real world. It stands to reason that the predictions from this type of distribution will be similarly constituted since they also represent our best subjective portrayal of that truth. One should fully expect, however, that actual exposure data and the distribution of that data should fit within the predicted distributions. If not, there was a serious error in the judgment that assigned the distribution of a Type # 2 predictor variable. A comparison of the distribution of these data with the predicted distribution could provide a reality check on the assumptions used for the Type # 2 uncertainties. Of course, if the industrial hygienist has a good data set, he or she does not need to perform a composite analysis of the elements of uncertainty, as occurred above.

References

1. **Burmaster, D.E., and K. von Stackelberg:** Using Monte Carlo Simulations in Public Health Risk Assessment: Estimating and Presenting Full Distributions of Risk. *J. Expos. Anal. Environ. Epidem. 1:*491-512.
2. **Thompson, K.M., D.E. Burmaster, and E.A.C. Crouch:** Monte Carlo Techniques for Quantitative Uncertainty Analysis in Public Health Risk Assessments. *Risk Analysis 12:*53-63 (1992).
3. **Burmaster, D.E., and R.H. Harris:** The Magnitude of Compounding Conservatisms in Superfund Risk Assessments. *Risk Analysis 13(2):*131 (1993).

4. **U.S. Environmental Protection Agency:** *Use of Monte Carlo Simulation in Risk Assessment*. Philadelphia, Pa.: U.S. Environmental Protection Agency/Region III, 1994.
5. **Fehrenbacher, M.C., and A.A. Hummel:** Evaluation of the Mass Balance Model Used by the Environmental Protection Agency for Estimating Inhalation Exposure to New Chemical Substances. *Am. Ind. Hyg. Assoc. J. 57(6):*526-536 (1996).
6. "Exposure Guidelines for Exposure Assessment," *Federal Register 57:*(29 May 1992). p. 22888.
7. **Bronowski, J:** *The Ascent of Man.* London: Warner Books, 1973. p. 232.
8. **Decisioneering, Inc.:** "Crystal Ball." Aurora, Colo.: Decisioneering, Inc, 1996. [Software.]
9. **Palisade:** "@Risk." Newfield, N.Y.: Palisade, 1996. [Software.]

Appendix IV

Descriptive Statistics

Descriptive statistics are used to summarize data — typically their central tendency (mean, median, and geometric mean) and their spread (range, minimum and maximum, standard deviation, and geometric standard deviation).

Calculating these summary statistics helps us organize our monitoring data to begin understanding the exposures they represent. Many industrial hygiene data sets can be interpreted simply by comparing the OEL with descriptive statistics. When most of the data are clustered well below or well above the OEL, the industrial hygienist can generally make a decision on workplace acceptability by using descriptive statistics and professional judgment. When the range of data approaches or includes the OEL, inferential statistics can be useful for decision making.

The following descriptive statistics should be calculated routinely for all monitoring data. With a programmable calculator or computer spreadsheet, they are easy to compute.

- number of samples (n)
- maximum (max)
- minimum (min)
- range
- percent above OEL (% > OEL)
- mean ($\overline{x}$)
- median
- standard deviation (s)
- mean of the logtransformed data ($\overline{y}$)
- standard deviation of the logtransformed data (s_y)
- geometric mean (GM)
- geometric standard deviation (GSD)

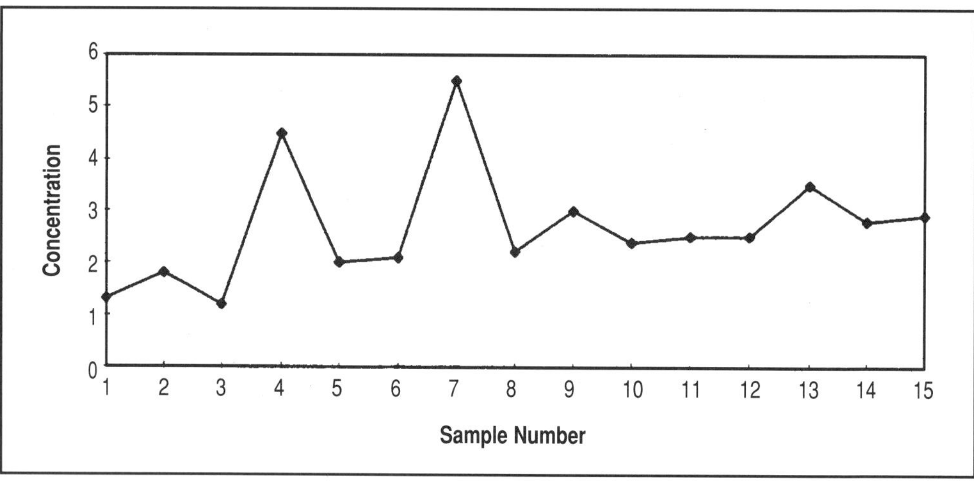

Figure IV.1 — Sequential plot.

It also may be useful to make a simple sequential plot of the data (earliest samples first; see Figure IV.1). A plot such as this can indicate trends in exposure over time (nonstationary distribution).

Calculating the Descriptive Statistics

n
max
min

The number of samples, the maximum value, and the minimum value can be determined through observation of the data.

range
percent above OEL (% >OEL)
mean

Calculation of the range, percent above the OEL, and sample mean is straightforward:

$$\text{range} = \max - \min \tag{1}$$

$$\% > \text{OEL} = \frac{\text{number of samples} > \text{OEL}}{\text{total number of samples}} \times 100 \tag{2}$$

$$\bar{x} = \frac{\text{sum of all the data}}{\text{number of samples}} = \frac{\Sigma x_i}{n} \tag{3}$$

median

The median can also be determined by examination of the sorted data. If n is odd, then the median is simply the middle value in the data. If n is even, then the median is the average of the two middle values in the data.

standard deviation

Calculating the standard deviation of the data is less intuitive. Luckily, many inexpensive calculators now offer a standard deviation function so you do not have to compute the following formula by hand:

$$s = \sqrt{\frac{\Sigma(x_i - \bar{x})^2}{n - 1}} \tag{4}$$

mean and standard deviation of logtransformed data

The mean of the logtransformed data and the standard deviation of the logtransformed data can be calculated for the ln (log_e) or the log (log_{10}) transformation of the original data. [This text will use ln (log_e) consistently.]

$$y_i = \log(x_i) \text{ or } y_i = \ln(x_i) \tag{5}$$

mean of the logtransformed data =

$$\bar{y} = \frac{\Sigma y_i}{n} \tag{6}$$

standard deviation of the logtransformed data = s_y

$$s_y = \sqrt{\frac{\Sigma(y_i - \bar{y})^2}{n - 1}} \tag{7}$$

GM
GSD

Once the mean and standard deviation of the logtransformed data have been determined, calculating the geometric mean (GM) and the geometric standard deviation (GSD) is a simple step:

$$GM = \text{antilog}\ (\bar{y}) = e^{\bar{y}} \text{ or } 10^{\bar{y}} \tag{8}$$

$$GSD = \text{antilog}\ (s_y) = e^{s_y} \text{ or } 10^{s_y} \tag{9}$$

Example

Calculate descriptive statistics for the following monitoring results: 1.3, 1.8, 1.2, 4.5, 2, 2.1, 5.5, 2.2, 3, 2.4, 2.5, 2.5, 3.5, 2.8, and 2.9 (OEL = 5 mg/m^3).

(Note: Those using a spreadsheet or statistical software to work the examples in this book might get slightly different answers than those printed due to rounding errors in the written examples).

Table IV.1 — Example Data

x_i Monitoring data (mg/m³)	$(x_i - \bar{x})^2$	$y_i = \ln(x_i)$ Logtransformed data	$(y_i - \bar{y})^2$
1.3	1.904	0.262364	0.416725
1.8	0.774	0.587787	0.102477
1.2	2.190	0.182322	0.526473
4.5	3.312	1.504077	0.355420
2	0.462	0.693147	0.046122
2.1	0.336	0.741937	0.027546
5.5	7.952	1.704748	0.634957
2.2	0.230	0.788457	0.014268
3	0.102	1.098612	0.036369
2.4	0.078	0.875469	0.001052
2.5	0.032	0.916291	0.000070
2.5	0.032	0.916291	0.000070
3.5	0.672	1.252763	0.118926
2.8	0.014	1.029619	0.014814
2.9	0.048	1.064711	0.024588
$\Sigma x_i = 40.2$ mg/m³	$\Sigma(x_i - \bar{x})^2 = 18.14$	$\Sigma y_i = 13.62$	$\Sigma(y_i - \bar{y})^2 = 2.320$

number of samples: By observation = 15
maximum: By observation = 5.5 mg/m³
minimum: By observation = 1.2 mg/m³
range: range = maximum - minimum
= 5.5 - 1.2 = 4.3 mg/m³

percent above OEL:
By observation: number of samples > OEL = 1

$$\% > \text{OEL} = \frac{\text{number of samples} > \text{OEL}}{\text{total number of samples}} \times 100$$

$$\% > \text{OEL} = \frac{1}{15} \times 100 = 6.7\%$$

mean:

$$\bar{x} = \frac{\Sigma x_i}{n}$$

$$\bar{x} = \frac{40.2}{15} = 2.7 \text{ mg/m}^3$$

median:
By observation — find the 8th value by rank: 2.5 mg/m³

standard deviation:

To calculate the standard deviation we must first calculate the sum of the squared deviation of each value from the mean (see Column 2 in Table IV.1). We then calculate the standard deviation as:

$$s = \sqrt{\frac{\Sigma(x_i - \overline{x})^2}{n - 1}}$$

$$s = \sqrt{\frac{18.14}{15 - 1}}$$

$$s = 1.1 \text{ mg/m}^3$$

mean and standard deviation of ln(data):

We must first perform a logtransformation of the data ($y_i = \ln(x_i)$ in Column 3 of Table IV.1). We then calculate the mean and standard deviation of the transformed data:

mean of ln(data):

$$\overline{y} = \frac{\Sigma y_i}{n}$$

$$\overline{y} = \frac{13.62}{15} = 0.91$$

standard deviation of ln(data):

$$s_y = \sqrt{\frac{\Sigma(y_i - \overline{y})^2}{n - 1}}$$

$$s_y = \sqrt{\frac{2.320}{15 - 1}}$$

$$s_y = 0.41$$

geometric mean (GM) and geometric standard deviation (GSD):

Calculating the GM and the GSD is straightforward once the mean and standard deviation of the logtransformed data have been calculated.

GM:

$GM = \text{antilog}\ (\overline{y}) = e^{\overline{y}} = e^{0.91} = 2.5 \text{ mg/m}^3$

GSD:

$GSD = \text{antilog}\ (s_y) = e^{s_y} = e^{0.41} = 1.5$

Appendix V

Probability Plotting and Measures of Goodness-of-Fit

Probability Plotting

When reviewing monitoring data for an SEG, consider making a probability plot. Probability plots are useful for several reasons:

- They indicate whether the exposure profile can reasonably be approximated by a lognormal or normal distribution.
- They can help identify potential outliers that may indicate that the SEG has not been well-defined.
- They are a simple and convenient method for forming a picture of the exposure profile indicated by the monitoring results. They provide direct estimates of the distribution geometric mean (GM), geometric standard deviation (GSD), and various percentiles (e.g., 95th percentile). This estimation can be performed even when some of the monitoring data results are below the analytical detection limit.

Checking the Assumption of Normality or Lognormality

If data form a straight line when plotted on lognormal or normal probability paper, that is evidence they come from a single population that is lognormally or normally distributed. Perfectly straight lines are rare and are not a necessity. On the other hand, probability plotting is not a goodness-of-fit test, only an indicator of whether the proper distribution shape has been chosen.

Checking the SEG

If data do not form an approximately straight line when plotted on probability paper, that indicates the monitoring data might not come from a lognormal or normal distribution. If so, consider using nonparametric statistics. The absence of a straight line might also be evidence that the data do not represent a single SEG. If so, the data representing the exposures for individual workers or tasks should be divided into two or more data sets (i.e., two or more SEGs) and analyzed separately.

Estimating Exposure Profile Parameters

If the plotted data adhere reasonably well to a straight line, a variety of exposure distribution parameters can be estimated directly from the probability plot:

- Any percentile of interest can be read directly off the plot. For example, the 95th percentile of the exposure distribution can be estimated by finding the concentration that corresponds to 95% on the graph.
- The geometric mean is equal to the concentration corresponding to the 50% point (in other words, GM = 50th percentile).
- The geometric standard deviation can be calculated either by dividing the 84% concentration by the 50% concentration or by dividing the 50% concentration by the 16% concentration (in other words, GSD = 84th percentile/50th percentile = 50th percentile/16th percentile).
- The percentage of the exposure distribution that exceeds the OEL can also be estimated from the probability plot. Simply find the percentage that corresponds to the OEL concentration on the graph.

Making a Probability Plot

There are several types of probability paper. The two most often used for industrial hygiene monitoring data are lognormal probability paper and normal probability paper. Both have a probability (or probit) scale on one axis with the median (50th percentile) at the midpoint and percentage units that widen as they move away from the 50% point in both directions. The other axis is either log (lognormal) or linear (normal) for plotting the concentration data.

The procedure for constructing a probability plot is:

1. Rank order the data, lowest to highest (see Table V.1).
2. Rank each value from 1 (lowest) to n (highest).
3. Calculate the plotting position for each value. Statisticians have developed a variety of computational formulas and tables for determining the plotting positions of the ranked data. The following formula is easy to calculate and will be adequate for most industrial hygiene applications: plotting position = rank/(n + 1).

Table V.1 — Probability Plotting

Monitoring data (mg/m³)	*Ranked data (mg/m³)*	*r = rank*	*Plotting position*
1.3	1.2	1	0.0625
1.8	1.3	2	0.125
1.2	1.8	3	0.1875
4.5	2	4	0.25
2	2.1	5	0.3125
2.1	2.2	6	0.375
5.5	2.4	7	0.4375
2.2	2.5	8	0.5
3	2.5	9	0.5625
2.4	2.8	10	0.625
2.5	2.9	11	0.6875
2.5	3	12	0.75
3.5	3.5	13	0.8125
2.8	4.5	14	0.875
2.9	5.5	15	0.9375

4. Plot the concentrations against the plotting positions (see Figure V.1).
5. "Eyeball" a best-fit line through the plotted data.
6. Determine whether the data provide a reasonable fit for the straight line. If so, this is evidence they are lognormally or normally distributed. If not, the assumption of lognormality or normality may have to be abandoned. If the data cannot be found to fit some other distribution, nonparametric statistical methods must be used.
7. If the data form a reasonable fit to a straight line, estimate the distribution GM, GSD, and percentiles of interest off the best-fit line (see Figure V.2).

Missing Data

One notable benefit of probability plotting is that the exposure distribution can be modeled even when some of the monitoring data are less-than detection limit values. Those values are simply ranked along with the other monitoring data and plotting positions calculated for each of the values — including the less-than values. The plot is then made in the usual fashion except that the less-than values are excluded when determining the best-fit line.

If, for example, our data set had a limit of detection of 1.9, three of the sample results would have been below the detection limit. We could use probability plotting to help form a picture of the distribution even though these samples at first seem unusable. We would order the data and calculate plotting positions in the usual fashion (see Table V.2).

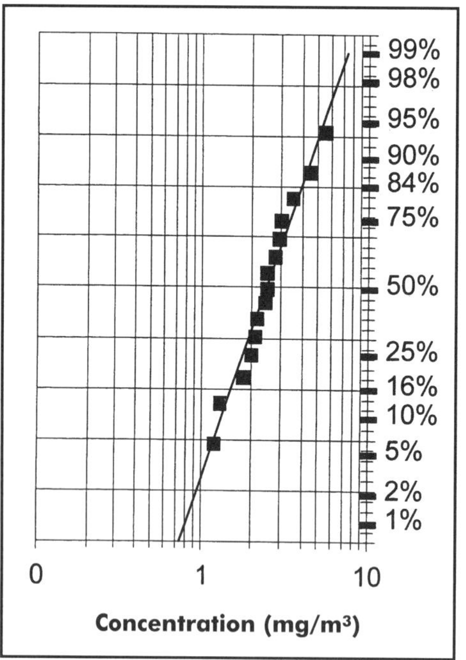

Figure V.1 — Logprobability plot and least-squares best-fit line.

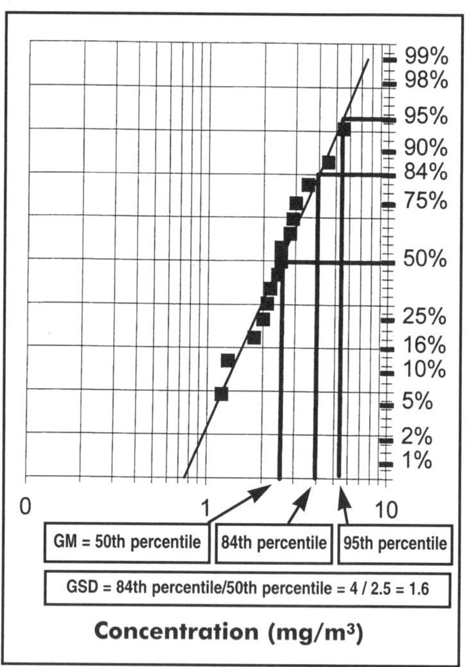

Figure V.2 — GM and GSD determined from logprobability plot and least-squares best-fit line.

Table V.2 — Probability Plotting to Handle Less-Than Values

Monitoring data (mg/m³)	*Ranked data (mg/m³)*	*r = rank*	*Plotting position*
<1.9	<1.9	1	0.0625
<1.9	<1.9	2	0.125
<1.9	<1.9	3	0.1875
4.5	2	4	0.25
2	2.1	5	0.3125
2.1	2.2	6	0.375
5.5	2.4	7	0.4375
2.2	2.5	8	0.5
3	2.5	9	0.5625
2.4	2.8	10	0.625
2.5	2.9	11	0.6875
2.5	3	12	0.75
3.5	3.5	13	0.8125
2.8	4.5	14	0.875
2.9	5.5	15	0.9375

The data would then be plotted in the usual manner and a best-fit line eyeballed through the points — excluding those points that represent the less-than values (see Figure V.3). The distribution GM, GSD, and percentiles of interest could then be estimated off the best-fit line.

W-test for Distribution Goodness-of-Fit

Various techniques for determining how well data fit a specific distribution are available. The Shapiro and Wilk Test (known usually as the W-test) is a method for determining whether sample data have been drawn from a normal distribution, or — if applied to the logtransformed sample data — a lognormal distribution. Although the computations involved are fairly intensive, the W-test is one of the most powerful tests for determining goodness-of-fit for normal or lognormal data when n is fairly small ($n \le 50$).[1] The W-test is a preferred mechanism for checking the assumption of normality or lognormality when a personal computer is available.

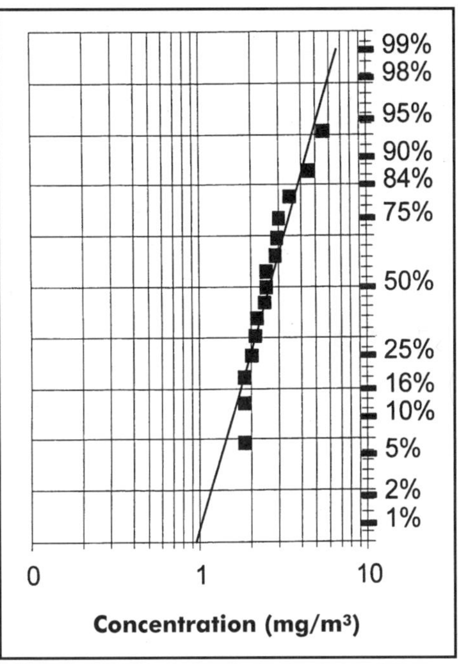

Figure V.3 — Logprobability plot and least-squares best-fit line. The lowest three points are for concentrations less than 1.9 mg/m³.

The W-test is performed as follows:

1. Order the data, smallest to largest.
2. Calculate k: $k = n/2$ if n is even; $k = (n - 1)/2$ if n is odd
3. Calculate the W statistic:

$$W = \frac{\left[\sum_{i=1}^{k} a_i (x_{[n-i+1]} - x_{[i]})\right]^2}{s^2(n-1)} \qquad (1)$$

where:

a_i is found in Table V.3.

4. The data are from a normal (or lognormal if applied to the logtransformed data) population if W is greater than the percentile given in Table V.4.

Table V.3 — Coefficients a_i for the Shapiro and Wilk W-test for Normality

i \ n	2	3	4	5	6	7	8	9	10
1	0.7071	0.7071	0.6872	0.6646	0.6431	0.6233	0.6052	0.5888	0.5739
2	-	0.0000	0.1677	0.2413	0.2806	0.3031	0.3164	0.3244	0.3291
3	-	-	-	0.0000	0.0875	0.1401	0.1743	0.1976	0.2141
4	-	-	-	-	-	0.0000	0.0561	0.0947	0.1224
5	-	-	-	-	-	-	-	0.0000	0.0399

i \ n	11	12	13	14	15	16	17	18	19	20
1	0.5601	0.5475	0.5359	0.5251	0.5150	0.5056	0.4968	0.4886	0.4808	0.4734
2	0.3315	0.3325	0.3325	0.3318	0.3306	0.3290	0.3273	0.3253	0.3232	0.3211
3	0.2260	0.2347	0.2412	0.2460	0.2495	0.2521	0.2540	0.2553	0.2561	0.2565
4	0.1429	0.1586	0.1707	0.1802	0.1878	0.1939	0.1988	0.2027	0.2059	0.2085
5	0.0695	0.0922	0.1099	0.1240	0.1353	0.1447	0.1524	0.1587	0.1641	0.1686
6	0.0000	0.0303	0.0539	0.0727	0.0880	0.1005	0.1109	0.1197	0.1271	0.1334
7	-	-	0.0000	0.0240	0.0433	0.0593	0.0725	0.0837	0.0932	0.1013
8	-	-	-	-	0.0000	0.0196	0.0359	0.0496	0.0612	0.0711
9	-	-	-	-	-	-	0.0000	0.0163	0.0303	0.0422
10	-	-	-	-	-	-	-	-	0.0000	0.0140

i \ n	21	22	23	24	25	26	27	28	29	30
1	0.4643	0.4590	0.4542	0.4493	0.4450	0.4407	0.4366	0.4328	0.4291	0.4254
2	0.3185	0.3156	0.3126	0.3098	0.3069	0.3043	0.3018	0.2992	0.2968	0.2944
3	0.2578	0.2571	0.2563	0.2554	0.2543	0.2533	0.2522	0.2510	0.2499	0.2487
4	0.2119	0.2131	0.2139	0.2145	0.2148	0.2151	0.2152	0.2151	0.2150	0.2148
5	0.1736	0.1764	0.1787	0.1807	0.1822	0.1836	0.1848	0.1857	0.1864	0.1870
6	0.1399	0.1443	0.1480	0.1512	0.1539	0.1563	0.1584	0.1601	0.1616	0.1630
7	0.1092	0.1150	0.1201	0.1245	0.1283	0.1316	0.1346	0.1372	0.1395	0.1415
8	0.0804	0.0878	0.0941	0.0997	0.1046	0.1089	0.1128	0.1162	0.1192	0.1219
9	0.0530	0.0618	0.0696	0.0764	0.0823	0.0876	0.0923	0.0965	0.1002	0.1036
10	0.0263	0.0368	0.0459	0.0539	0.0610	0.0672	0.0728	0.0778	0.0822	0.0862
11	0.0000	0.0122	0.0228	0.0321	0.0403	0.0476	0.0540	0.0598	0.0650	0.0697
12	-	-	0.0000	0.0107	0.0200	0.0284	0.0358	0.0424	0.0483	0.0537
13	-	-	-	-	0.0000	0.0094	0.0178	0.0253	0.0320	0.0381
14	-	-	-	-	-	-	0.0000	0.0084	0.0159	0.0227
15	-	-	-	-	-	-	-	-	0.0000	0.0076

i \ n	31	32	33	34	35	36	37	38	39	40
1	0.4220	0.4188	0.4156	0.4127	0.4096	0.4068	0.4040	0.4015	0.3989	0.3964
2	0.2921	0.2898	0.2876	0.2854	0.2834	0.2813	0.2794	0.2774	0.2755	0.2737
3	0.2475	0.2462	0.2451	0.2439	0.2427	0.2415	0.2403	0.2391	0.2380	0.2368
4	0.2145	0.2141	0.2137	0.2132	0.2127	0.2121	0.2116	0.2110	0.2104	0.2098
5	0.1874	0.1878	0.1880	0.1882	0.1883	0.1883	0.1883	0.1881	0.1880	0.1878
6	0.1641	0.1651	0.1660	0.1667	0.1673	0.1678	0.1683	0.1686	0.1689	0.1691
7	0.1433	0.1449	0.1463	0.1475	0.1487	0.1496	0.1505	0.1513	0.1520	0.1526
8	0.1243	0.1265	0.1284	0.1301	0.1317	0.1331	0.1344	0.1356	0.1366	0.1376
9	0.1066	0.1093	0.1118	0.1140	0.1160	0.1179	0.1196	0.1211	0.1225	0.1237
10	0.0899	0.0931	0.0961	0.0988	0.1013	0.1036	0.1056	0.1075	0.1092	0.1108
11	0.0739	0.0777	0.0812	0.0844	0.0873	0.0900	0.0924	0.0947	0.0967	0.0986
12	0.0585	0.0629	0.0669	0.0706	0.0739	0.0770	0.0798	0.0824	0.0848	0.0870
13	0.0435	0.0485	0.0530	0.0572	0.0610	0.0645	0.0677	0.0706	0.0733	0.0759
14	0.0289	0.0344	0.0395	0.0441	0.0484	0.0523	0.0559	0.0592	0.0622	0.0651
15	0.0144	0.0206	0.0262	0.0314	0.0361	0.0404	0.0444	0.0481	0.0515	0.0546
16	0.0000	0.0068	0.0131	0.0187	0.0239	0.0287	0.0331	0.0372	0.0409	0.0444
17	-	-	0.0000	0.0062	0.0119	0.0172	0.0220	0.0264	0.0305	0.0343
18	-	-	-	-	0.0000	0.0057	0.0110	0.0158	0.0203	0.0244
19	-	-	-	-	-	-	0.0000	0.0053	0.0101	0.0146
20	-	-	-	-	-	-	-	-	0.0000	0.0049

Source: From Shapiro and Wilk, 1965.

Table V.3 — Coefficients a_i for the Shapiro and Wilk W-test for Normality (continued)

i \ n	41	42	43	44	45	46	47	48	49	50
1	0.3940	0.3917	0.3894	0.3872	0.3850	0.3830	0.3808	0.3789	0.3770	0.3751
2	0.2719	0.2701	0.2684	0.2667	0.2651	0.2635	0.2620	0.2604	0.2589	0.2574
3	0.2357	0.2345	0.2334	0.2323	0.2313	0.2302	0.2291	0.2281	0.2271	0.2260
4	0.2091	0.2085	0.2078	0.2072	0.2065	0.2058	0.2052	0.2045	0.2038	0.2032
5	0.1876	0.1874	0.1871	0.1868	0.1865	0.1862	0.1859	0.1855	0.1851	0.1847
6	0.1693	0.1694	0.1695	0.1695	0.1695	0.1695	0.1695	0.1693	0.1692	0.1691
7	0.1531	0.1535	0.1539	0.1542	0.1545	0.1548	0.1550	0.1551	0.1553	0.1554
8	0.1384	0.1392	0.1398	0.1405	0.1410	0.1415	0.1420	0.1423	0.1427	0.1430
9	0.1249	0.1259	0.1269	0.1278	0.1286	0.1293	0.1300	0.1306	0.1312	0.1317
10	0.1123	0.1136	0.1149	0.1160	0.1170	0.1180	0.1189	0.1197	0.1205	0.1212
11	0.1004	0.1020	0.1035	0.1049	0.1062	0.1073	0.1085	0.1095	0.1105	0.1113
12	0.0891	0.0909	0.0927	0.0943	0.0959	0.0972	0.0986	0.0998	0.1010	0.1020
13	0.0782	0.0804	0.0824	0.0842	0.0860	0.0876	0.0892	0.0906	0.0919	0.0932
14	0.0677	0.0701	0.0724	0.0745	0.0765	0.0783	0.0801	0.0817	0.0832	0.0846
15	0.0575	0.0602	0.0628	0.0651	0.0673	0.0694	0.0713	0.0731	0.0748	0.0764
16	0.0476	0.0506	0.0534	0.0560	0.0584	0.0607	0.0628	0.0648	0.0667	0.0685
17	0.0379	0.0411	0.0442	0.0471	0.0497	0.0522	0.0546	0.0568	0.0588	0.0608
18	0.0283	0.0318	0.0352	0.0383	0.0412	0.0439	0.0465	0.0489	0.0511	0.0532
19	0.0188	0.0227	0.0263	0.0296	0.0328	0.0357	0.0385	0.0411	0.0436	0.0459
20	0.0094	0.0136	0.0175	0.0211	0.0245	0.0277	0.0307	0.0335	0.0361	0.0386
21	0.0000	0.0045	0.0087	0.0126	0.0163	0.0197	0.0229	0.0259	0.0288	0.0314
22	-	-	0.0000	0.0042	0.0081	0.0118	0.0153	0.0185	0.0215	0.0244
23	-	-	-	-	0.0000	0.0039	0.0076	0.0111	0.0143	0.0174
24	-	-	-	-	-	-	0.0000	0.0037	0.0071	0.0104
25	-	-	-	-	-	-	-	-	0.0000	0.0035

Table V.4 — Quantiles of the Shapiro and Wilk W-test for Normality (Values of *W* such that 100% (p) of the Distribution of W is less than W_p)

n	$W_{0.01}$	$W_{0.02}$	$W_{0.05}$	$W_{0.10}$	$W_{0.50}$
3	0.753	0.756	0.767	0.789	0.959
4	0.687	0.707	0.748	0.792	0.935
5	0.686	0.715	0.762	0.806	0.927
6	0.713	0.743	0.788	0.826	0.927
7	0.730	0.760	0.803	0.838	0.928
8	0.749	0.778	0.818	0.851	0.932
9	0.764	0.791	0.829	0.859	0.935
10	0.781	0.806	0.842	0.869	0.938
11	0.792	0.817	0.850	0.876	0.940
12	0.805	0.828	0.859	0.883	0.943
13	0.814	0.837	0.866	0.889	0.945
14	0.825	0.846	0.874	0.895	0.947
15	0.835	0.855	0.881	0.901	0.950
16	0.844	0.863	0.887	0.906	0.952
17	0.851	0.869	0.892	0.910	0.954
18	0.858	0.874	0.897	0.914	0.956
19	0.863	0.879	0.901	0.917	0.957
20	0.868	0.884	0.905	0.920	0.959
21	0.873	0.888	0.908	0.923	0.960
22	0.878	0.892	0.911	0.926	0.961
23	0.881	0.895	0.914	0.928	0.962
24	0.884	0.898	0.916	0.930	0.963
25	0.888	0.901	0.918	0.931	0.964
26	0.891	0.904	0.920	0.933	0.965
27	0.894	0.906	0.923	0.935	0.965
28	0.896	0.908	0.924	0.936	0.966
29	0.898	0.910	0.926	0.937	0.966
30	0.900	0.912	0.927	0.939	0.967
31	0.902	0.914	0.929	0.940	0.967
32	0.904	0.915	0.930	0.941	0.968
33	0.906	0.917	0.931	0.942	0.968
34	0.908	0.919	0.933	0.943	0.969
35	0.910	0.920	0.934	0.944	0.969
36	0.912	0.922	0.935	0.945	0.970
37	0.914	0.924	0.936	0.946	0.970
38	0.916	0.925	0.938	0.947	0.971
39	0.917	0.927	0.939	0.948	0.971
40	0.919	0.928	0.940	0.949	0.972
41	0.920	0.929	0.941	0.950	0.972
42	0.922	0.930	0.942	0.951	0.972
43	0.923	0.932	0.943	0.951	0.973
44	0.924	0.933	0.944	0.952	0.973
45	0.926	0.934	0.945	0.953	0.973
46	0.927	0.935	0.945	0.953	0.974
47	0.928	0.936	0.946	0.954	0.974
48	0.929	0.937	0.947	0.954	0.974
49	0.929	0.937	0.947	0.955	0.974
50	0.930	0.938	0.947	0.955	0.974

The null hypothesis of a normal distribution is rejected at the α significance level if the calculated *W* is less than W_α.

Source: From Shapiro and Wilk, 1965.

Example: W-test of Normal Distribution of Sample Data

Perform a W-test to determine how well the following monitoring data fit a normal distribution: 1.3, 1.8, 1.2, 4.5, 2, 2.1, 5.5, 2.2, 3, 2.4, 2.5, 2.5, 3.5, 2.8, 2.9 (all units are mg/m^3).

Table V.5 — W-test of Normal Distribution of Sample Data

*Monitoring data**	*Ranked data**	*i = rank*	$x_{[n-i+1]}$	x_i	$x_{[n-i+1]} - x_i$	*a from Table V.3*	$a(x_{[n-i+1]} - x_i)$
1.3	1.2	1	5.5	1.2	4.3	0.5150	2.2145
1.8	1.3	2	4.5	1.3	3.2	0.3306	1.05792
1.2	1.8	3	3.5	1.8	1.7	0.2495	0.42415
4.5	2	4	3	2	1	0.1878	0.1878
2	2.1	5	2.9	2.1	0.8	0.1353	0.10824
2.1	2.2	6	2.8	2.2	0.6	0.0880	0.0528
5.5	2.4	7	2.5	2.4	0.1	0.0433	0.00433
2.2	2.5	8					sum = **4.04974**
3	2.5	9					
2.4	2.8	10					
2.5	2.9	11					
2.5	3	12					
3.5	3.5	13					
2.8	4.5	14					
2.9	5.5	15					

* Units are in mg/m^3

k = (15-1)/2 = 7

W = (4.04974)^2/(s^2 (n - 1))

W = (4.04974)^2/(1.14^2 (15 - 1))

W = 0.904

Compare to p = 0.05 value from Table V.4: 0.881

0.904 >0.881; therefore, do not reject the hypothesis that distribution is normal.

Example: W-test of Lognormal Distribution of Sample Data

Perform a W-test to determine how well the following monitoring data fit a lognormal distribution: 1.3, 1.8, 1.2, 4.5, 2, 2.1, 5.5, 2.2, 3, 2.4, 2.5, 2.5, 3.5, 2.5 (all units are mg/m^3).

Table V.6 — W-test of Lognormal Distribution of Sample Data

x_i = Monitoring data (mg/m^3)	Ranked data (mg/m^3)	y_i = ln of Ranked monitoring data	i = Rank	$y_{[n-i+1]}$	y_i	$y_{[n-i+1]} - y_i$	a from Table V.3	$a(y_{[n-i+1]} - y_i)$
1.3	1.2	0.182	1	1.70	0.182	1.52	0.5150	0.78405
1.8	1.3	0.262	2	1.50	0.262	1.238	0.3306	0.41051
1.2	1.8	0.588	3	1.25	0.588	0.662	0.2495	0.16591
4.5	2	0.693	4	1.10	0.693	0.407	0.1878	0.07615
2	2.1	0.742	5	1.06	0.742	0.318	0.1353	0.04367
2.1	2.2	0.788	6	1.03	0.788	0.242	0.0880	0.02122
5.5	2.4	0.875	7	0.916	0.875	0.041	0.0433	0.00177
2.2	2.5	0.916	8					sum = **1.503279**
3	2.5	0.916	9					
2.4	2.8	1.03	10					
2.5	2.9	1.06	11					
2.5	3	1.10	12					
3.5	3.5	1.25	13					
2.8	4.5	1.50	14					
2.9	5.5	1.70	15					

$k = (15 - 1)/2 = 7$

$W = (1.503279)^2/(s_y^2\ (n - 1))$

$W = (1.503279)^2/(0.407^2\ (15 - 1))$

$W = 0.974$

Compare to $p = 0.05$ value from Table V.4: 0.881

$0.974 > 0.881$; therefore, do not reject the hypothesis that distribution is lognormal.

References

1. **Gilbert, R.O.:** *Statistical Methods for Environmental Pollution Monitoring*. New York: Van Nostrand Reinhold, 1987.

Appendix VI

Examining the Arithmetic Mean: Mean Estimates and Confidence Intervals

Understanding the mean of the exposure profile may be important when judging exposures (as discussed in Chapters 3, 6, and 7). An example would be those instances when several short-term measurements are used to characterize a daily average, or when several day-long TWA measurements are being used to estimate the long-term average of a day-to-day exposure profile. Epidemi-ologists are often interested in the long-term arithmetic mean exposure as an indicator of long-term dose.

You may need to make a judgment for an agent that is principally a chronic toxin and for which you have found or developed an LTA–OEL. If so, the tools described in this appendix would help in estimating the exposure profile's arithmetic mean and in using confidence limits to quantify uncertainty in that arithmetic mean estimate. *Remember that the best predictor of dose is the exposure distribution's arithmetic mean, not the geometric mean.*

The general technique is to:

1. Estimate the exposure distribution's arithmetic mean.
2. Characterize the uncertainty in the arithmetic mean's point estimate by calculating confidence limits for the true mean.
3. Examine the arithmetic mean's point estimate and true mean confidence limit(s) in light of an LTA–OEL or other information to make a judgment on the exposure profile.

Note that if these techniques are applied to random short-term (e.g., grab) samples on one person within one shift, the results can be compared with the appropriate single-shift TWA (generally the 8-hour TWA).

To be conservatively protective of worker health, the upper confidence limit (UCL) for the arithmetic mean estimate is

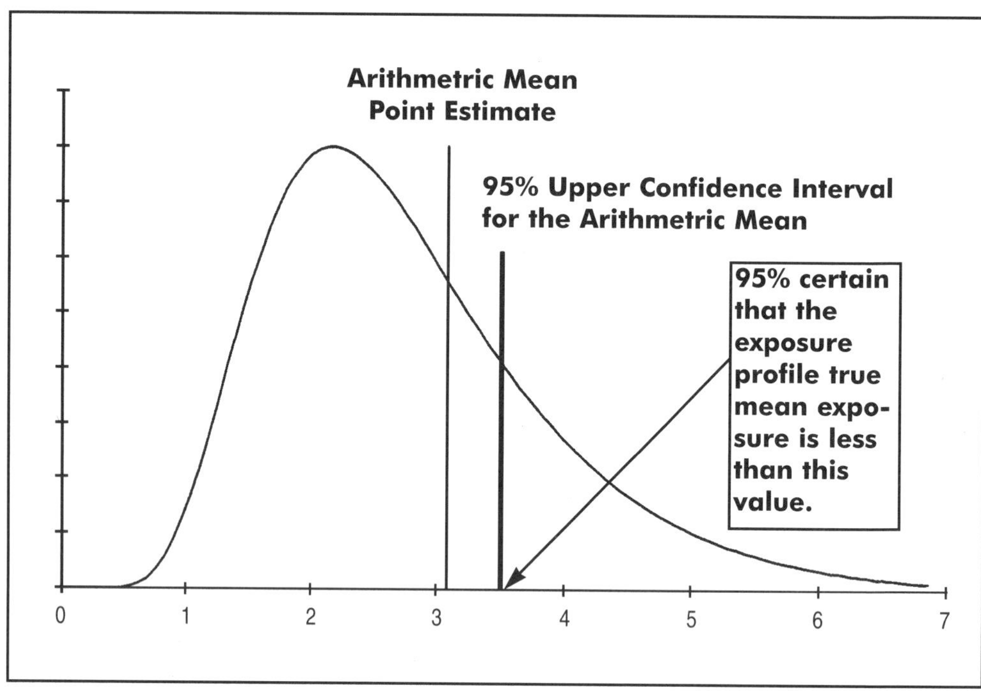

Figure VI.1 — 95% upper confidence interval for arithmetic mean.

emphasized in this text. The industrial hygienists can examine the UCL with some chosen degree of certainty that the true arithmetic mean is less-than or equal-to that UCL. For example, if the arithmetic mean's one-sided 95% upper confidence limit ($UCL_{1,95\%}$) is calculated and found to be below the LTA–OEL, the industrial hygienist would be at least 95% sure that the exposure profile's true mean was below the LTA–OEL.

For completeness, the text also provides formulas for calculating the lower confidence limit (LCL). In most instances, however, "spending" statistical power to characterize the LCL for the arithmetic mean estimate contributes little to the judgment on the exposure profile's acceptability. Most of the time, industrial hygienists want an answer to the question "How high could the true average exposure be?" rather than "How low could it be?"

It is common practice, of course, to calculate a two-sided confidence limit. This requires that statistical power be spent at both ends of the distribution so that the boundaries at each end are pushed further out to gain the same degree of confidence. If you were to combine the one-sided 95% UCL and the one-sided 95% LCL into a two-sided limit, you would be 90% sure the exposure profile's true mean was between the two values. Usually you are better off to decide which boundary (upper or lower) is most important to understand. You would then place all of the statistical power into characterizing the single boundary most important to the judgment.

Probability Plotting and Goodness-of-Fit

The statistical tools given here are parametric methods: they rely on an assumption about the shape of the underlying population distribution (e.g., whether it is lognormal or normal). As discussed in Chapter 7, before calculating any arithmetic mean estimates and confidence intervals using these parametric techniques, examine the monitoring data using the probability plotting and goodness-of-fit techniques discussed in Appendix V.

Empirical evidence is strong that most exposure distributions are right-skewed and can be reasonably approximated by the lognormal distribution. If the probability plotting and goodness-of-fit techniques verify a lognormal distribution, the tools for lognormal distributions should be used — even if the same data also seem to fit a normal distribution.

If the data do not seem to fit a lognormal distribution, but they do seem to fit a normal distribution, the tools for normally distributed data should be used. If the data do not seem to fit either the normal or lognormal distribution, neither of these parametric techniques should be used. Instead, you should examine the data carefully to determine whether the SEG has been properly defined or whether there has been some systematic change to the underlying exposure distribution while the monitoring data were being gathered. If no reason can be found for splitting the data so that it represents two or more SEG exposure profiles that fit either the lognormal or the normal distribution, you might have to limit yourself to using descriptive (Appendix IV) and nonparametric (Appendix VIII) statistics to aid your exposure judgment.

Characterizing the Arithmetic Mean of a Lognormal Distribution

If you believe the exposure distribution is reasonably approximated by a lognormal distribution, as is usually the case, there are several methods for estimating the arithmetic mean of the lognormal distribution and for calculating confidence limits. Several techniques are discussed in this appendix.

Easy to Calculate but Less Accurate

- *Sample Mean and t-Distribution Confidence Limits:* The simple mean of the sample is an unbiased estimator of the true mean of the lognormal distribution and has the advantage of being easy to calculate. However, it can be more variable than other estimates, particularly for larger sample sizes and larger distribution GSDs.[1,2] It is preferred over the maximum likelihood estimate (MLE; see below) for small sample sizes (less than 15–20 samples). When the sample size is large (n > 30) a simple t-distribution confidence interval can be calculated for the sample mean point estimate.[3]

- *Maximum Likelihood Estimate and Confidence Limits:* The MLE of the lognormal distribution arithmetic mean is easy to calculate and, for larger sample sizes, less variable than the sample mean. A confidence interval can be easily calculated for this point estimate. Generally, however, the confidence interval calculated using this method underestimates variability and will be too narrow (i.e., it will not be as wide as the exact interval).[4]

Accurate but More Difficult to Calculate

- *Minimum Variance Unbiased Estimate (MVUE) — Point Estimate Only:* The MVUE of the true arithmetic mean of a lognormal distribution is unbiased and has minimum variance. It is therefore always the preferred point estimate; however, it is difficult to compute without a computer or programmable calculator.
- *Land's "Exact" Confidence Limits — Confidence Limits Only:* Land's procedure is preferred because it calculates exact confidence limits for the true arithmetic mean of a lognormal distribution.[2,4] Recently, procedures have been developed that greatly simplify the use of this technique.[2] If a computer or programmable calculator is available, this method should always be used for calculating confidence limits.

Which To Use — Point Estimate of the True Mean of the Lognormal Distribution

If a computer or programmable calculator is available, the MVUE should be used as the preferred point estimate of the true mean of the lognormal distribution. If not, the sample mean should be used if the GSD is small (<2) or there are few samples (<15–20). The MLE should be used if there is no computer or programmable calculator available and the sample size is large (>15–20 measurements).

Which To Use — Confidence Limits for the True Mean of the Lognormal Distribution

Land's method should always be used for calculating exact confidence limits for the true mean if a programmable calculator or computer is available. If a computer is not available, calculate the confidence limits using the MLE method. Remember, however, that this will tend to underestimate the true upper confidence limit. Also, when many monitoring results are available (>30), the easy-to-calculate sample mean and t-distribution confidence interval may be chosen.

Specific Techniques

Sample Mean and t-Distribution Confidence Limit

Use the sample mean as a point estimate for the exposure distribution arithmetic mean when there is no computer or programmable calculator available and there are few samples (<15–20) and a small GSD (<2).

Developed for use with normal distributions, the simple t-distribution confidence interval procedure also works well for many non-normal distributions (including the lognormal distribution) when sample sizes are large. The usual rule-of-thumb is that this procedure works well when the sample size exceeds 30 or the underlying GSD is *known* to be less than about 1.5.

Whenever you have reason to believe the exposure distribution is better characterized by a normal distribution than a lognormal distribution, this sample mean and t-distribution method should be used instead of the other techniques described in this appendix.

The procedure is as follows:

Step 1: Calculate the sample mean (x) and sample standard deviation (s). [Note: These should have been calculated with descriptive statistics, as outlined in Appendix IV.]

Step 2: Calculate the confidence limits.

$$CL = x \pm t\,(s/\sqrt{n}) \qquad (1)$$

where:

The value of t can be looked up in a table such as Table VI.1.

TABLE VI.1 — Percentiles of the t-Distribution[A]

df	$t_{.60}$	$t_{.70}$	$t_{.80}$	$t_{.90}$	$t_{.95}$	$t_{.975}$	$t_{.95}$	$t_{.995}$
1	.325	.727	1.376	3.078	6.314	12.706	31.821	63.657
2	.289	.617	1.061	1.886	2.920	4.303	6.965	9.925
3	.277	.584	.978	1.638	2.353	3.182	4.541	5.841
4	.271	.569	.941	1.533	2.132	2.776	3.747	4.604
5	.267	.559	.920	1.476	2.015	2.571	3.365	4.032
6	.265	.553	.906	1.440	1.943	2.447	3.143	3.707
7	.263	.549	.896	1.415	1.895	2.365	2.998	3.499
8	.262	.546	.889	1.397	1.860	2.306	2.896	3.355
9	.261	.543	.883	1.383	1.833	2.262	2.821	3.250
10	.260	.542	.879	1.372	1.812	2.228	2.764	3.169
11	.260	.540	.876	1.363	1.796	2.201	2.718	3.106
12	.259	.539	.873	1.356	1.782	2.179	2.681	3.055
13	.259	.538	.870	1.350	1.771	2.160	2.650	3.012
14	.258	.537	.868	1.345	1.761	2.145	2.624	2.977
15	.258	.536	.866	1.341	1.753	2.131	2.602	2.947
16	.258	.535	.865	1.337	1.746	2.120	2.583	2.921
17	.257	.534	.863	1.333	1.740	2.110	2.567	2.898
18	.257	.534	.862	1.330	1.734	2.101	2.552	2.878
19	.257	.533	.861	1.328	1.729	2.093	2.539	2.861
20	.257	.533	.860	1.325	1.725	2.086	2.528	2.845
21	.257	.532	.859	1.323	1.721	2.080	2.518	2.831
22	.256	.532	.858	1.321	1.717	2.074	2.508	2.819
23	.256	.532	.858	1.319	1.714	2.069	2.500	2.807
24	.256	.531	.857	1.318	1.711	2.064	2.492	2.797
25	.256	.531	.856	1.316	1.708	2.060	2.485	2.787
26	.256	.531	.856	1.315	1.706	2.056	2.479	2.779
27	.256	.531	.855	1.314	1.703	2.052	2.473	2.771
28	.256	.530	.855	1.313	1.701	2.048	2.467	2.763
29	.256	.530	.854	1.311	1.699	2.045	2.462	2.756
30	.256	.530	.854	1.310	1.697	2.042	2.457	2.750
40	.255	.529	.851	1.303	1.684	2.021	2.423	2.704
60	.254	.527	.848	1.296	1.671	2.000	2.390	2.660
120	.254	.526	.845	1.289	1.658	1.980	2.358	2.617
∞	.253	.524	.842	1.282	1.645	1.960	2.326	2.576

[A]From **National Bureau of Standards:** Experimental Statistics. In *National Bureau of Standards Handbook 91*. Washington, D.C.: National Bureau of Standards, 1966.

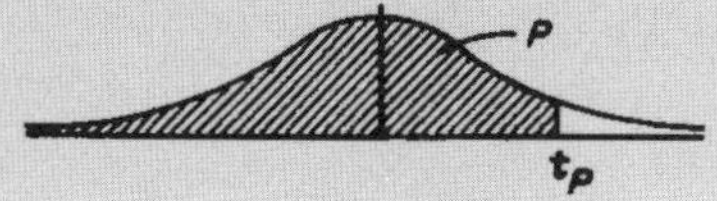

$$UCL_{1,95\%} = \bar{x} + t_{0.95}\,(s/\sqrt{n}) \quad (2)$$

$$LCL_{1,95\%} = \bar{x} - t_{0.95}\,(s/\sqrt{n}) \quad (3)$$

Step 3: Compare the UCL to the LTA–OEL.

Maximum Likelihood Estimate and Confidence Limits for the Arithmetic Mean of a Lognormal Distribution

The MLE of the arithmetic mean is not too difficult to calculate and is therefore useful when there is no programmable calculator or computer available. It may be a better point estimate than the sample mean when there are more than 15–20 samples or a high GSD.

Although easy to calculate, in many cases this technique is known to underestimate variability. Therefore the computed UCL should be interpreted cautiously because it will often be lower that the exact UCL. The technique is as follows:

Step 1: Calculate the mean ($\bar{y}$) and standard deviation (s_y) of the logtransformed data where y = ln(x). [Note: These should have been calculated with descriptive statistics (see Appendix IV).]

Step 2: Calculate the MLE.

$$MLE = \exp\left(\bar{y} + \frac{1}{2}\left(\frac{n-1}{n}\right)s_y^2\right) \quad (4)$$

Step 3: Calculate the UCL (and/or LCL) for the MLE.

$$CL = \exp\left(\ln MLE \pm t\,\frac{s_y\sqrt{n-1}}{n}\right) \quad (5)$$

Step 4: Compare the UCL to the LTA–OEL.

Minimum Variance Unbiased Estimate of the Arithmetic Mean of a Lognormal Distribution

The MVUE is the preferred point estimate of the arithmetic mean of a lognormal distribution. It should be used routinely unless there is no programmable calculator or computer available.

The MVUE is calculated iteratively. Calculation using five terms will give results correct to three significant figures for sample sizes from 5 to 500 and GSDs from 2 to 5.[1]

Step 1: Calculate the mean ($\bar{y}$) and standard deviation (s_y) of the logtransformed data where y = ln(x). [Note: These should have been calculated with descriptive statistics (see Appendix IV).]

Step 2: Calculate the MVUE.

MVUE =

$$\exp(\bar{y})\left[1+\frac{(n-1)}{n}l+\frac{(n-1)^3}{n^2(n+1)}\frac{l^2}{2!}+\frac{(n-1)^5}{n^3(n+1)(n+3)}\frac{l^3}{3!}\cdots\right] \quad (6)$$

where: $l = \frac{s_y^2}{2}$

Land's "Exact" Estimate of the Arithmetic Mean Confidence Limits for a Lognormal Distribution

Land's exact method provides the most accurate and least-biased estimate of the arithmetic mean confidence limits. This method is preferred and should be used whenever possible.

For purposes of the example in this text, a graphical technique developed by Hewett and Ganser should be used for interpolating one of the parameters needed for the calculation.[1] Hewett and Ganser also developed equations to approximate the curves in the graphs; these equations can be entered into a spreadsheet or programmable calculator. If one of these tools is available, that technique is preferred.

The technique for determining Land's exact confidence limits for the arithmetic mean is:

Step 1: Calculate the mean ($\bar{y}$) and standard deviation (s_y) of the logtransformed data where y = ln(x). [Note: These should have been calculated with descriptive statistics (see Appendix IV).]

Step 2: Obtain the C-factor for Land's formula (C(s_y, n, 0.05) for 95% LCL and C(s_y, n, 0.95) for 95% UCL). Land's C-factors can be obtained from Land's tables.[5] Land's tables almost always require interpolation between the tabular values of s_y. An alternative procedure is to read the appropriate C-factors from Figures VI.2 and VI.3.[2]

Step 3: Calculate the 95% UCL (or 95% LCL).

$$CL = \exp\left[\ln(\hat{u}) + C\frac{s_y}{\sqrt{n-1}}\right] \quad (7)$$

where: $\hat{u} = \exp(\bar{y} + \frac{1}{2} s_y^2)$

Step 4: Compare the 95% UCL to the LTA–OEL.

Example

Estimate the arithmetic mean and its 95% UCL for the day-to-day exposure distribution from which the following air monitoring data were obtained. For illustrative purposes, an LTA–OEL of 5 mg/m³ is assumed.

Table VI.2 — Example Air Monitoring Data

x_i monitoring data (mg/m³)	$(x_i - \bar{x})^2$	$y_i = \ln(x_i)$ Logtransformed data	$(y_i - \bar{y})^2$
1.3	1.904	0.262364	0.416725
1.8	0.774	0.587787	0.102477
1.2	2.190	0.182322	0.526473
4.5	3.312	1.504077	0.35542
2	0.462	0.693147	0.046122
2.1	0.336	0.741937	0.027546
5.5	7.952	1.704748	0.634957
2.2	0.230	0.788457	0.014268
3	0.102	1.098612	0.036369
2.4	0.078	0.875469	0.001052
2.5	0.032	0.916291	0.00007
2.5	0.032	0.916291	0.00007
3.5	0.672	1.252763	0.118926
2.8	0.014	1.029619	0.014814
2.9	0.048	1.064711	0.024588

Descriptive Statistics:

Number of samples:	15
Maximum (mg/m³):	5.5
Minimum (mg/m³):	1.2
Range:	4.3
Percent above OEL:	6.7
Mean (mg/m³):	2.7
Median (mg/m³):	2.5
Standard deviation (mg/m³):	1.14
Mean of ln(data):	0.91
SD of ln(data):	0.41
GM (mg/m³):	2.5
GSD:	1.5

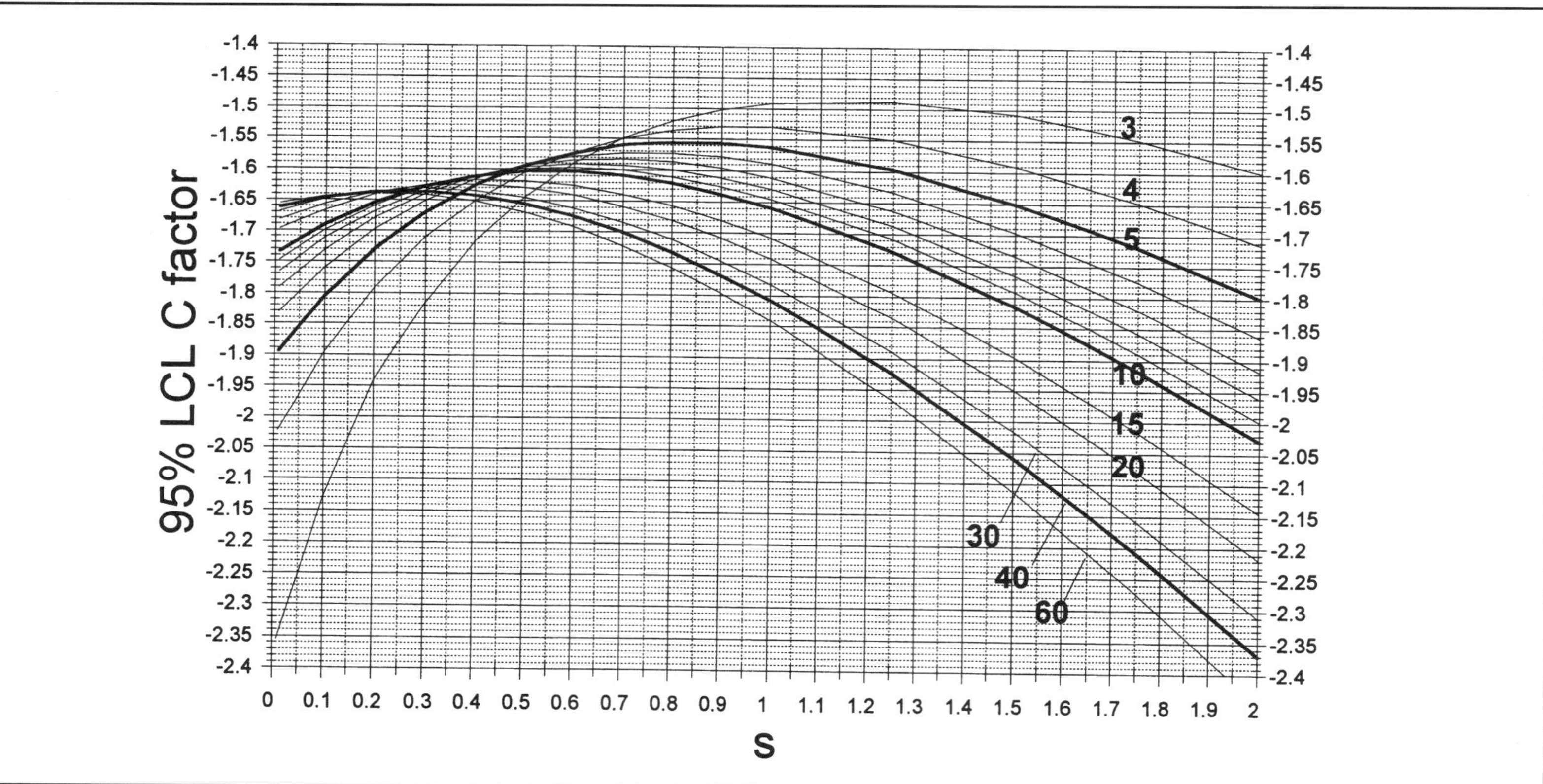

Figure VI.2 — Land's LCL C-factor, as a function of S and sample size. C(S; n, α) may be read from the y axis for each combination of S and sample size and used to calculate the 95% LCL for the sample mean of lognormally distributed data. [From **Hewett, P., and G.H. Ganser:** Simple Procedures for Calculating Confidence Intervals Around the Sample Mean and Exceedance Fraction Derived from Lognormally Distributed Data. *Appl. Occup. Environ. Hyg. 12(2)*:132-142 (1997). Reprinted with permission of the American Conference of Governmental Industrial Hygienists.]

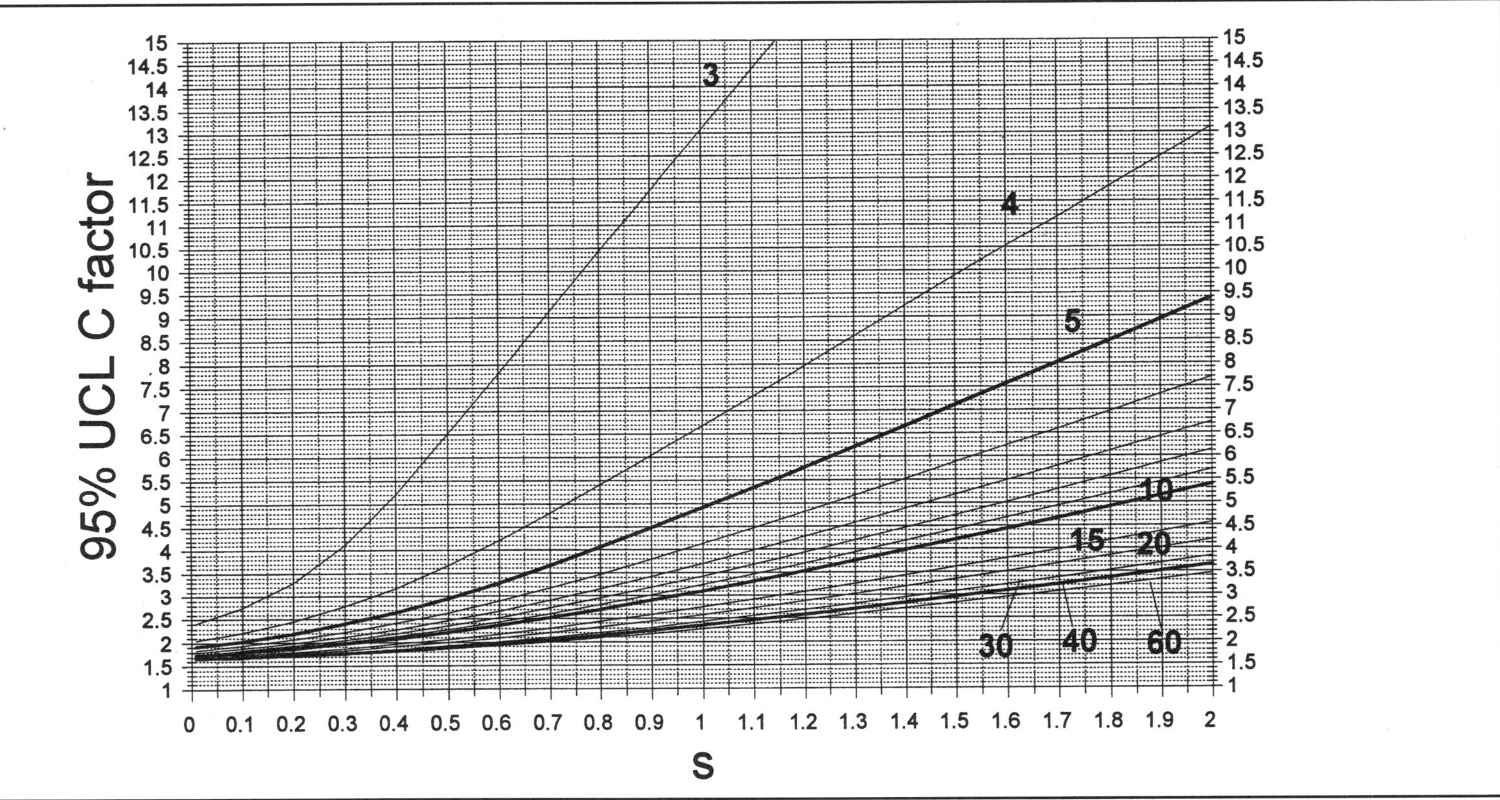

Figure VI.3 — Land's UCL C-factor, as a function of S and sample size. C(S; n, 1 – α) may be read from the y axis for each combination of S and sample size and used to calculate the 95% UCL for the sample mean of lognormally distributed data. [From **Hewett, P., and G.H. Ganser:** Simple Procedures for Calculating Confidence Intervals Around the Sample Mean and Exceedance Fraction Derived from Lognormally Distributed Data. *Appl. Occup. Environ. Hyg. 12(2)*:132-142 (1997). Reprinted with permission of the American Conference of Governmental Industrial Hygienists.]

Arithmetic Mean Estimates and $UCL_{1,95\%}$

Sample Mean and t-Distribution Confidence Limit

$\bar{x} = 2.7$ mg/m^3 (mean of the sample data calculated as part of descriptive statistics)

$$UCL_{1,95\%} = \bar{x} + t_{0.95}\,(s/\sqrt{n})$$

$t_{0.95} = 1.761$ (see Table VI.1, d.f. = n - 1 = 15 - 1 = 14)

$$UCL_{1,95\%} = 2.7 + 1.761\,(1.14/\sqrt{15})$$

$$UCL_{1,95\%} = 3.2 \text{ mg/m}^3$$

MLE Estimate

$$MLE = \exp\left(\bar{y} + \frac{1}{2}\left(\frac{n-1}{n}\right)s_y^2\right)$$

$$MLE = \exp\left(0.91 + \frac{1}{2}\left(\frac{15-1}{15}\right)0.41^2\right)$$

$= 2.7$ mg/m^3

MLE Upper Confidence Limit

$$UCL_{1,95\%} = \exp\left(\ln MLE + t_{0.95}\frac{s_y\sqrt{n-1}}{n}\right)$$

$$UCL_{1,95\%} = \exp\left(\ln 2.7 + 1.761\frac{0.41\sqrt{15-1}}{15}\right)$$

$= 3.2$ mg/m^3

MVUE Point Estimate of the Lognormal Distribution Arithmetic Mean

MVUE =

$$\exp(\bar{y})\left[1 + \frac{(n-1)}{n}l + \frac{(n-1)^3}{n^2(n+1)}\frac{l^2}{2!} + \frac{(n-1)^5}{n^3(n+1)(n+3)}\frac{l^3}{3!} \cdots\right]$$

where $l = \frac{s_y^2}{2}$ $\quad l = \frac{0.41^2}{2}$ $\quad l = 0.084$

Computed to five terms:

$$\text{MVUE} = \exp(\bar{y})\left[1+\frac{(n-1)}{n}l+\frac{(n-1)^3}{n^2(n+1)}\frac{l^2}{2!}+\frac{(n-1)^5}{n^3(n+1)(n+3)}\frac{l^3}{3!}+\frac{(n-1)^7}{n^4(n+1)(n+3)(n+5)}\frac{l^4}{4!}+\frac{(n-1)^9}{n^5(n+1)(n+3)(n+5)(n+7)}\frac{l^5}{5!}\right]$$

$$\text{MVUE} = \exp(0.91)\left[1+\frac{(15-1)}{15}0.084+\frac{(15-1)^3}{15^2(15+1)}\frac{0.084^2}{2!}+\frac{(15-1)^5}{15^3(15+1)(15+3)}\frac{0.084^3}{3!}+\frac{(15-1)^7}{15^4(15+1)(15+3)(15+5)}\frac{0.084^4}{4!}+\frac{(15-1)^9}{15^5(15+1)(15+3)(15+5)(15+7)}\frac{0.084^5}{5!}\right]$$

$\text{MVUE} =$
$\exp(0.91)[1 + 0.0784 + 0.00268912 + 0.00005466 + 0.00000075 + 0.00000001]$

$\text{MVUE} = 2.68 \text{ mg/m}^3$

Land's Exact Upper Confidence Limit:

$$\text{UCL}_{1,95\%} = \exp\left(\ln(\hat{u}) + C\frac{s_y}{\sqrt{n-1}}\right)$$

where:

$\hat{u} = \exp(\bar{y} + \frac{1}{2} s_y^2)$

$\hat{u} = \exp(0.91 + \frac{1}{2} 0.41^2)$

$= 2.7 \text{ mg/m}^3$

Determine $C(s_y, n, 0.95)$ from the graphs in Figure VI.3.

$C(0.41, 15, 0.95) \cong 1.9$

$$\text{UCL}_{1,95\%} = \exp\left(\ln(2.7) + 1.9\frac{0.41}{\sqrt{15-1}}\right)$$

$= 3.3 \text{ mg/m}^3$

In this example, all three methods for estimating the arithmetic mean achieved nearly the same result (2.7 mg/m^3). Still, our best point estimate of the arithmetic mean generally is the MVUE.

In this example, the $UCL_{1,95\%}$ calculated by the sample mean t-distribution, the MLE, and Land's exact methods are fairly close. Generally, however, the MLE method will underestimate the exact UCL, and the sample t-distribution method should be reserved for sample sizes greater than 30. Land's method, therefore, is preferred.

Land's exact 95% UCL of 3.3 mg/m^3 means we can be 95% confident that the true arithmetic mean exposure for the exposure profile is less than 3.3 mg/m^3. Because that is less than the 5 mg/m^3 LTA–OEL, we are at least 95% confident the arithmetic mean exposure is below the LTA–OEL.

References

1. **Attfield, M.D., and P. Hewett:** Exact Expressions for the Bias and Variance of Estimators of the Mean of a Lognormal Distribution. *Am. Ind. Hyg. Assoc. J. 53(7):*432- 435 (1992).
2. **Hewett, P., and G.H. Ganser:** Simple Procedures for Calculating Confidence Intervals Around the Sample Mean and Exceedance Fraction Derived from Lognormally Distributed Data. *Appl. Occup. Environ. Hyg. 12(2):*132-142 (1997).
3. **Hawkins, N.C., S.K. Norwood, and J.C. Rock:** *A Strategy for Occupational Exposure Assessment.* Akron, Ohio: American Industrial Hygiene Association, 1991.
4. **Armstrong, B.G.:** Confidence Intervals for Arithmetic Means of Lognormally Distributed Exposures. *Am. Ind. Hyg. Assoc. J. 53(8):*481-485 (1992).
5. **Land, C.E.:** Standard Confidence Limits for Linear Functions of the Normal Mean and Variance. *J. Am. Statist. Assoc. 68:*344 (1993).

Appendix VII

Examining the Upper Tail of an Exposure Profile: Tolerance Limits and Exceedance Tests

Understanding the upper tail of an exposure profile is important when the industrial hygienist must 1) characterize the health risk associated with exposure to an acute toxin; or 2) demonstrate compliance with OELs that are set (or interpreted) as upper limits to a daily TWA exposure.

These situations (and others) demand an understanding of the rightmost tip of the exposure distribution. In this appendix, we present parametric tools that can be used to characterize the upper tail of the exposure profile to aid in a judgment about the exposure acceptability. Nonparametric tolerance limit tools, for examining data that do not fit a distribution, are explained in Appendix VIII.

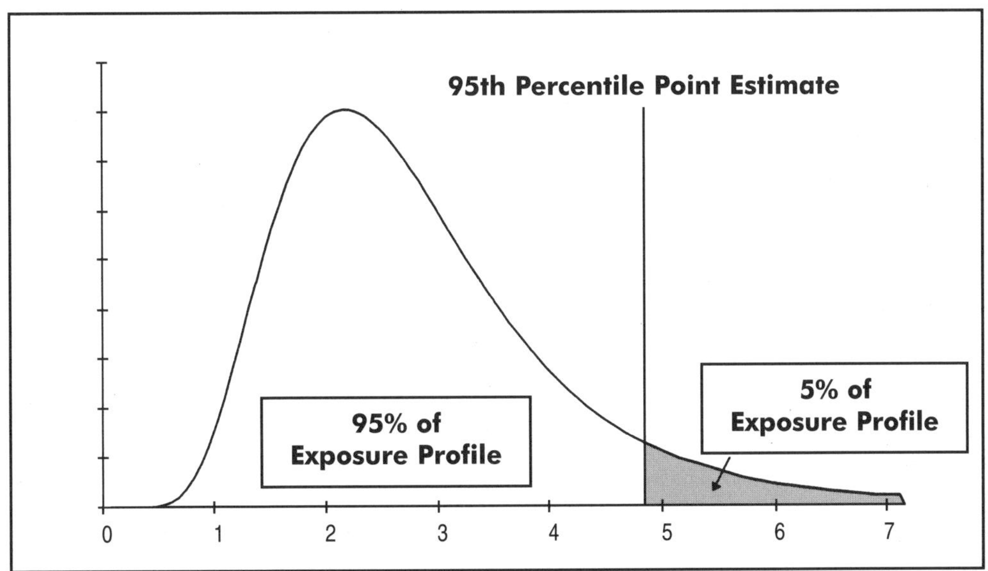

Figure VII.1 — 95% percentile.

Percentiles and Upper Tolerance Limits

The first set of tools is the point estimate of an upper percentile in the exposure distribution and its upper confidence limit — or, as it is more commonly called, the distribution's upper tolerance limit (UTL).

Using this technique, the industrial hygienist picks an upper percentile as the minimum proportion of the exposure distribution that must fall below the OEL for the exposure profile to be considered acceptable. That upper percentile can then be estimated and compared with the OEL.

The uncertainty in the percentile point estimate can be characterized by calculating the UTL for the distribution. One can then state with known confidence that the UTL is greater than a known proportion of the distribution.

One problem with tolerance limits is the low power available with small sample sizes. This results in very large confidence limits around the percentile estimate (the tolerance limits differ considerably from the percentile) when the number of samples is small. This is illustrated in Table VII.1, which shows the sample sizes needed to be 95% confident that the 95th percentile is less than the OEL.

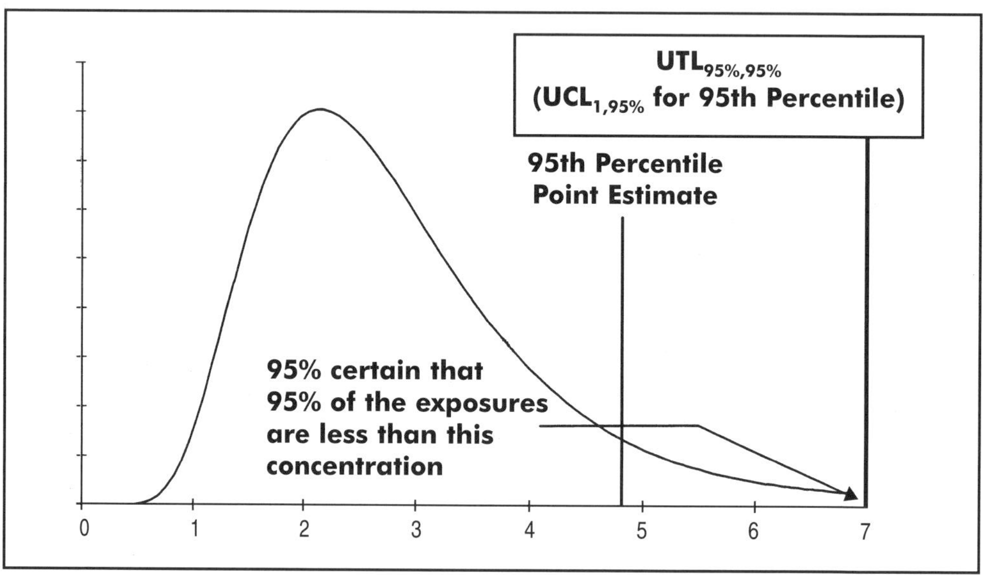

Figure VII.2 — Upper tolerance limit.

Table VII.1 — Sample Size Needed for Using $UTL_{95\%,95\%}$ to Show 95% Confidence that the 95th Percentile is below the OEL (Power = 0.80)

	Sample size (n)				
True 95th percentile/OEL	*GSD = 2.03*	*GSD = 2.72*	*GSD = 3.4*	*GSD = 4.11*	*GSD = 4.86*
0.67	58	107	154	202	249
0.5	24	42	59	76	93
0.4	16	27	37	47	57
0.33	13	20	28	35	42

Adapted from **Lyles, R.H., and L.L. Kupper:** On Strategies for Comparing Occupational Exposure Data to Limits. *Am. Ind. Hyg. Assoc. J. 57(1)*:6-15 (1996).

Exceedance Fraction

The second set of useful statistical tools determines the proportion of the exposure profile that exceeds a given value, such as an OEL. This is called the exceedance fraction.

A point estimate of the OEL exceedance fraction is calculated. The uncertainty in the exceedance fraction is then characterized by calculating a confidence limit for the point estimate. Using this technique the industrial hygienist is able to determine, with known confidence, the percentage of exposures in the exposure profile that exceeds the OEL.

Probability Plots and Goodness-of-Fit

The techniques presented in this appendix are parametric statistical tools. They require the industrial hygienist to know the shape of the exposure distribution, whether lognormal or normal. Before using these tools to estimate parameters of the exposure distribution, it is important that the distribution shape assumption be verified using the techniques outlined in Appendix V.

One way to get an initial characterization of the upper tail of an exposure distribution is to pick point estimates directly off the "eyeballed" best-fit line through the plotted data on a probability plot. Both upper percentiles and the percent of a distribution above or below an OEL can be estimated in this manner (see Appendix V for more detail).

Percentile Estimates

Upper percentiles for a lognormal distribution can be estimated as follows:

Step 1: Calculate the mean ($\bar{y}$) and standard deviation (s_y) of the logtransformed data where $y = \ln(x)$. [Note: These should have been calculated with descriptive statistics, as outlined in Appendix IV).]

Step 2: Percentile = $\exp(\bar{y} + Z\ s_y)$ (1)

where:

Z = standard normal variable for the proportion of interest (see Table VII.2).

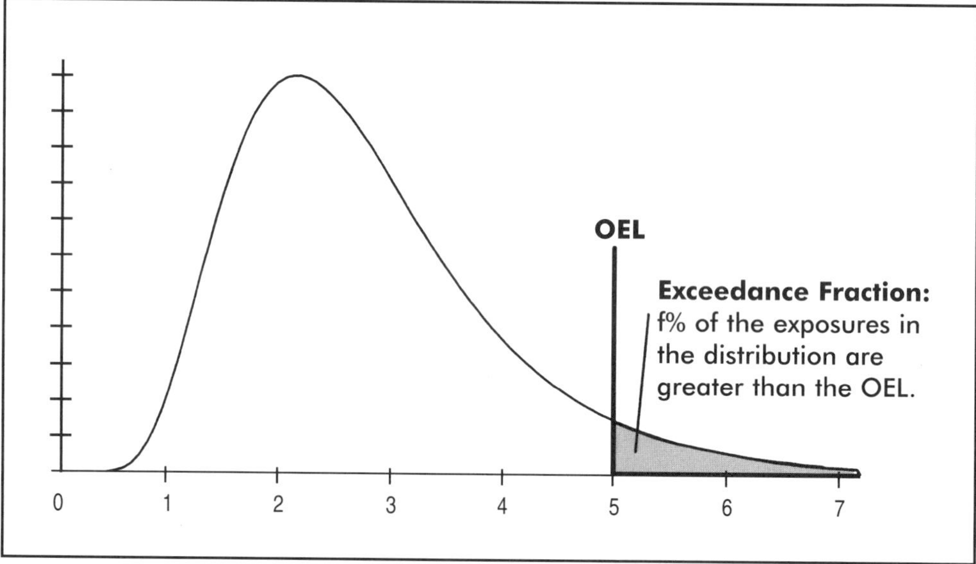

Figure VII.3 — Exceedance fraction.

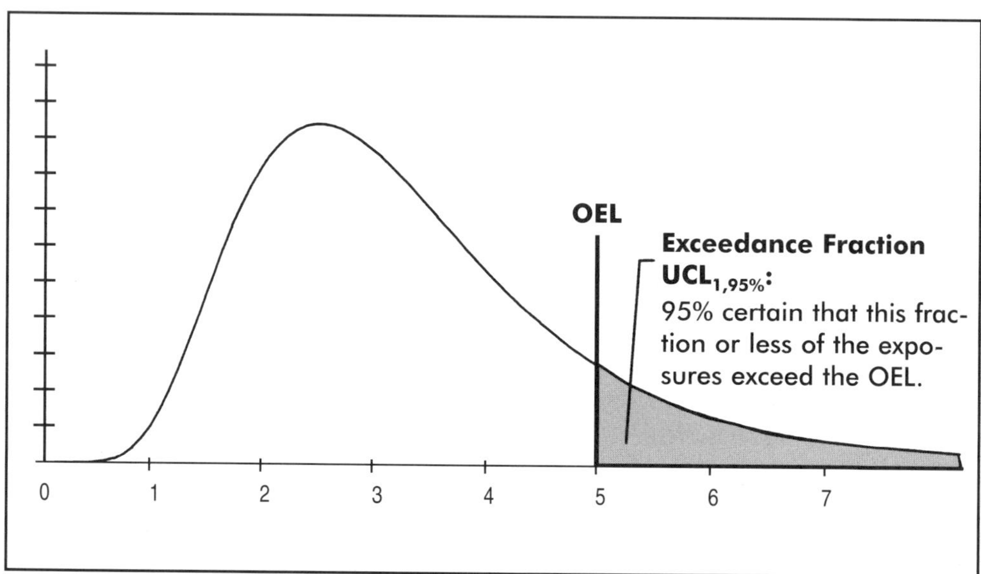

Figure VII.4 — Exceedance fraction upper confidence level.

TABLE VII.2 — Cumulative Normal Distribution — Values of P[A]

z_p	.00	.01	.02	.03	.04	.05	.06	.07	.08	.09
.0	.5000	.5040	.5080	.5120	.5160	.5199	.5239	.5279	.5319	.5359
.1	.5398	.5438	.5478	.5517	.5557	.5596	.5636	.5675	.5714	.5753
.2	.5793	.5832	.5871	.5910	.5948	.5987	.6026	.6064	.6103	.6141
.3	.6179	.6217	.6255	.6293	.6331	.6368	.6406	.6443	.6480	.6517
.4	.6554	.6591	.6628	.6664	.6700	.6736	.6772	.6808	.6844	.6879
.5	.6915	.6950	.6985	.7019	.7054	.7088	.7123	.7157	.7190	.7224
.6	.7257	.7291	.7324	.7357	.7389	.7422	.7454	.7486	.7517	.7549
.7	.7580	.7611	.7642	.7673	.7704	.7734	.7764	.7794	.7823	.7852
.8	.7881	.7910	.7939	.7967	.7995	.8023	.8051	.8078	.8106	.8133
.9	.8159	.8186	.8212	.8238	.8264	.8289	.8315	.8340	.8365	.8389
1.0	.8413	.8438	.8461	.8485	.8508	.8531	.8554	.8577	.8599	.8621
1.1	.8643	.8665	.8686	.8708	.8729	.8749	.8770	.8790	.8810	.8830
1.2	.8849	.8869	.8888	.8907	.8925	.8944	.8962	.8980	.8997	.9015
1.3	.9032	.9049	.9066	.9082	.9099	.9115	.9131	.9147	.9162	.9177
1.4	.9192	.9207	.9222	.9236	.9251	.9265	.9279	.9292	.9306	.9319
1.5	.9332	.9345	.9357	.9370	.9382	.9394	.9406	.9418	.9429	.9441
1.6	.9452	.9463	.9474	.9484	.9495	.9505	.9515	.9525	.9535	.9545
1.7	.9554	.9564	.9573	.9582	.9591	.9599	.9608	.9616	.9625	.9633
1.8	.9641	.9649	.9656	.9664	.9671	.9678	.9686	.9693	.9699	.9706
1.9	.9713	.9719	.9726	.9732	.9738	.9744	.9750	.9756	.9761	.9767
2.0	.9772	.9778	.9783	.9788	.9793	.9798	.9803	.9808	.9812	.9817
2.1	.9821	.9826	.9830	.9834	.9838	.9842	.9846	.9850	.9854	.9857
2.2	.9861	.9864	.9868	.9871	.9875	.9878	.9881	.9884	.9887	.9890
2.3	.9893	.9896	.9898	.9901	.9904	.9906	.9909	.9911	.9913	.9916
2.4	.9918	.9920	.9922	.9925	.9927	.9929	.9931	.9932	.9934	.9936
2.5	.9938	.9940	.9941	.9943	.9945	.9946	.9948	.9949	.9951	.9952
2.6	.9953	.9955	.9956	.9957	.9959	.9960	.9961	.9962	.9963	.9964
2.7	.9965	.9966	.9967	.9968	.9969	.9970	.9971	.9972	.9973	.9974
2.8	.9974	.9975	.9976	.9977	.9977	.9978	.9979	.9979	.9980	.9981
2.9	.9981	.9982	.9982	.9983	.9984	.9984	.9985	.9985	.9986	.9986
3.0	.9987	.9987	.9987	.9988	.9988	.9989	.9989	.9989	.9990	.9990
3.1	.9990	.9991	.9991	.9991	.9992	.9992	.9992	.9992	.9993	.9993
3.2	.9993	.9993	.9994	.9994	.9994	.9994	.9994	.9995	.9995	.9995
3.3	.9995	.9995	.9995	.9996	.9996	.9996	.9996	.9996	.9996	.9997
3.4	.9997	.9997	.9997	.9997	.9997	.9997	.9997	.9997	.9997	.9998

[A]Values of P corresponding to z_p for the normal curve. z is the standard normal variable. The value of P for $-z_p$ equals one minus the value of P for $+z_p$, e.g., the P for −1.62 equals 1 − .9474 = .0526.

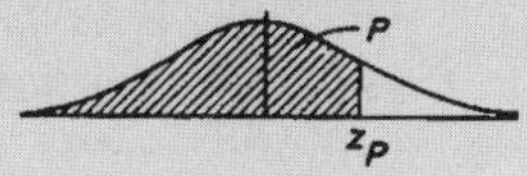

Upper percentiles for a normal distribution can be estimated in a similar fashion:

Step 1: Calculate the mean ($\bar{x}$) and standard deviation (s) of the monitoring data.

Step 2: Percentile = $\bar{x} + Z\ s$ (2)

Upper Tolerance Limits

Upper tolerance limits are simply upper confidence limits calculated for distribution percentiles. An upper percentile (typically the 95th percentile) of the exposure distribution is chosen and the uncertainty in that percentile estimate is quantified by calculating a confidence limit (typically the 95% UCL).

The $UTL_{95\%,95\%}$ is the 95% UCL for the distribution's 95th percentile: for an exposure profile, it is the exposure level that we are 95% sure is greater than 95% of the exposures in the distribution. If the OEL is greater than the $UTL_{95\%,95\%}$ we are at least 95% sure that 95% of the exposures are less than the OEL.

The UTL for a lognormal distribution is calculated as follows:

Step 1: Calculate the mean ($\bar{y}$) and standard deviation (s_y) of the logtransformed data where y = ln(x). [Note: These should have been calculated with descriptive statistics (see Appendix IV).]

Step 2: UTL = $\exp(\bar{y} + K\ s_y)$ (3)

where:

K = factor for tolerance limits determined from Table VII.3 as a function of the probability (confidence, γ), proportion (percentile, P), and number of samples (n).

The UTL for a normal distribution is calculated as follows:

Step 1: Calculate the mean ($\bar{x}$) and standard deviation (s) of the monitoring data.

Step 2: UTL = $\bar{x} + K\ s$ (4)

TABLE VII.3 — Factors for One-Sided Tolerance Limits for Normal Distributions[A,B]

	γ = 0.75					γ = 0.90				
n \ P	0.75	0.90	0.95	0.99	0.999	0.75	0.90	0.95	0.99	0.999
3	1.464	2.501	3.152	4.396	5.805	2.602	4.258	5.310	7.340	9.651
4	1.256	2.134	2.680	3.726	4.910	1.972	3.187	3.957	5.437	7.128
5	1.152	1.961	2.463	3.421	4.507	1.698	2.742	3.400	4.666	6.112
6	1.087	1.860	2.336	3.243	4.273	1.540	2.494	3.091	4.242	5.556
7	1.043	1.791	2.250	3.126	4.118	1.435	2.333	2.894	3.972	5.201
8	1.010	1.740	2.190	3.042	4.008	1.360	2.219	2.755	3.783	4.955
9	0.984	1.702	2.141	2.977	3.924	1.302	2.133	2.649	3.641	4.772
10	0.964	1.671	2.103	2.927	3.858	1.257	2.065	2.568	3.532	4.629
11	0.947	1.646	2.073	2.885	3.804	1.219	2.012	2.503	3.444	4.515
12	0.933	1.624	2.048	2.851	3.760	1.188	1.966	2.448	3.371	4.420
13	0.919	1.606	2.026	2.822	3.722	1.162	1.928	2.403	3.310	4.341
14	0.909	1.591	2.007	2.796	3.690	1.139	1.895	2.363	3.257	4.274
15	0.899	1.577	1.991	2.776	3.661	1.119	1.866	2.329	3.212	4.215
16	0.891	1.566	1.977	2.756	3.637	1.101	1.842	2.299	3.172	4.164
17	0.883	1.554	1.964	2.739	3.615	1.085	1.820	2.272	3.136	4.118
18	0.876	1.544	1.951	2.723	3.595	1.071	1.800	2.249	3.106	4.078
19	0.870	1.536	1.942	2.710	3.577	1.058	1.781	2.228	3.078	4.041
20	0.865	1.528	1.933	2.697	3.561	1.046	1.765	2.208	3.052	4.009
21	0.859	1.520	1.923	2.686	3.545	1.035	1.750	2.190	3.028	3.979
22	0.854	1.514	1.916	2.675	3.532	1.025	1.736	2.174	3.007	3.952
23	0.849	1.508	1.907	2.665	3.520	1.016	1.724	2.159	2.987	3.927
24	0.845	1.502	1.901	2.656	3.509	1.007	1.712	2.145	2.969	3.904
25	0.842	1.496	1.895	2.647	3.497	0.999	1.702	2.132	2.952	3.882
30	0.825	1.475	1.869	2.613	3.454	0.966	1.657	2.080	2.884	3.794
35	0.812	1.458	1.849	2.588	3.421	0.942	1.623	2.041	2.833	3.730
40	0.803	1.445	1.834	2.568	3.395	0.923	1.598	2.010	2.793	3.679
45	0.795	1.435	1.821	2.552	3.375	0.908	1.577	1.986	2.762	3.638
50	0.788	1.426	1.811	2.538	3.358	0.894	1.560	1.965	2.735	3.604

[A]From **National Bureau of Standards:** Experimental Statistics. In *National Bureau of Standards Handbook 91*. Washington, D.C.: National Bureau of Standards, 1966.

[B]Factors K such that the probability is γ that at least a proportion P of the distribution will be less than $\bar{X} + Ks$ (or greater than $\bar{X} - Ks$), where $\bar{X}$ and s are estimates of the mean and the standard deviation computed from a sample size of n.

TABLE VII.3 — Factors for One-Sided Tolerance Limits for Normal Distributions (continued)

	γ = 0.95					γ = 0.99				
n \ P	0.75	0.90	0.95	0.99	0.999	0.75	0.90	0.95	0.99	0.999
3	3.804	6.158	7.655	10.552	13.857	—	—	—	—	—
4	2.619	4.163	5.145	7.042	9.215	—	—	—	—	—
5	2.149	3.407	4.202	5.741	7.501	—	—	—	—	—
6	1.895	3.006	3.707	5.062	6.612	2.849	4.408	5.409	7.334	9.550*
7	1.732	2.755	3.399	4.641	6.061	2.490	3.856	4.730	6.411	8.348
8	1.617	2.582	3.188	4.353	5.686	2.252	3.496	4.287	5.811	7.566
9	1.532	2.454	3.031	4.143	5.414	2.085	3.242	3.971	5.389	7.014
10	1.465	2.355	2.911	3.981	5.203	1.954	3.048	3.739	5.075	6.603
11	1.411	2.275	2.815	3.852	5.036	1.854	2.897	3.557	4.828	6.284
12	1.366	2.210	2.736	3.747	4.900	1.771	2.773	3.410	4.633	6.032
13	1.329	2.155	2.670	3.659	4.787	1.702	2.677	3.290	4.472	5.826
14	1.296	2.108	2.614	3.585	4.690	1.645	2.592	3.189	4.336	5.651
15	1.268	2.068	2.566	3.520	4.607	1.596	2.521	3.102	4.224	5.507
16	1.242	2.032	2.523	3.463	4.534	1.553	2.458	3.028	4.124	5.374
17	1.220	2.001	2.486	3.415	4.471	1.514	2.405	2.962	4.038	5.268
18	1.200	1.974	2.453	3.370	4.415	1.481	2.357	2.906	3.961	5.167
19	1.183	1.949	2.423	3.331	4.364	1.450	2.315	2.855	3.893	5.078
20	1.167	1.926	2.396	3.295	4.319	1.424	2.275	2.807	3.832	5.003
21	1.152	1.905	2.371	3.262	4.276	1.397	2.241	2.768	3.776	4.932
22	1.138	1.887	2.350	3.233	4.238	1.376	2.208	2.729	3.727	4.866
23	1.126	1.869	2.329	3.206	4.204	1.355	2.179	2.693	3.680	4.806
24	1.114	1.853	2.309	3.181	4.171	1.336	2.154	2.663	3.638	4.755
25	1.103	1.838	2.292	3.158	4.143	1.319	2.129	2.632	3.601	4.706
30	1.059	1.778	2.220	3.064	4.022	1.249	2.029	2.516	3.446	4.508
35	1.025	1.732	2.166	2.994	3.934	1.195	1.957	2.431	3.334	4.364
40	0.999	1.697	2.126	2.941	3.866	1.154	1.902	2.365	3.250	4.255
45	0.978	1.669	2.092	2.897	3.811	1.122	1.857	2.313	3.181	4.168
50	0.961	1.646	2.065	2.863	3.766	1.096	1.821	2.269*	3.124	4.096

Exceedance Fractions

An exceedance fraction is an estimate of the proportion of the exposure distribution that is greater than some exposure level, such as an OEL. The uncertainty in the exceedance fraction point estimate (f) is characterized by calculating a confidence interval.

Exceedance Fraction Point Estimate

The equation for the exceedance fraction for a lognormal distribution has an odd format:

$$f = P(c > OEL) = P\left(Z > \frac{\ln OEL - \bar{y}}{s_y}\right) \qquad (5)$$

If this were stated in words, it would read: "The exceedance fraction equals the probability (P) that a concentration (c) in the exposure profile is greater than the OEL. This equals the probability that a Z-value (Z) from the distribution exceeds the calculated Z-value corresponding to the position of the OEL in the distribution [$(\ln \text{OEL} - \bar{y})/s_y$]."

Equation (5) is used in three steps:

Step 1: Calculate the Z-value corresponding to the position of the OEL in the exposure distribution:

$$Z_{OEL} = \frac{\ln OEL - \bar{y}}{s_y} \qquad (6)$$

Step 2: Look up the proportion of a normal distribution corresponding to Z_{OEL} in a Z-Table (see Table VII.2)

P = proportion of normal distribution corresponding to Z_{OEL} (7)

Step 3: Subtract the proportion from 1 to determine the exceedance fraction:

$$f = 1 - P \qquad (8)$$

Confidence Intervals for the Exceedance Fraction

The following procedure calculates the one-sided 95% confidence limits for the exceedance fraction.[2] Together, the upper and lower confidence limits form a two-sided 90% confidence interval. The procedure consists of two steps:

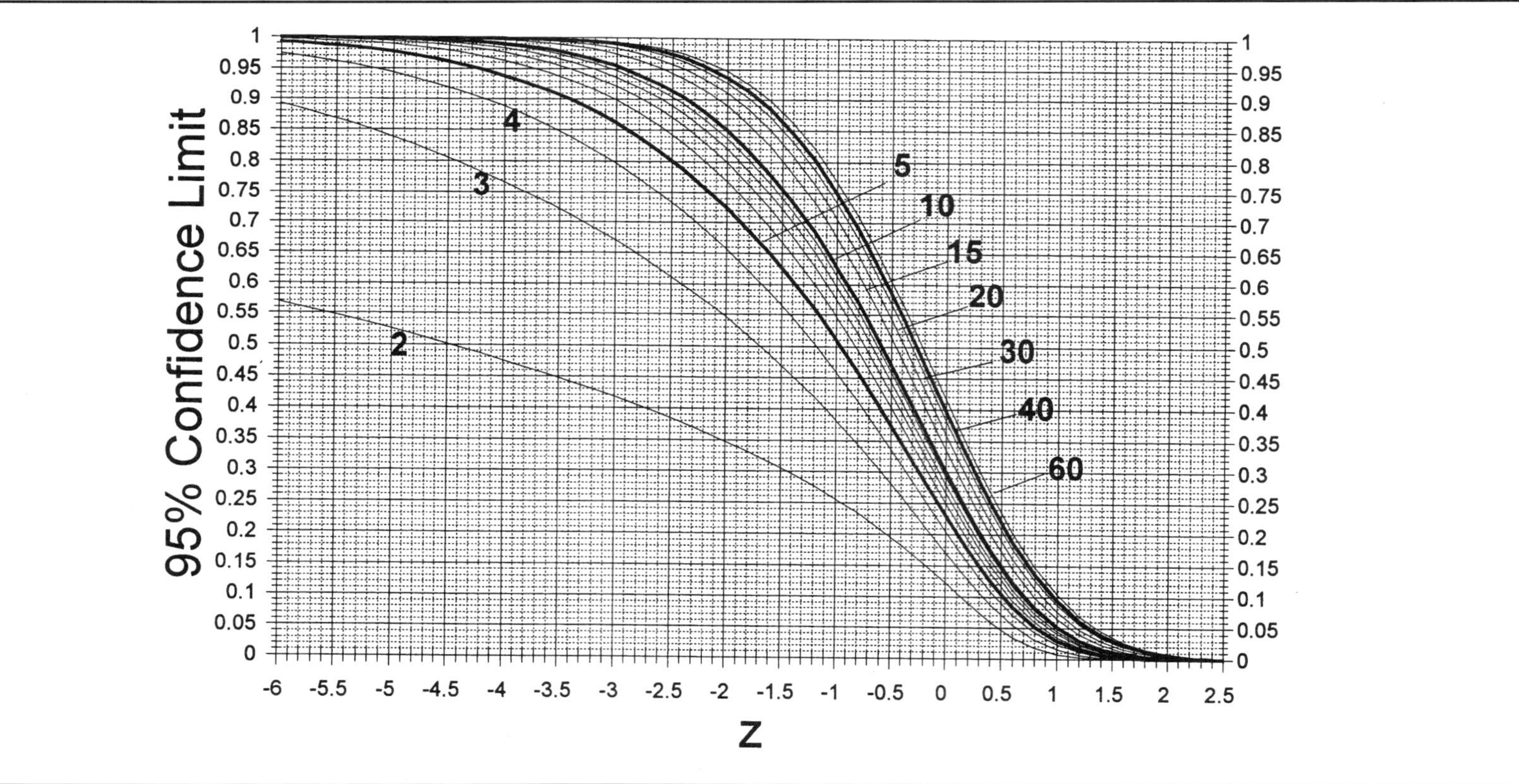

Figure VII.5 — Confidence limit for the exceedance fraction (f) vs. the calculated z-value. Using z and the sample size, read the 95th percentile LCL from the y axis. Using negative z and the sample size, read the corresponding y axis value. The 95th percentile UCL is the complement of this value (complement = 1 – value). [From **Hewett, P., and G.H. Ganser:** Simple Procedures for Calculating Confidence Intervals Around the Sample Mean and Exceedance Fraction Derived from Lognormally Distributed Data. *Appl. Occup. Environ. Hyg. 12(2)*:132-142 (1997). Reprinted with permission of the American Conference of Governmental Industrial Hygienists.]

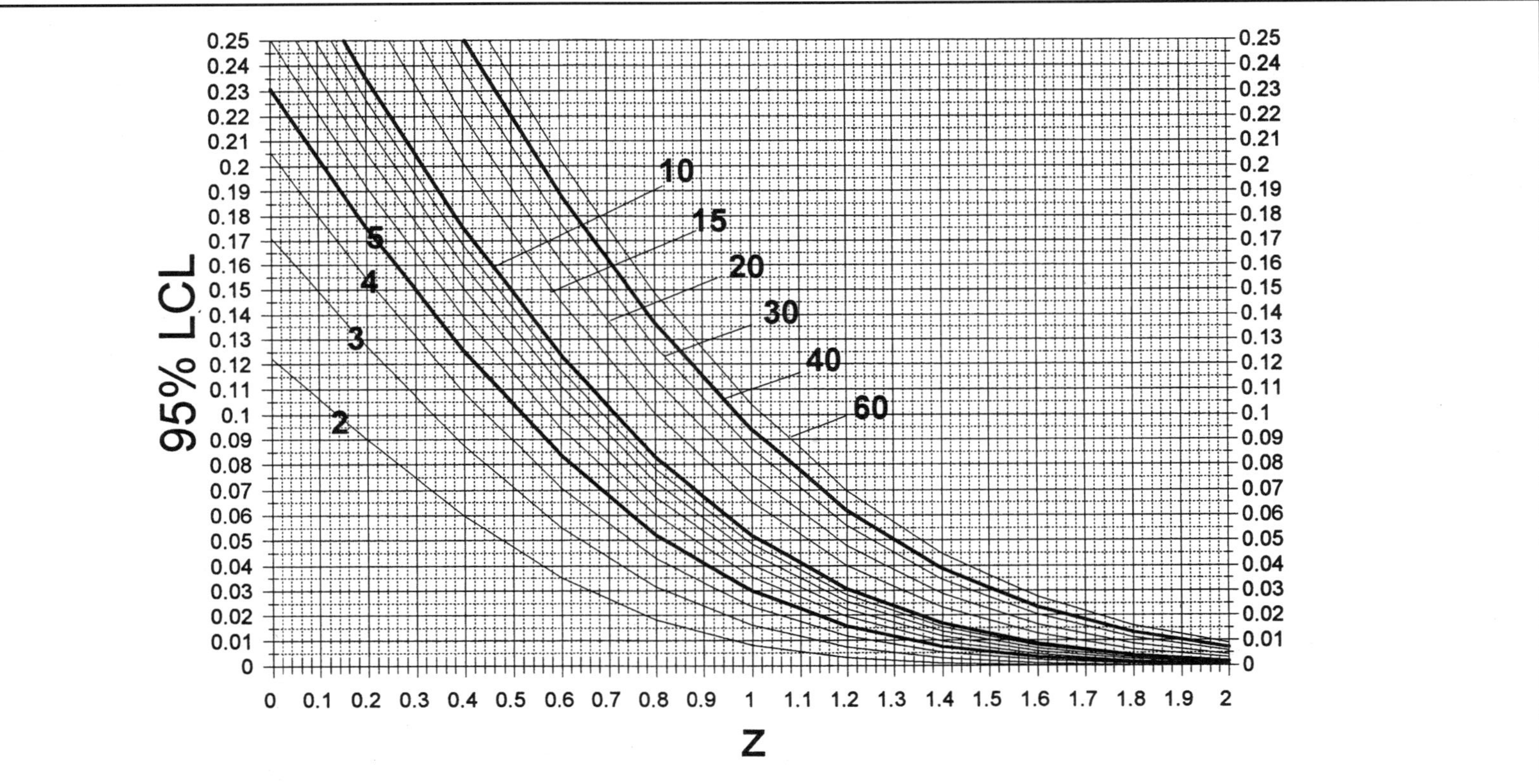

Figure VII.6 — 95th percentile LCL for the exceedance fraction (f) vs. the calculated z-value. Using z and the sample size, read the 95th percentile LCL from the y axis. [From **Hewett, P., and G.H. Ganser:** Simple Procedures for Calculating Confidence Intervals Around the Sample Mean and Exceedance Fraction Derived from Lognormally Distributed Data. *Appl. Occup. Environ. Hyg. 12(2)*:132-142 (1997). Reprinted with permission of the American Conference of Governmental Industrial Hygienists.]

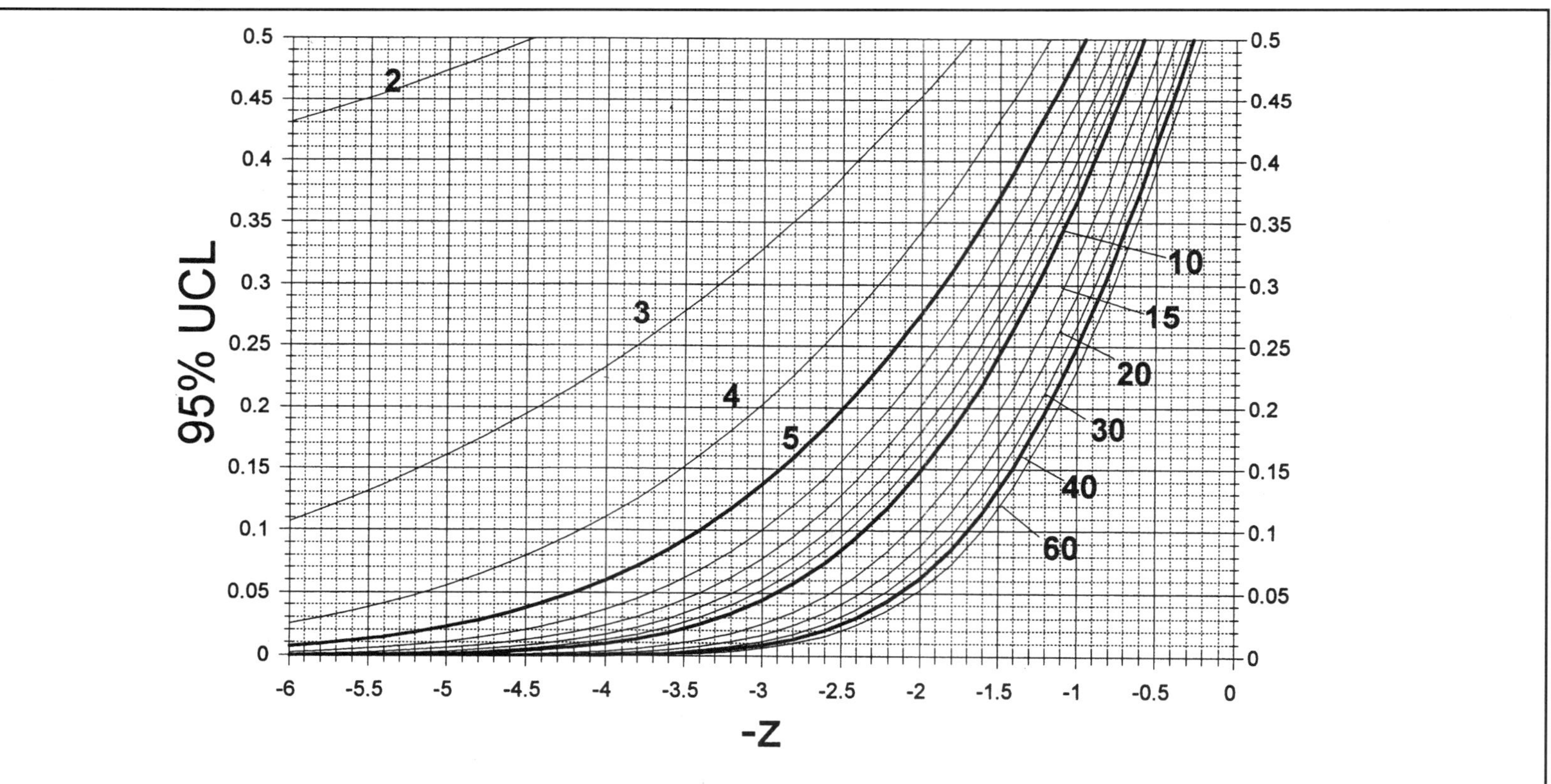

Figure VII.7 — 95th percentile UCL for the exceedance fraction (f) vs. the negative of the calculated z-value. Using -z and the sample size, read the 95th percentile UCL from the y axis. [From **Hewett, P., and G.H. Ganser:** Simple Procedures for Calculating Confidence Intervals Around the Sample Mean and Exceedance Fraction Derived from Lognormally Distributed Data. *App. Occup. Environ. Hyg. 12(2)*:132-142 (1997). Reprinted with permission of the American Conference of Governmental Industrial Hygienists.]

Step 1: Calculate Z_{OEL} (the same value used to obtain the point estimate of the exceedance fraction):

$$Z_{OEL} = \frac{\ln OEL - \overline{y}}{s_y}$$

Step 2: Using Z_{OEL} and the sample size, n, read the confidence limit from Figure VII.5. This represents the 95% LCL for f.

Using *negative* Z_{OEL} and n read the confidence limit from Figure VII.5. The 95% UCL for f is the complement of this value (complement = 1 - value).

For most data sets, Figures VII.6 and VII.7 should be used. These figures cover only a portion of Figure VII.5 and will often result in more accurate estimates of the LCL and UCL, respectively. Note that in Figure VII.7 the 95% UCL is read directly from the y-axis.

Example

Calculate the 95th percentile, the $UTL_{95\%,95\%}$, the exceedance fraction, and the exceedance fraction confidence interval to form a picture of the upper tail of the lognormal exposure profile represented by the following monitoring data. The OEL is 5 mg/m^3.

Monitoring data (mg/m^3):

1.3	2.1	2.5
1.8	5.5	2.5
1.2	2.2	3.5
4.5	3	2.8
2	2.4	2.9

Descriptive Statistics:

Number of samples	15
Maximum (mg/m^3)	5.5
Minimum (mg/m^3)	1.2
Range	4.3
% > OEL	6.7
Mean (mg/m^3)	2.7
Median (mg/m^3)	2.5
Standard deviation (mg/m^3)	1.14
Mean of ln(data)	0.91

SD of ln(data)	0.41
GM (mg/m^3)	2.5
GSD	1.5

Percentile — Lognormal Distribution:

$$\text{Percentile} = \exp(\bar{y} + Z\, s_y)$$

Choose Z for the 95th percentile (P = 0.95; see Table VII.2): $Z_{0.95} = 1.645$

$$\begin{aligned}\text{Percentile} &= \exp(0.91 + 1.645 \bullet 0.41)\\ &= 4.88\ mg/m^3\end{aligned}$$

The most likely estimate of the 95th percentile concentration is 4.88 mg/m^3. We would expect 95% of all exposures in the exposure profile to be less than 4.88 mg/m^3. This is below the OEL of 5 mg/m^3; however, there is uncertainty associated with the percentile estimate — to quantify that uncertainty, we can calculate an upper tolerance limit.

Upper Tolerance Limit — Lognormal Distribution:

$$UTL = \exp(\bar{y} + K\, s_y)$$

Choose K for 95% confidence in the 95th percentile and n = 15 (see Table VII.3) — $K_{95\%,95\%} = 2.566$:

$$\begin{aligned}UTL_{95\%,95\%} &= \exp(0.91 + 2.566 \bullet 0.41)\\ &= 7.11\ mg/m^3\end{aligned}$$

We can be 95% confident that 95% of the exposures in the exposure distribution are less than 7.11 mg/m^3. This is greater than our OEL of 5 mg/m^3. Therefore, we are *not* 95% certain that the exposure is less than the OEL 95% of the time.

To answer the question "What fraction of the time do we expect the exposures in this exposure profile to exceed the OEL?" we calculate the exceedance fraction.

Exceedance Fraction — Lognormal Distribution:

Step 1: Calculate the Z-value corresponding to the position of the OEL in the exposure distribution:

$$Z_{OEL} = \frac{\ln OEL - y}{s_y}$$

$$Z_{OEL} = \frac{\ln 5 - 0.91}{0.41}$$

$$= 1.706$$

Step 2: Look up the proportion of a normal distribution corresponding to $Z_{OEL} = 1.706$ in Table VII.2 — P = 0.9564.

Step 3: Subtract the proportion from 1 to determine the exceedance fraction:

$$f = 1 - P$$

$$f = 1 - 0.9564$$

$$= 0.044 \text{ (or } 4.4\%)$$

Our most likely estimate is that 4.4% of the exposures in the exposure profile will exceed the OEL; however, there is some error associated with that estimate — to quantify the confidence in the exceedance fraction estimate, we can calculate confidence limits.

Confidence Limits for the Exceedance Fraction:

Step 1: Calculate Z_{OEL} (the same value used to obtain the point estimate of the exceedance fraction):

$$Z_{OEL} = \frac{\ln OEL - y}{s_y}$$

$$Z_{OEL} = \frac{\ln 5 - 0.91}{0.41}$$

$$= 1.706$$

Step 2: Using Z_{OEL} and the sample size (n) read the confidence limit from Figure VII.5. This represents the 95% LCL for f:

95% LCL (Z_{OEL}, *n*): 0.02

95% LCL for f = 0.02 (or 2%)

Using *negative* Z_{OEL} and *n*, read the confidence limit from Figure VII.5:

95% UCL ($-Z_{OEL}$, *n*): 0.85

The 95% UCL for f is the complement of this value (complement = 1 - value):

95% UCL for f = 1 - 0.85 = 0.15 (or 15%)

We are 95% certain that the exposures exceed the 5 mg/m^3 OEL 15% of the time or less.

References

1. **Lyles, R.H., and L.L. Kupper:** On Strategies for Comparing Occupational Exposure Data to Limits. *Am. Ind. Hyg. Assoc. J. 57(1):*6-15 (1996).
2. **Hewett, P., and G.H. Ganser:** Simple Procedures for Calculating Confidence Intervals Around the Sample Mean and Exceedance Fraction Derived from Lognormally Distributed Data. *Appl. Occup. Environ. Hyg. 12(2):*132-142 (1997).

Appendix VIII

Distribution-Free Tolerance Limits

For those data sets that pass the W-test by demonstrating adequate fit to lognormal or normal parameters, the lognormal or normal parametric tests described in Appendices VI and VII provide good statistical power.* That power is not free, however. It is available only under the assumption that the data are drawn randomly from an appropriate distribution. If the population of exposures is not distributed parametrically, the statistical power is illusory and decisions based on small numbers of samples are suspect.

If you are unable to identify the distribution for your SEG's exposure profile, and you are reasonably confident the data represent a single SEG, you should consider the nonparametric procedures presented in this appendix. These procedures can be applied to any set of data drawn randomly from any continuous distribution to produce conservative exposure assessment statistics.

Quick answers to important questions are provided in Tables VIII.1 and VIII.2 — one before the monitoring campaign starts, and two for interpreting the resulting data:

1. How many samples are required to obtain desired confidence?
2. Given 50 or more samples, what is the confidence (γ) that a proportion (P) of the sampled population is below the mth largest sample?
3. What is the confidence (γ) that a proportion (P) of the sampled population lies between the minimum and maximum value of n samples?

*Software now makes it practical to obtain improved statistical power by testing for and using parametric distributions other than the normal and lognormal distributions.

Using Table VIII.1 to Determine the Number of Samples Needed

Generally, nonparametric distribution-free methods require at least 30 samples to achieve reasonable statistical power. This is in contrast with the need for six or more samples to achieve similar power from a normally or lognormally distributed population.

It is shown in Table VIII.1 that with fewer than 50 samples one has little confidence in upper percentile estimates when no population distribution can be inferred. For nonparametric data, it is almost impossible to achieve a 95%,95% upper tolerance limit ($UTL_{95\%,95\%}$) when there are less than 60 samples. In Table VIII.2, it is shown that 40 samples are required to achieve 92% confidence that 90% of the population is between the largest and smallest sample. Translated into industrial hygiene terms, this means the largest of 40 samples must be less than the OEL to obtain at least 92% confidence that 90% of all exposures are below the OEL. Numerical examples follow to help clarify these concepts.

Example VIII.1: How many samples are required to obtain 95% confidence ($\gamma = 0.95$) that 95% of the sampled population of exposures (P = 0.95) are less than the largest sample?

Enter Table VIII.1 in the column for which $\gamma = 0.95$ and P = 0.95. Move down the column to the smallest value of n for which m = 1. Find that n = 60 samples are required.

Example VIII.2: If the largest sample is above the OEL and seems to be an outlier, how many samples must be taken to achieve 95% confidence that 95% of the sampled population is less than the second largest sample?

Move further down the same column ($\gamma = 0.95$ and P = 0.95) to find the smallest value of n for which m = 2. Find that n = 95 samples are required.

One-Sided Nonparametric Tolerance Limit Test Using Table VIII.1

Example VIII.3: Suppose 54 of 55 sampled exposures are smaller than the OEL. What conclusions can an industrial hygienist draw without making any assumptions about the distribution of exposures?

In this example, the second largest sample is less than the OEL, so m = 2. Enter Table VIII.1 in the row labeled n = 55, the number of samples available. Find locations where m = 2 and interpolate between columns if necessary. The following

Table VIII.1 — Table for Distribution-Free Tolerance Limits (One-Sided)[A,B]

	$\gamma = 0.75$				$\gamma = 0.90$				$\gamma = 0.95$				$\gamma = 0.99$			
n\P	.75	.90	.95	.99	.75	.90	.95	.99	.75	.90	.95	.99	.75	.90	.95	.99
50	10	3	1	—	9	2	1	—	8	2	—	—	6	1	—	—
55	12	4	2	—	10	3	1	—	9	2	—	—	7	1	—	—
60	13	4	2	—	11	3	1	—	10	2	1	—	8	1	—	—
65	14	5	2	—	12	4	1	—	11	3	1	—	9	2	—	—
70	15	5	2	—	13	4	1	—	12	3	1	—	10	2	—	—
75	16	6	2	—	14	4	1	—	13	3	1	—	10	2	—	—
80	17	6	3	—	15	5	2	—	14	4	1	—	11	2	—	—
85	19	7	3	—	16	5	2	—	15	4	1	—	12	3	—	—
90	20	7	3	—	17	5	2	—	16	5	1	—	13	3	1	—
95	21	7	3	—	18	6	2	—	17	5	2	—	14	3	1	—
100	22	8	3	—	20	6	2	—	18	5	2	—	15	4	1	—
110	24	9	4	—	22	7	3	—	20	6	2	—	17	4	1	—
120	27	10	4	—	24	8	3	—	22	7	2	—	19	5	1	—
130	29	11	5	—	26	9	3	—	25	8	3	—	21	6	2	—
140	31	12	5	1	28	10	4	—	27	8	3	—	23	6	2	—
150	34	12	6	1	31	10	4	—	29	9	3	—	26	7	2	—
170	39	14	7	1	35	12	5	—	33	11	4	—	30	9	3	—
200	46	17	8	1	42	15	6	—	40	13	5	—	36	11	4	—
300	70	26	12	2	65	23	10	1	63	22	9	1	58	19	7	—
400	94	36	17	3	89	32	15	2	86	30	13	1	80	27	11	—
500	118	45	22	3	113	41	19	2	109	39	17	2	103	35	14	1
600	143	55	26	4	136	51	23	3	133	48	21	2	126	44	18	1
700	167	65	31	5	160	60	28	4	156	57	26	3	149	52	22	2
800	192	74	36	6	184	69	32	5	180	66	30	4	172	61	26	2
900	216	84	41	7	208	79	37	5	204	75	35	4	195	70	30	3
1000	241	94	45	8	233	88	41	6	228	85	39	5	219	79	35	3

[A] Largest values of *m* such that one may assert with confidence at least γ that 100*P* percent of a population lies below the *m*th largest (or above the *m*th smallest) of a random sample of *n* from that population (no assumption of normality required).

[B] From **National Bureau of Standards:** Experimental Statistics. In *National Bureau of Standards Handbook 91*. Washington, D.C.: National Bureau of Standards, 1966.

statements are supported by this data:

- There is 75% confidence that 95% of the exposures are less than the second largest sample (and less than the OEL).
- There is 90% confidence that about 92% of the exposures are less than the second largest sample.
- There is 95% confidence that 90% of the exposures are less than the second largest sample.

Two-Sided Nonparametric Tolerance Interval Using Table VIII.2.

When all of the exposure measurements are below the OEL, Table VIII.2 can be used for answering the following occupational health question: What proportion of exposures are below

Table VIII.2 — Confidence Associated with a Tolerance Limit Statement[A,B]

n	*P* = .75	*P* = .90	*P* = .95	*P* = .99
3	.16	.03	.01	.00
4	.26	.05	.01	.00
5	.37	.08	.02	.00
6	.47	.11	.03	.00
7	.56	.15	.04	.00
8	.63	.19	.06	.00
9	.70	.23	.07	.00
10	.76	.26	.09	.00
11	.80	.30	.10	.01
12	.84	.34	.12	.01
13	.87	.38	.14	.01
14	.90	.42	.15	.01
15	.92	.45	.17	.01
16	.94	.49	.19	.01
17	.95	.52	.21	.01
18	.96	.55	.23	.01
19	.97	.58	.25	.02
20	.98	.61	.26	.02
25	.99	.73	.36	.03
30	1.00	.82	.45	.04
40	—	.92	.60	.06
50	—	.97	.72	.09
60	—	.99	.81	.12
70	—	.99	.87	.16
80	—	1.00	.91	.19
90	—	—	.94	.23
100	—	—	.96	.26

[A] Confidence γ with which one may assert that 100*P* percent of the population lies between the largest and smallest of a random sample of *n* from that population (continuous distribution assumed).
[B] From **National Bureau of Standards:** Experimental Statistics. In *National Bureau of Standards Handbook 91.* Washington, D.C.: National Bureau of Standards, 1966.

the OEL? Table VIII.2 is more useful than Table VIII.1 for the smaller sample sizes that are more typical in industrial hygiene.

Example VIII.4: Using Table VIII.2, what conclusions about workplace exposures are supported if 15 of 15 samples are smaller than the OEL?

Enter Table VIII.2 in the row for which n = 15. Read the confidence levels associated with each proportion:

- There is 92% confidence that 75% of the exposures are less than the OEL.
- There is 45% confidence that 90% of the exposures are less than the OEL.
- There is only 17% confidence that 95% of the exposures are less than the OEL.

Example VIII.5: Suppose the number of samples is doubled from the previous example. What statistical statements can be made when 30 of 30 samples are less than the OEL?

Enter Table VIII.2 in the row for which n = 30. Read the confidence levels associated with each proportion:

- There is nearly 100% confidence that 75% of the exposures are less than the OEL.
- There is 82% confidence that 90% of the exposures are less than the OEL.
- There is only 45% confidence that 95% of the exposures are less than the OEL.

Note that example VIII.5 quantifies the earlier assertion that at least 30 samples are required to obtain reasonable confidence about exposures in a nonparametrically distributed SEG. Note also that an acceptable workplace is one in which 30 of 30 randomly collected samples lie below the OEL. Nevertheless, such data by themselves do not justify a professional judgment that fewer than 5% of all exposures exceed the standard, which might be a surprise to an industrial hygienist not familiar with statistical analysis tools.

Example VIII.6: How many samples are required to obtain 95% confidence that 95% of the measured exposures are between the smallest and largest observed exposures?

Enter Table VIII.2 in the column labeled P = 0.95 and proceed down the column to $\gamma = 0.95$. Interpolate to estimate that it takes n = 95 samples to achieve the desired confidence.

Summary

The purpose of this appendix is to make distribution-free statistics readily available and easy to use. For the industrial hygienists, they are a valuable aid to quantifying professional judgment. Conclusions supported by distribution-free tolerance interval tests are truly robust since they do not depend on assumptions about the distributional form of the sampled workplace exposure population.

The distribution-free or nonparametric tolerance interval tests summarized in this appendix can be applied to every exposure data set. The resulting estimate of the confidence with which one can assert that a proportion of exposures in an SEG are below the OEL can be an important tool for aiding the exposure judgment. Higher confidence levels are achieved only with additional assumptions about the distribution of exposures in the SEG. Then, if the data pass appropriate goodness-of-fit tests for parametric distributions,* parametric tolerance interval tests can be used.

Beyond that, the industrial hygienist is encouraged to examine closely each workplace producing exposure data that fail the goodness-of-fit tests for parametric distributions. Often, this indicates a workplace with equipment, training, or procedures that are out of statistical control. Exposures in these situations usually can be reduced by enlightened management interventions.

*Normal and lognormal distributions are especially "nice" for tolerance interval testing, which is described in Appendix VII.

Appendix IX

Analysis of Variance for Refining Similar Exposure Groups

A method for analyzing the homogeneity of critical SEGs is described in this appendix. As discussed in Chapter 7, critical SEGs are those where potential misclassification of individual workers in the SEG presents the most risk. Critical SEGs are generally those with exposure profiles near but below the OEL. If an individual worker assigned to a critical SEG has an exposure profile with significantly higher exposures than other workers in the SEG, then that individual worker may be exposed to an unacceptable health risk even though the SEG was judged "acceptable."

The method quantifies variability in exposure levels among workers in an SEG.(1) It is based on a statistical model termed the "within-between lognormal model," and the analysis of sample exposure data in the framework of this model is known as the "analysis of variance," or ANOVA.

The variability in an SEG can be split into two parts: within-worker variability and between-worker variability (see Figure IX-1A). Within-worker variability can be represented by the variability in each of the individual worker exposure profiles that make up the SEG exposure profile (see Figure IX-1B).

Each of those individual worker exposure profiles has an arithmetic mean. Those arithmetic mean exposures can be aggregated to form a distribution of average exposures for workers in the SEG (see Figure IX-1C). The variability of this distribution of average exposures for workers in the SEG represents between-worker variability. The degree to which the individual exposure distribution arithmetic mean values differ depends on the homogeneity of the SEG. In a perfectly homogenous SEG the mean values would all be identical.

ANOVA is used to compare the SEG's between-worker variability with its within-worker variability. If the magnitude of the

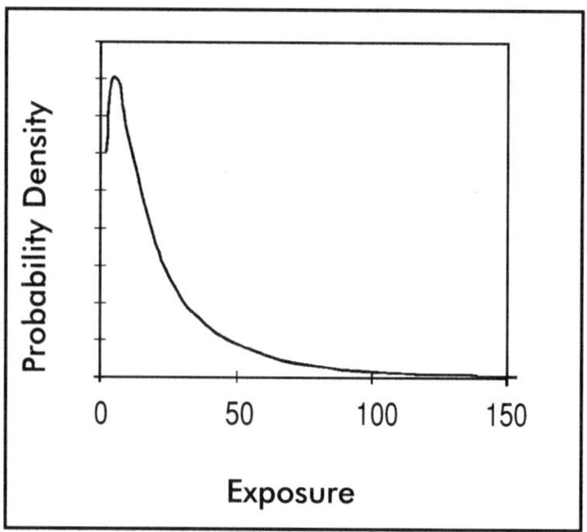

Figure IX.1a — SEG exposure profile.

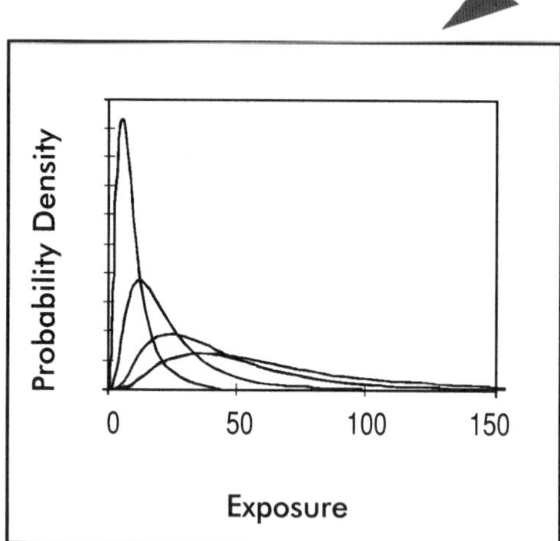

Figure IX.1b — Individual worker exposure profiles.

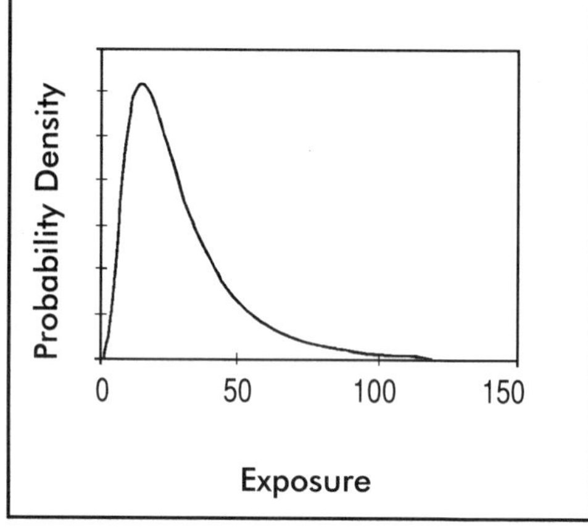

Figure IX.1c — Distribution of worker arithmetic mean exposures.

between-worker variability is large enough to be distinguished from the within-worker variability, it is evident there are significant differences in mean exposures between individual workers in the SEG. The SEGs should then be examined more carefully through additional exposure monitoring and/or observation to determine whether workers might appropriately be reclassified into one or more additional SEGs.

This appendix is organized as follows: First, the within-between lognormal model is summarized. Next, the computations involved in an ANOVA are described. Finally, a worked example for some hypothetical data is presented.

The Within-Between Lognormal Model

The following assumptions usually are made when applying the ANOVA model:

- Each worker in the SEG experiences a lognormal distribution of 8-hour TWA exposure values;
- The GSD values are the same for each worker's distribution, but the arithmetic mean value is different;
- The arithmetic mean values for each worker represent the long-term average (LTA) exposure level, such that the worker's cumulative exposure is the product of his or her LTA exposure level and the number of workdays; and
- The arithmetic mean exposure values for different workers are lognormally distributed.

Given the conditions that 1) every worker has lognormally distributed 8-hour TWA exposures with the same GSD value, and 2) arithmetic mean exposure values for different workers are lognormally distributed, a third condition follows: the mixture or aggregate of all the 8-hour TWA exposure values experienced by all workers in the population forms a total distribution that is also lognormal. A mathematical statement of this model is:

$$C_{ij} = \mu \bullet B_i \bullet W_j \qquad (1)$$

where:

C_{ij} equals 8-hour TWA experienced by the ith worker on the jth day
μ equals grand mean exposure level in the group
B represents variability *between* workers in LTA exposure levels
W represents *within*-worker variability in day-to-day 8-hour TWA values.

The grand mean μ is considered fixed (constant), while factors B and W are lognormal variables.

The ANOVA Method

The appropriate data for ANOVA are obtained by randomly selecting at least three workers, randomly selecting at least three workdays for each chosen worker, and monitoring the 8-hour TWA on all these days. Larger sample sizes (e.g., selecting six workers) are preferred because they provide more precise estimates of model parameters. Decisions on the best sample size involve a balance between cost and precision, are often complex, and are beyond the scope of this appendix. For more detailed information on ANOVA the reader should consult a statistics text, such as *Statistics for Research*[2] or *Applied Linear Statistical Models*.[3]

The ANOVA permits a statistical test of the null hypothesis that all workers have the same LTA exposure level. If this null hypothesis is rejected, ANOVA results provide an estimate of the extent of variability between workers in LTA exposure levels.

Notation

- There are k number of workers selected from the population of workers.
- There are n_i number of exposure values measured for the ith worker selected, where $i = 1,2,\ldots,k$.
- N is the total number of measured exposure values, where

  $$N = \sum_{i=1}^{k} n_i$$

  A "balanced" design signifies that all the n_i are equal, or $n_1 = n_2 = \ldots = n_k$, and this constant number of exposure measurements per worker is designated n.
- x_{ij} denotes the jth measured 8-hour TWA value for the ith worker in the sample, where $j = 1,2,\ldots,n_i$.
- $y_{ij} = \ln x_{ij}$ is the logtransformed value (using natural logarithms to the base e) of x_{ij}.
- $\bar{y}_i$ is the mean logtransformed exposure value for the ith worker, where $\bar{y}_i = \sum_{j=1}^{n_i} \frac{y_{ij}}{n_i} = \sum_{j=1}^{n_i} \frac{\ln x_{ij}}{n_i}$
- $\bar{y}_T$ is the grand mean logtransformed exposure value, where

  $$\bar{y}_T = \sum_{i=1}^{k} \sum_{j=1}^{n_i} \frac{y_{ij}}{N} \qquad (2)$$

  When a balanced design is used,

  $$\bar{y}_T = \sum_{i=1}^{k} \frac{\bar{y}_i}{k} \qquad (3)$$

Mechanics of the ANOVA

(Note: A worked example follows:)

Step 1. Logtransform each exposure value (i.e., change x_{ij} to y_{ij}).

Step 2. For each worker in the sample, compute $\bar{y}_i$, the mean of the worker's logtransformed exposure values. Because there are k number of workers in the sample, there are k number of $\bar{y}_i$ values.

Step 3. Compute the grand mean logtransformed exposure value, $\bar{y}_T$, using equation (2) or (3)

Step 4. Compute the within-group sum of squares, denoted SSW, where:

$$SSW = \sum_{i=1}^{k} \sum_{j=1}^{n_i} (y_{ij} - \bar{y}_i)^2 \qquad (4)$$

The number of "degrees of freedom" for SSW equals *N - k*.

Step 5. Compute the within-group mean square, denoted MSW, where:

$$MSW = \frac{SSW}{N - k} \qquad (5)$$

Step 6. Compute the between-group sum of squares, denoted SSB, where:

$$SSB = \sum_{i=1}^{k} n_i(\bar{y}_i - \bar{y}_T)^2 \qquad (6)$$

The number of "degrees of freedom" for SSB equals *k* - 1.

Step 7. Compute the between-group mean square, denoted MSB, where:

$$MSB = \frac{SSB}{k - 1} \qquad (7)$$

Step 8. To test whether there is significant variability between LTA exposure levels for these workers, compute the F-statistic, which is the ratio of MSB to MSW:

$$F_{v_1,v_2} = \frac{MSB}{MSW} \qquad (8)$$

where:

$v_1 = k - 1$, which is the number of degrees of freedom associated with the numerator

$v_2 = N - k$, which is the number of degrees of freedom associated with the denominator

Step 9. Choose the desired confidence level for the test (e.g., 95% confidence). The confidence level is the complement of the acceptable probability of making a Type I error in the F-test procedure; a Type I error signifies that one would conclude there are differences between workers when there truly are no differences. The symbol α is typically used to denote the acceptable Type I error probability (where α is treated as a decimal fraction rather than a percent), so the confidence level can be denoted $1 - \alpha$ in terms of a decimal fraction rather than a percent.

Consult the table of F values (see Table IX.1). Locate the F value associated with the desired confidence level ($1 - \alpha$) and the appropriate degrees of freedom for the numerator (v_1) and the denominator (v_2). If the computed F-statistic is greater than the corresponding tabled F value, one should conclude that there is significant variability in LTA exposure values between workers in the population from which the sample was drawn. If the computed F-statistic is less than the corresponding F value in the table, one cannot technically conclude there is significant variability between workers. Keep in mind, however, that small sample sizes tend to impart low *power* to the F-test procedure. In the present context, power is the probability of correctly concluding there is exposure variability between workers when such variability truly exists.

Step 10. The values of MSW and MSB can be used to estimate parameters of the within-between lognormal model. Three important parameters are μ, GSD[B], and GSD[W].

a. $\widehat{\text{GSD[W]}} = \exp(\sqrt{\text{MSW}})$ (9)

$$\text{b. } \widehat{GSD[B]} = \exp\left(\sqrt{\frac{MSB - MSW}{n_O}}\right) \quad (10)$$

where:

$$n_O = \frac{N - \sum_{i=1}^{k} (n_i^2/N)}{k - 1} \quad (11)$$

Note that for a balanced design, $n_O = n$.

$$\text{c. } \hat{u} = [\exp(\overline{y}_T)]\left[\exp\left(\frac{\ln^2\widehat{GSD[W]} + \ln^2\widehat{GSD[B]}}{2}\right)\right] \quad (12)$$

Table IX.1 — Percentiles of the *F* Distribution

Entry is $F\ (A;\ v_1, v_2)$ where $P\{F(v_1, v_2) \leq F(A;\ v_1, v_2)\} = A$

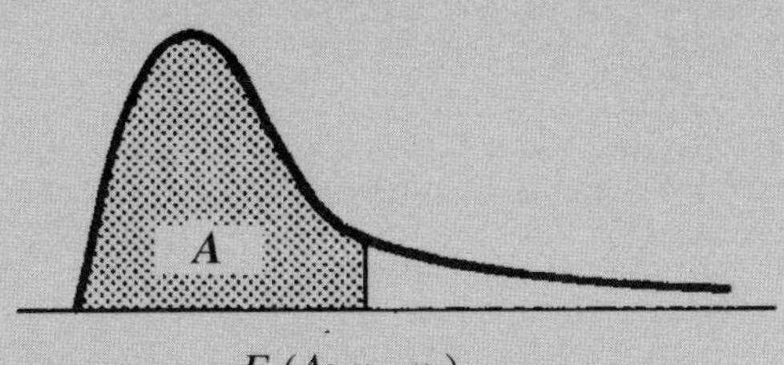

$F\ (A;\ v_1, v_2)$

$$F\ (A;\ v_1, v_2) = \frac{1}{F\ (1 - A;\ v_1, v_2)}$$

From **Neter, J., W. Wasserman, and M.H. Kutner:** *Applied Linear Statistical Models,* 3rd Ed. Homewood, Ill.: Richard D. Irwin, Inc., 1990. Reprinted with permission of the McGraw-Hill Companies.

Table IX.1 — Percentiles of the *F* Distribution (continued)

Den. df	*A*	1	2	3	4	5	6	7	8	9
		Numerator df								
1	.50	1.00	1.50	1.71	1.82	1.89	1.94	1.98	2.00	2.03
	.90	39.9	49.5	53.6	55.8	57.2	58.2	58.9	59.4	59.9
	.95	161	200	216	225	230	234	237	239	241
	.975	648	800	864	900	922	937	948	957	963
	.99	4,052	5,000	5,403	5,625	5,764	5,859	5,928	5,981	6,022
	.995	16,211	20,000	21,615	22,500	23,056	23,437	23,715	23,925	24,091
	.999	405,280	500,000	540,380	562,500	576,400	585,940	592,870	598,140	602,280
2	.50	0.667	1.00	1.13	1.21	1.25	1.28	1.30	1.32	1.33
	.90	8.53	9.00	9.16	9.24	9.29	9.33	9.35	9.37	9.38
	.95	18.5	19.0	19.2	19.2	19.3	19.3	19.4	19.4	19.4
	.975	38.5	39.0	39.2	39.2	39.3	39.3	39.4	39.4	39.4
	.99	98.5	99.0	99.2	99.2	99.3	99.3	99.4	99.4	99.4
	.995	199	199	199	199	199	199	199	199	199
	.999	998.5	999.0	999.2	999.2	999.3	999.3	999.4	999.4	999.4
3	.50	0.585	0.881	1.00	1.06	1.10	1.13	1.15	1.16	1.17
	.90	5.54	5.46	5.39	5.34	5.31	5.28	5.27	5.25	5.24
	.95	10.1	9.55	9.28	9.12	9.01	8.94	8.89	8.85	8.81
	.975	17.4	16.0	15.4	15.1	14.9	14.7	14.6	14.5	14.5
	.99	34.1	30.8	29.5	28.7	28.2	27.9	27.7	27.5	27.3
	.995	55.6	49.8	47.5	46.2	45.4	44.8	44.4	44.1	43.9
	.999	167.0	148.5	141.1	137.1	134.6	132.8	131.6	130.6	129.9
4	.50	0.549	0.828	0.941	1.00	1.04	1.06	1.08	1.09	1.10
	.90	4.54	4.32	4.19	4.11	4.05	4.01	3.98	3.95	3.94
	.95	7.71	6.94	6.59	6.39	6.26	6.16	6.09	6.04	6.00
	.975	12.2	10.6	9.98	9.60	9.36	9.20	9.07	8.98	8.90
	.99	21.2	18.0	16.7	16.0	15.5	15.2	15.0	14.8	14.7
	.995	31.3	26.3	24.3	23.2	22.5	22.0	21.6	21.4	21.1
	.999	74.1	61.2	56.2	53.4	51.7	50.5	49.7	49.0	48.5
5	.50	0.528	0.799	0.907	0.965	1.00	1.02	1.04	1.05	1.06
	.90	4.06	3.78	3.62	3.52	3.45	3.40	3.37	3.34	3.32
	.95	6.61	5.79	5.41	5.19	5.05	4.95	4.88	4.82	4.77
	.975	10.0	8.43	7.76	7.39	7.15	6.98	6.85	6.76	6.68
	.99	16.3	13.3	12.1	11.4	11.0	10.7	10.5	10.3	10.2
	.995	22.8	18.3	16.5	15.6	14.9	14.5	14.2	14.0	13.8
	.999	47.2	37.1	33.2	31.1	29.8	28.8	28.2	27.6	27.2
6	.50	0.515	0.780	0.886	0.942	0.977	1.00	1.02	1.03	1.04
	.90	3.78	3.46	3.29	3.18	3.11	3.05	3.01	2.98	2.96
	.95	5.99	5.14	4.76	4.53	4.39	4.28	4.21	4.15	4.10
	.975	8.81	7.26	6.60	6.23	5.99	5.82	5.70	5.60	5.52
	.99	13.7	10.9	9.78	9.15	8.75	8.47	8.26	8.10	7.98
	.995	18.6	14.5	12.9	12.0	11.5	11.1	10.8	10.6	10.4
	.999	35.5	27.0	23.7	21.9	20.8	20.0	19.5	19.0	18.7
7	.50	0.506	0.767	0.871	0.926	0.960	0.983	1.00	1.01	1.02
	.90	3.59	3.26	3.07	2.96	2.88	2.83	2.78	2.75	2.72
	.95	5.59	4.74	4.35	4.12	3.97	3.87	3.79	3.73	3.68
	.975	8.07	6.54	5.89	5.52	5.29	5.12	4.99	4.90	4.82
	.99	12.2	9.55	8.45	7.85	7.46	7.19	6.99	6.84	6.72
	.995	16.2	12.4	10.9	10.1	9.52	9.16	8.89	8.68	8.51
	.999	29.2	21.7	18.8	17.2	16.2	15.5	15.0	14.6	14.3

Table IX.1 — Percentiles of the *F* Distribution (continued)

Den. df	A	10	12	15	20	24	30	60	120	∞
		Numerator df								
1	.50	2.04	2.07	2.09	2.12	2.13	2.15	2.17	2.18	2.20
	.90	60.2	60.7	61.2	61.7	62.0	62.3	62.8	63.1	63.3
	.95	242	244	246	248	249	250	252	253	254
	.975	969	977	985	993	997	1,001	1,010	1,014	1,018
	.99	6,056	6,106	6,157	6,209	6,235	6,261	6,313	6,339	6,366
	.995	24,224	24,426	24,630	24,836	24,940	25,044	25,253	25,359	25,464
	.999	605,620	610,670	615,760	620,910	623,500	626,100	631,340	633,970	636,620
2	.50	1.34	1.36	1.38	1.39	1.40	1.41	1.43	1.43	1.44
	.90	9.39	9.41	9.42	9.44	9.45	9.46	9.47	9.48	9.49
	.95	19.4	19.4	19.4	19.4	19.5	19.5	19.5	19.5	19.5
	.975	39.4	39.4	39.4	39.4	39.5	39.5	39.5	39.5	39.5
	.99	99.4	99.4	99.4	99.4	99.5	99.5	99.5	99.5	99.5
	.995	199	199	199	199	199	199	199	199	200
	.999	999.4	999.4	999.4	999.4	999.5	999.5	999.5	999.5	999.5
3	.50	1.18	1.20	1.21	1.23	1.23	1.24	1.25	1.26	1.27
	.90	5.23	5.22	5.20	5.18	5.18	5.17	5.15	5.14	5.13
	.95	8.79	8.74	8.70	8.66	8.64	8.62	8.57	8.55	8.53
	.975	14.4	14.3	14.3	14.2	14.1	14.1	14.0	13.9	13.9
	.99	27.2	27.1	26.9	26.7	26.6	26.5	26.3	26.2	26.1
	.995	43.7	43.4	43.1	42.8	42.6	42.5	42.1	42.0	41.8
	.999	129.2	128.3	127.4	126.4	125.9	125.4	124.5	124.0	123.5
4	.50	1.11	1.13	1.14	1.15	1.16	1.16	1.18	1.18	1.19
	.90	3.92	3.90	3.87	3.84	3.83	3.82	3.79	3.78	3.76
	.95	5.96	5.91	5.86	5.80	5.77	5.75	5.69	5.66	5.63
	.975	8.84	8.75	8.66	8.56	8.51	8.46	8.36	8.31	8.26
	.99	14.5	14.4	14.2	14.0	13.9	13.8	13.7	13.6	13.5
	.995	21.0	20.7	20.4	20.2	20.0	19.9	19.6	19.5	19.3
	.999	48.1	47.4	46.8	46.1	45.8	45.4	44.7	44.4	44.1
5	.50	1.07	1.09	1.10	1.11	1.12	1.12	1.14	1.14	1.15
	.90	3.30	3.27	3.24	3.21	3.19	3.17	3.14	3.12	3.11
	.95	4.74	4.68	4.62	4.56	4.53	4.50	4.43	4.40	4.37
	.975	6.62	6.52	6.43	6.33	6.28	6.23	6.12	6.07	6.02
	.99	10.1	9.89	9.72	9.55	9.47	9.38	9.20	9.11	9.02
	.995	13.6	13.4	13.1	12.9	12.8	12.7	12.4	12.3	12.1
	.999	26.9	26.4	25.9	25.4	25.1	24.9	24.3	24.1	23.8
6	.50	1.05	1.06	1.07	1.08	1.09	1.10	1.11	1.12	1.12
	.90	2.94	2.90	2.87	2.84	2.82	2.80	2.76	2.74	2.72
	.95	4.06	4.00	3.94	3.87	3.84	3.81	3.74	3.70	3.67
	.975	5.46	5.37	5.27	5.17	5.12	5.07	4.96	4.90	4.85
	.99	7.87	7.72	7.56	7.40	7.31	7.23	7.06	6.97	6.88
	.995	10.2	10.0	9.81	9.59	9.47	9.36	9.12	9.00	8.88
	.999	18.4	18.0	17.6	17.1	16.9	16.7	16.2	16.0	15.7
7	.50	1.03	1.04	1.05	1.07	1.07	1.08	1.09	1.10	1.10
	.90	2.70	2.67	2.63	2.59	2.58	2.56	2.51	2.49	2.47
	.95	3.64	3.57	3.51	3.44	3.41	3.38	3.30	3.27	3.23
	.975	4.76	4.67	4.57	4.47	4.42	4.36	4.25	4.20	4.14
	.99	6.62	6.47	6.31	6.16	6.07	5.99	5.82	5.74	5.65
	.995	8.38	8.18	7.97	7.75	7.65	7.53	7.31	7.19	7.08
	.999	14.1	13.7	13.3	12.9	12.7	12.5	12.1	11.9	11.7

Table IX.1 — Percentiles of the *F* Distribution (continued)

Den. df	α	Numerator df 1	2	3	4	5	6	7	8	9
8	.50	0.499	0.757	0.860	0.915	0.948	0.971	0.988	1.00	1.01
	.90	3.46	3.11	2.92	2.81	2.73	2.67	2.62	2.59	2.56
	.95	5.32	4.46	4.07	3.84	3.69	3.58	3.50	3.44	3.39
	.975	7.57	6.06	5.42	5.05	4.82	4.65	4.53	4.43	4.36
	.99	11.3	8.65	7.59	7.01	6.63	6.37	6.18	6.03	5.91
	.995	14.7	11.0	9.60	8.81	8.30	7.95	7.69	7.50	7.34
	.999	25.4	18.5	15.8	14.4	13.5	12.9	12.4	12.0	11.8
9	.50	0.494	0.749	0.852	0.906	0.939	0.962	0.978	0.990	1.00
	.90	3.36	3.01	2.81	2.69	2.61	2.55	2.51	2.47	2.44
	.95	5.12	4.26	3.86	3.63	3.48	3.37	3.29	3.23	3.18
	.975	7.21	5.71	5.08	4.72	4.48	4.32	4.20	4.10	4.03
	.99	10.6	8.02	6.99	6.42	6.06	5.80	5.61	5.47	5.35
	.995	13.6	10.1	8.72	7.96	7.47	7.13	6.88	6.69	6.54
	.999	22.9	16.4	13.9	12.6	11.7	11.1	10.7	10.4	10.1
10	.50	0.490	0.743	0.845	0.899	0.932	0.954	0.971	0.983	0.992
	.90	3.29	2.92	2.73	2.61	2.52	2.46	2.41	2.38	2.35
	.95	4.96	4.10	3.71	3.48	3.33	3.22	3.14	3.07	3.02
	.975	6.94	5.46	4.83	4.47	4.24	4.07	3.95	3.85	3.78
	.99	10.0	7.56	6.55	5.99	5.64	5.39	5.20	5.06	4.94
	.995	12.8	9.43	8.08	7.34	6.87	6.54	6.30	6.12	5.97
	.999	21.0	14.9	12.6	11.3	10.5	9.93	9.52	9.20	8.96
12	.50	0.484	0.735	0.835	0.888	0.921	0.943	0.959	0.972	0.981
	.90	3.18	2.81	2.61	2.48	2.39	2.33	2.28	2.24	2.21
	.95	4.75	3.89	3.49	3.26	3.11	3.00	2.91	2.85	2.80
	.975	6.55	5.10	4.47	4.12	3.89	3.73	3.61	3.51	3.44
	.99	9.33	6.93	5.95	5.41	5.06	4.82	4.64	4.50	4.39
	.995	11.8	8.51	7.23	6.52	6.07	5.76	5.52	5.35	5.20
	.999	18.6	13.0	10.8	9.63	8.89	8.38	8.00	7.71	7.48
15	.50	0.478	0.726	0.826	0.878	0.911	0.933	0.949	0.960	0.970
	.90	3.07	2.70	2.49	2.36	2.27	2.21	2.16	2.12	2.09
	.95	4.54	3.68	3.29	3.06	2.90	2.79	2.71	2.64	2.59
	.975	6.20	4.77	4.15	3.80	3.58	3.41	3.29	3.20	3.12
	.99	8.68	6.36	5.42	4.89	4.56	4.32	4.14	4.00	3.89
	.995	10.8	7.70	6.48	5.80	5.37	5.07	4.85	4.67	4.54
	.999	16.6	11.3	9.34	8.25	7.57	7.09	6.74	6.47	6.26
20	.50	0.472	0.718	0.816	0.868	0.900	0.922	0.938	0.950	0.959
	.90	2.97	2.59	2.38	2.25	2.16	2.09	2.04	2.00	1.96
	.95	4.35	3.49	3.10	2.87	2.71	2.60	2.51	2.45	2.39
	.975	5.87	4.46	3.86	3.51	3.29	3.13	3.01	2.91	2.84
	.99	8.10	5.85	4.94	4.43	4.10	3.87	3.70	3.56	3.46
	.995	9.94	6.99	5.82	5.17	4.76	4.47	4.26	4.09	3.96
	.999	14.8	9.95	8.10	7.10	6.46	6.02	5.69	5.44	5.24
24	.50	0.469	0.714	0.812	0.863	0.895	0.917	0.932	0.944	0.953
	.90	2.93	2.54	2.33	2.19	2.10	2.04	1.98	1.94	1.91
	.95	4.26	3.40	3.01	2.78	2.62	2.51	2.42	2.36	2.30
	.975	5.72	4.32	3.72	3.38	3.15	2.99	2.87	2.78	2.70
	.99	7.82	5.61	4.72	4.22	3.90	3.67	3.50	3.36	3.26
	.995	9.55	6.66	5.52	4.89	4.49	4.20	3.99	3.83	3.69
	.999	14.0	9.34	7.55	6.59	5.98	5.55	5.23	4.99	4.80

Table IX.1 — Percentiles of the *F* Distribution (continued)

Den. df	A	Numerator df 10	12	15	20	24	30	60	120	∞
8	.50	1.02	1.03	1.04	1.05	1.06	1.07	1.08	1.08	1.09
	.90	2.54	2.50	2.46	2.42	2.40	2.38	2.34	2.32	2.29
	.95	3.35	3.28	3.22	3.15	3.12	3.08	3.01	2.97	2.93
	.975	4.30	4.20	4.10	4.00	3.95	3.89	3.78	3.73	3.67
	.99	5.81	5.67	5.52	5.36	5.28	5.20	5.03	4.95	4.86
	.995	7.21	7.01	6.81	6.61	6.50	6.40	6.18	6.06	5.95
	.999	11.5	11.2	10.8	10.5	10.3	10.1	9.73	9.53	9.33
9	.50	1.01	1.02	1.03	1.04	1.05	1.05	1.07	1.07	1.08
	.90	2.42	2.38	2.34	2.30	2.28	2.25	2.21	2.18	2.16
	.95	3.14	3.07	3.01	2.94	2.90	2.86	2.79	2.75	2.71
	.975	3.96	3.87	3.77	3.67	3.61	3.56	3.45	3.39	3.33
	.99	5.26	5.11	4.96	4.81	4.73	4.65	4.48	4.40	4.31
	.995	6.42	6.23	6.03	5.83	5.73	5.62	5.41	5.30	5.19
	.999	9.89	9.57	9.24	8.90	8.72	8.55	8.19	8.00	7.81
10	.50	1.00	1.01	1.02	1.03	1.04	1.05	1.06	1.06	1.07
	.90	2.32	2.28	2.24	2.20	2.18	2.16	2.11	2.08	2.06
	.95	2.98	2.91	2.84	2.77	2.74	2.70	2.62	2.58	2.54
	.975	3.72	3.62	3.52	3.42	3.37	3.31	3.20	3.14	3.08
	.99	4.85	4.71	4.56	4.41	4.33	4.25	4.08	4.00	3.91
	.995	5.85	5.66	5.47	5.27	5.17	5.07	4.86	4.75	4.64
	.999	8.75	8.45	8.13	7.80	7.64	7.47	7.12	6.94	6.76
12	.50	0.989	1.00	1.01	1.02	1.03	1.03	1.05	1.05	1.06
	.90	2.19	2.15	2.10	2.06	2.04	2.01	1.96	1.93	1.90
	.95	2.75	2.69	2.62	2.54	2.51	2.47	2.38	2.34	2.30
	.975	3.37	3.28	3.18	3.07	3.02	2.96	2.85	2.79	2.72
	.99	4.30	4.16	4.01	3.86	3.78	3.70	3.54	3.45	3.36
	.995	5.09	4.91	4.72	4.53	4.43	4.33	4.12	4.01	3.90
	.999	7.29	7.00	6.71	6.40	6.25	6.09	5.76	5.59	5.42
15	.50	0.977	0.989	1.00	1.01	1.02	1.02	1.03	1.04	1.05
	.90	2.06	2.02	1.97	1.92	1.90	1.87	1.82	1.79	1.76
	.95	2.54	2.48	2.40	2.33	2.29	2.25	2.16	2.11	2.07
	.975	3.06	2.96	2.86	2.76	2.70	2.64	2.52	2.46	2.40
	.99	3.80	3.67	3.52	3.37	3.29	3.21	3.05	2.96	2.87
	.995	4.42	4.25	4.07	3.88	3.79	3.69	3.48	3.37	3.26
	.999	6.08	5.81	5.54	5.25	5.10	4.95	4.64	4.48	4.31
20	.50	0.966	0.977	0.989	1.00	1.01	1.01	1.02	1.03	1.03
	.90	1.94	1.89	1.84	1.79	1.77	1.74	1.68	1.64	1.61
	.95	2.35	2.28	2.20	2.12	2.08	2.04	1.95	1.90	1.84
	.975	2.77	2.68	2.57	2.46	2.41	2.35	2.22	2.16	2.09
	.99	3.37	3.23	3.09	2.94	2.86	2.78	2.61	2.52	2.42
	.995	3.85	3.68	3.50	3.32	3.22	3.12	2.92	2.81	2.69
	.999	5.08	4.82	4.56	4.29	4.15	4.00	3.70	3.54	3.38
24	.50	0.961	0.972	0.983	0.994	1.00	1.01	1.02	1.02	1.03
	.90	1.88	1.83	1.78	1.73	1.70	1.67	1.61	1.57	1.53
	.95	2.25	2.18	2.11	2.03	1.98	1.94	1.84	1.79	1.73
	.975	2.64	2.54	2.44	2.33	2.27	2.21	2.08	2.01	1.94
	.99	3.17	3.03	2.89	2.74	2.66	2.58	2.40	2.31	2.21
	.995	3.59	3.42	3.25	3.06	2.97	2.87	2.66	2.55	2.43
	.999	4.64	4.39	4.14	3.87	3.74	3.59	3.29	3.14	2.97

Table IX.1 — Percentiles of the *F* Distribution (continued)

Den. df	A	Numerator df 1	2	3	4	5	6	7	8	9
30	.50	0.466	0.709	0.807	0.858	0.890	0.912	0.927	0.939	0.948
	.90	2.88	2.49	2.28	2.14	2.05	1.98	1.93	1.88	1.85
	.95	4.17	3.32	2.92	2.69	2.53	2.42	2.33	2.27	2.21
	.975	5.57	4.18	3.59	3.25	3.03	2.87	2.75	2.65	2.57
	.99	7.56	5.39	4.51	4.02	3.70	3.47	3.30	3.17	3.07
	.995	9.18	6.35	5.24	4.62	4.23	3.95	3.74	3.58	3.45
	.999	13.3	8.77	7.05	6.12	5.53	5.12	4.82	4.58	4.39
60	.50	0.461	0.701	0.798	0.849	0.880	0.901	0.917	0.928	0.937
	.90	2.79	2.39	2.18	2.04	1.95	1.87	1.82	1.77	1.74
	.95	4.00	3.15	2.76	2.53	2.37	2.25	2.17	2.10	2.04
	.975	5.29	3.93	3.34	3.01	2.79	2.63	2.51	2.41	2.33
	.99	7.08	4.98	4.13	3.65	3.34	3.12	2.95	2.82	2.72
	.995	8.49	5.80	4.73	4.14	3.76	3.49	3.29	3.13	3.01
	.999	12.0	7.77	6.17	5.31	4.76	4.37	4.09	3.86	3.69
120	.50	0.458	0.697	0.793	0.844	0.875	0.896	0.912	0.923	0.932
	.90	2.75	2.35	2.13	1.99	1.90	1.82	1.77	1.72	1.68
	.95	3.92	3.07	2.68	2.45	2.29	2.18	2.09	2.02	1.96
	.975	5.15	3.80	3.23	2.89	2.67	2.52	2.39	2.30	2.22
	.99	6.85	4.79	3.95	3.48	3.17	2.96	2.79	2.66	2.56
	.995	8.18	5.54	4.50	3.92	3.55	3.28	3.09	2.93	2.81
	.999	11.4	7.32	5.78	4.95	4.42	4.04	3.77	3.55	3.38
∞	.50	0.455	0.693	0.789	0.839	0.870	0.891	0.907	0.918	0.927
	.90	2.71	2.30	2.08	1.94	1.85	1.77	1.72	1.67	1.63
	.95	3.84	3.00	2.60	2.37	2.21	2.10	2.01	1.94	1.88
	.975	5.02	3.69	3.12	2.79	2.57	2.41	2.29	2.19	2.11
	.99	6.63	4.61	3.78	3.32	3.02	2.80	2.64	2.51	2.41
	.995	7.88	5.30	4.28	3.72	3.35	3.09	2.90	2.74	2.62
	.999	10.8	6.91	5.42	4.62	4.10	3.74	3.47	3.27	3.10

Table IX.1 — Percentiles of the *F* Distribution (continued)

Den. df	1	Numerator df 10	12	15	20	24	30	60	120	∞
30	.50	0.955	0.966	0.978	0.989	0.994	1.00	1.01	1.02	1.02
	.90	1.82	1.77	1.72	1.67	1.64	1.61	1.54	1.50	1.46
	.95	2.16	2.09	2.01	1.93	1.89	1.84	1.74	1.68	1.62
	.975	2.51	2.41	2.31	2.20	2.14	2.07	1.94	1.87	1.79
	.99	2.98	2.84	2.70	2.55	2.47	2.39	2.21	2.11	2.01
	.995	3.34	3.18	3.01	2.82	2.73	2.63	2.42	2.30	2.18
	.999	4.24	4.00	3.75	3.49	3.36	3.22	2.92	2.76	2.59
60	.50	0.945	0.956	0.967	0.978	0.983	0.989	1.00	1.01	1.01
	.90	1.71	1.66	1.60	1.54	1.51	1.48	1.40	1.35	1.29
	.95	1.99	1.92	1.84	1.75	1.70	1.65	1.53	1.47	1.39
	.975	2.27	2.17	2.06	1.94	1.88	1.82	1.67	1.58	1.48
	.99	2.63	2.50	2.35	2.20	2.12	2.03	1.84	1.73	1.60
	.995	2.90	2.74	2.57	2.39	2.29	2.19	1.96	1.83	1.69
	.999	3.54	3.32	3.08	2.83	2.69	2.55	2.25	2.08	1.89
120	.50	0.939	0.950	0.961	0.972	0.978	0.983	0.994	1.00	1.01
	.90	1.65	1.60	1.55	1.48	1.45	1.41	1.32	1.26	1.19
	.95	1.91	1.83	1.75	1.66	1.61	1.55	1.43	1.35	1.25
	.975	2.16	2.05	1.95	1.82	1.76	1.69	1.53	1.43	1.31
	.99	2.47	2.34	2.19	2.03	1.95	1.86	1.66	1.53	1.38
	.995	2.71	2.54	2.37	2.19	2.09	1.98	1.75	1.61	1.43
	.999	3.24	3.02	2.78	2.53	2.40	2.26	1.95	1.77	1.54
∞	.50	0.934	0.945	0.956	0.967	0.972	0.978	0.989	0.994	1.00
	.90	1.60	1.55	1.49	1.42	1.38	1.34	1.24	1.17	1.00
	.95	1.83	1.75	1.67	1.57	1.52	1.46	1.32	1.22	1.00
	.975	2.05	1.94	1.83	1.71	1.64	1.57	1.39	1.27	1.00
	.99	2.32	2.18	2.04	1.88	1.79	1.70	1.47	1.32	1.00
	.995	2.52	2.36	2.19	2.00	1.90	1.79	1.53	1.36	1.00
	.999	2.96	2.74	2.51	2.27	2.13	1.99	1.66	1.45	1.00

Example

The following 8-hour TWA heptane (8-hour TWA–OEL = 400 ppm) exposure measurements have been taken using the 6/3 strategy (six workers, three exposure-days per worker):

Table IX.2 — Sample Data (x_{ij})

Person 1 (ppm)	Person 2 (ppm)	Person 3 (ppm)	Person 4 (ppm)	Person 5 (ppm)	Person 6 (ppm)
124	44	239	45	43	73
63	8	94	53	32	49
274	23	114	47	97	48

Number workers: k = 6
Total number of exposure values: N = 18

Step 1. Logtransform each exposure value:

Table IX.3 — Logtransformed Sample Data (y_{ij})

Person 1	Person 2	Person 3	Person 4	Person 5	Person 6
4.82	3.78	5.48	3.81	3.76	4.29
4.14	2.08	4.54	3.97	3.47	3.89
5.61	3.14	4.74	3.85	4.58	3.87
$\Sigma = 14.57$	$\Sigma = 9.00$	$\Sigma = 14.76$	$\Sigma = 11.63$	$\Sigma = 11.81$	$\Sigma = 12.05$
$n_1 = 3$	$n_2 = 3$	$n_3 = 3$	$n_4 = 3$	$n_5 = 3$	$n_6 = 3$

Step 2. Compute the mean of each worker's logtransformed exposure values:

Table IX.4 — Mean of Logtransformed Exposure Values

Person 1	Person 2	Person 3	Person 4	Person 5	Person 6
$\bar{y}_1 = 4.86$	$\bar{y}_2 = 3.00$	$\bar{y}_3 = 4.92$	$\bar{y}_4 = 3.88$	$\bar{y}_5 = 3.94$	$\bar{y}_6 = 4.02$

Step 3. Compute the grand mean of the logtransformed exposure values:

grand mean: $\bar{y}_T = 4.10$

Step 4. Compute the within-group sum of squares (SSW):

For each worker, calculate the sum of the squared deviations of each logtransformed exposure value from the worker's mean logtransformed exposure value, $\sum_{j=1}^{3} (y_{ij} - \bar{y}_i)^2$:

Table IX.5 — Squared Deviation of Logtransformed Exposure Values

Person 1 $(y_{1j}-\overline{y}_1)^2$	*Person 2* $(y_{2j}-\overline{y}_2)^2$	*Person 3* $(y_{3j}-\overline{y}_3)^2$	*Person 4* $(y_{4j}-\overline{y}_4)^2$	*Person 5* $(y_{5j}-\overline{y}_5)^2$	*Person 6* $(y_{6j}-\overline{y}_6)^2$
0.0016	0.6084	0.3136	0.0049	0.0324	0.0729
0.5184	0.8464	0.1444	0.0081	0.2209	0.0169
0.5625	0.0196	0.0324	0.0009	0.4096	0.0225
Σ = 1.0825	Σ = 1.4744	Σ = 0.4904	Σ = 0.0139	Σ = 0.6629	Σ = 0.1123

$$SSW = \sum_{i=1}^{6} \sum_{j=1}^{3} (y_{ij} - \overline{y}_i)^2$$

$$= 1.0825 + 1.4744 + 0.4904 + 0.0139 + 0.6629 + 0.1123$$

$$= 3.8364$$

Step 5. Compute the within-group mean square (MSW):

$$MSW = SSW/(N - k) = 3.8364/(18 - 6) = 0.3197$$

Step 6. Compute the between-group sum of squares (SSB):

Table IX.6 — Number of Measurements (n) and Mean Logtransformed Exposure for Each Person

Person 1	*Person 2*	*Person 3*	*Person 4*	*Person 5*	*Person 6*
$n_1 = 3$	$n_2 = 3$	$n_3 = 3$	$n_4 = 3$	$n_5 = 3$	$n_6 = 3$
$\overline{y}_1 = 4.86$	$\overline{y}_2 = 3.00$	$\overline{y}_3 = 4.92$	$\overline{y}_4 = 3.88$	$\overline{y}_5 = 3.94$	$\overline{y}_6 = 4.02$

$$SSB = \sum_{i=1}^{6} n_i(\overline{y}_i - \overline{y}_T)^2$$

grand mean: $\overline{y}_T = 4.10$

$$SSB = 3(4.86-4.10)^2 + 3(3.00-4.10)^2 + 3(4.92-4.10)^2 + 3(3.88-4.10)^2 + 3(3.94-4.10)^2 + 3(4.02-4.10)^2$$

$$= 1.7328 + 3.63 + 2.0172 + 0.1452 + 0.0768 + 0.0192 = 7.6212$$

Step 7. Compute the between-group mean square (MSB):

$$MSB = SSB/(k - 1) = 7.6212/(6 - 1) = 1.52424$$

Step 8. Compute the F-statistic:

$$F_{v_1,v_2} = MSB/MSW = 1.52424/\ 0.3197 = 4.76772$$

where:

$v_1 = k - 1 = 6 - 1 = 5$

$v_2 = N - k = 18 - 6 = 12$

Step 9. Compare to the critical F value from Table IX.1:

- Tabled $F_{0.95,\,5,\,12} = 3.11$ vs. Calculated $F_{5,\,12} = 4.76772$
- Calculated $F_{5,\,12} >$ Tabled $F_{0.95,\,5,\,12}$
- Therefore, conclude that there is significant exposure variability between workers.

Step 10. Estimate the GSD for within-worker variability in 8-hour TWA heptane exposure levels:

$$\widehat{GSD[W]} = \exp(\sqrt{MSW}) = \exp(\sqrt{0.3197}) = 1.76$$

- Estimate the GSD for between-worker variability in LTA heptane exposure levels:

$$\widehat{GSD[B]} = \exp\left(\sqrt{\frac{MSB - MSW}{n_O}}\right) = \exp\left(\sqrt{\frac{1.5242 - 0.3197}{3}}\right) = 1.88$$

- Estimate the group grand mean LTA exposure level:

$$\hat{u} = [\exp(\bar{y}_T)]\left[\exp\left(\frac{\ln^2\widehat{GSD[W]} + \ln^2\widehat{GSD[B]}}{2}\right)\right]$$

$$= [\exp(4.1)]\left[\exp\left(\frac{\ln^2 1.76 + \ln^2 1.88}{2}\right)\right] =$$

$$(60.3)(1.43) = 86.3 \text{ ppm}$$

This is an estimate of the arithmetic mean of the SEG. See Appendix VI for a discussion of other statistical methods for examining the arithmetic mean of an SEG exposure profile.

Table IX.7 — ANOVA: Single Factor

Summary

Groups	*Count*	*Sum*	*Average*	*Variance*
Person 1	3	14.57654	4.85884813	0.541336
Person 2	3	8.999125	2.99970846	0.74037
Person 3	3	14.75596	4.91865226	0.242668
Person 4	3	11.6271	3.87570067	0.007183
Person 5	3	11.80165	3.93388233	0.329821
Person 6	3	12.05348	4.01782692	0.055853

ANOVA

Source of variation	*SS*	*df*	*MS*	*F*	*P-value*	*F critical*
Between groups	7.624013	5	1.52480256	4.771892	0.012417	3.105875
Within groups	3.834461	12	0.31953839			
Total	11.45847	17				

NOTE: For users of Microsoft Excel®, the results shown in Table IX.7 were calculated for the same logtransformed data based on Excel's single-factor ANOVA function.

Discussion

Based on the results of the ANOVA analysis in the example above, we would conclude that workers in the group have significantly different mean exposure levels. We reach this conclusion because the calculated F-statistic (4.77) is greater than the critical F from Table IX.1 (3.11). Given an estimated GSD[B] of 1.88, there is a 12-fold range in the value of the mean exposure level among workers at the low and high ends of the SEG. [Note that if the GSD equals 1.88, the ratio of the values of the 97.5th percentile and the 2.5th percentile is 12.]

Significant variability in average exposures indicates that the workers might have been improperly grouped into an SEG. The SEG should be examined carefully, through observation or additional monitoring, to determine how workers might be reapportioned to two or more SEGs that would have low between-worker variability. Note that in many cases the refinement of SEGs might not be straightforward. Remember that the workers and days for monitoring were chosen randomly from a larger population of workers in the SEG. It may be quite difficult to determine how the SEG should be reapportioned without closer observation or significant further monitoring of additional workers.

As new information is gathered, workers may be placed into more homogeneous SEGs. The same ANOVA techniques can be used to compare the between-worker variability to the within-worker variability for those new SEGs.

References

1. **Oldham, P.D., and S.A. Roach:** A Sampling Procedure for Measuring Industrial Dust Exposure. *Br. J. Ind. Med. 9:*112-119 (1952).
2. **Dowdy, S., and S. Wearden:** *Statistics for Research.* New York: John Wiley & Sons, 1983.
3. **Neter, J., W. Wasserman, and M.H. Kutner:** *Applied Linear Statistical Models,* 3rd Ed. Homewood, Ill.: Richard D. Irwin, Inc., 1990.

Appendix X

Control Chart Analysis

The Objective of Control Chart Analysis

Control chart analysis is a statistical method used to evaluate whether a population of some variable is in "statistical control" (i.e., it does not change over time). As discussed in Chapter 7 (interpretation, decision making, and statistical tools) the assumption of a "stationary" population distribution is a fundamental aspect of performing most statistical tests.

Control charts may be applied to exposure data, concentration data, noise data, or contamination level data to make inferences on whether the population is in statistical control (i.e., stationary). They can also be used as a semiquantitative visual tool to examine trends over time and to demonstrate magnitudes of these variables relative to past levels or to some standard.

The process is in "statistical control" when repeated samples from the defined population behave as random samples from a stationary population distribution. The tools for using control charts rely exclusively on the sampled data. For control chart analysis, the assumption of randomly collected samples is again central to the analysis.

Information to Be Learned from Control Charts

Control charts provide a running graphical record of small subgroups of randomly collected data from the defined population. Several types of control charts can be applied:

- Average (or mean) chart;
- Range chart (surrogate for standard deviation); and
- Attribute chart (e.g., percent of exposure over the OEL; not covered in detail in this book).

Each chart provides unique information. The most commonly applied control chart methods use the mean and range charts on the same data sets. The mean chart provides indications of gross blunders (e.g., outliers), shifts in average exposure, slow trends over time, etc. The range chart provides some information on gross blunders (e.g., outliers), but it is most effective in helping to identify shifts in variability and fast fluctuations (cycles in the process).

Calculation of Control Chart Parameters

The calculation of control chart parameters is rather straightforward. A typical data set suited for control analysis has the following characteristics:

k sampling campaigns each of *n* random samples from the population.

Typically *n* may be from 5 to 10 samples. From this data set, the calculation of parameters follows these steps:

1. The sample mean and sample range for each of the *k* campaigns should be calculated.

$$\bar{X}_k = \sum_{i=1}^{n} X_{i,k}/n \qquad (1)$$

$$R_k = X_{max,k} - X_{min,k} \qquad (2)$$

2. The grand mean should be calculated by averaging the means of all k campaigns.

$$\bar{\bar{X}} = \sum_{i=1}^{k} \bar{X}_i \,/k \qquad (3)$$

3. The sample average range from the k campaigns should be calculated.

$$\bar{R} = \sum_{i=1}^{k} R_i \,/k \qquad (4)$$

4. The mean chart is drawn with the grand mean as centerline and the upper and lower confidence limits are calculated as follows using constants from a control chart table of control chart constants (see Table X.1).

$$\text{Centerline} = \bar{\bar{X}} \qquad (5)$$

$$UCL = \bar{\bar{X}} + A_2\bar{R} \quad (6)$$

$$LCL = \bar{\bar{X}} - A_2\bar{R} \quad (7)$$

$$A_2 = \frac{3}{d_2\sqrt{n}} \quad (8)$$

5. The range chart is constructed using the average range as the centerline and using the following equations and table constants to construct the upper and lower control limits.

$$\text{Centerline} = \bar{R} \quad (9)$$

$$UCL = D_4\bar{R} \quad (10)$$

$$LCL = D_3\bar{R} \quad (11)$$

6. Once the graphs have been drawn for the mean and range, the parameter estimates (mean and range) from each of the *k* campaigns should be plotted sequentially (vs. time). One should examine the plotted points on the chart to determine whether all points fall within the control limits. If they do not, some investigation of those that do not might be needed. The goal is to establish the baseline stationary distribution — there might be a need to omit outliers from the baseline data set.
7. New data sets of size *n* should have their means and ranges plotted on the chart sequentially. Do these new points fall within the control limits? If they do, one may decide that the process is in statistical control. If not, the outliers should be investigated. In many cases, values falling outside the control limits indicate that the process may be out of control, necessitating action to correct problems (e.g., if exposures are trending higher), or it may indicate that a new baseline is needed because the original data are no longer representative of the process.

Example

An example of control chart analysis of a given set of wipe testing data is provided here. These data, given in Table X.2, represent micrograms of agent per 100 cm^2 area wiped (standard procedures followed). There are seven campaigns each consisting of seven samples. The sample mean and range are calculated for each campaign as well as the grand mean and the

Table X.1 — Control Chart Constants[A]

	$\bar{X}$ Chart	R Chart		
	Factors for Control Limits	Factors for Central Line	Factors for Control Limits	
n^B	A_2^C	d_2^D	D_3^E	D_4^F
2	1.880	1.128	0	3.267
3	1.023	1.693	0	2.575
4	0.729	2.059	0	2.282
5	0.577	2.326	0	2.115
6	0.483	2.534	0	2.004
7	0.419	2.704	0.076	1.924
8	0.373	2.847	0.136	1.864
9	0.337	2.970	0.184	1.816
10	0.308	3.078	0.223	1.777
11	0.285	3.173	0.256	1.744
12	0.266	3.258	0.284	1.716
13	0.249	3.336	0.308	1.692
14	0.235	3.407	0.329	1.671
15	0.223	3.472	0.348	1.652
16	0.212	3.532	0.364	1.636
17	0.203	3.588	0.379	1.621
18	0.194	3.640	0.392	1.608
19	0.187	3.689	0.404	1.596
20	0.180	3.735	0.414	1.586
21	0.173	3.778	0.425	1.575
22	0.167	3.819	0.434	1.566
23	0.162	3.858	0.443	1.557
24	0.157	3.895	0.452	1.548
25	0.153	3.931	0.459	1.541

[A] Adapted from **National Bureau of Standards:** Experimental Statistics. In *National Bureau of Standards Handbook 91.* Washington, D.C.: National Bureau of Standards, 1996.
[B] n = Number of samples in a campaign.
[C] A_2 = Upper confidence limit and lower confidence limit factors for mean chart.
[D] d_2 = Factor for centerline.
[E] D_3 = Lower confidence limit factor for range chart.
[F] D_4 = Upper confidence limit factor for range chart.

average range. These summary parameters are combined as follows to find the parameters of the mean chart and range chart. The control chart parameters, centerline, UCL, and LCL are plotted for the mean chart and range chart (see Figures X.1 and X.2, respectively). Sample mean and range values should be plotted sequentially after the control charts are constructed.

$\bar{X}$ Chart: Centerline = 29.2 µg
UCL = 29.2 + (0.419) (61.3) = 54.9 µg
LCL = 29.2 - (0.419) (61.3) = 3.5 µg

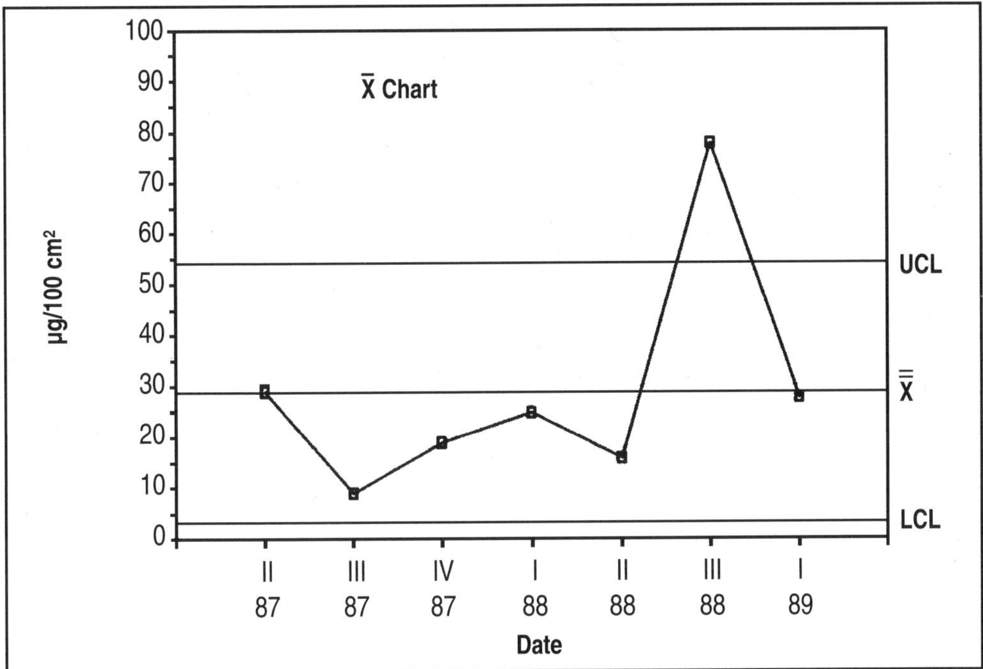

Figure X.1 — Mean chart developed as an example of control chart analysis of a given set of wipe-testing data.

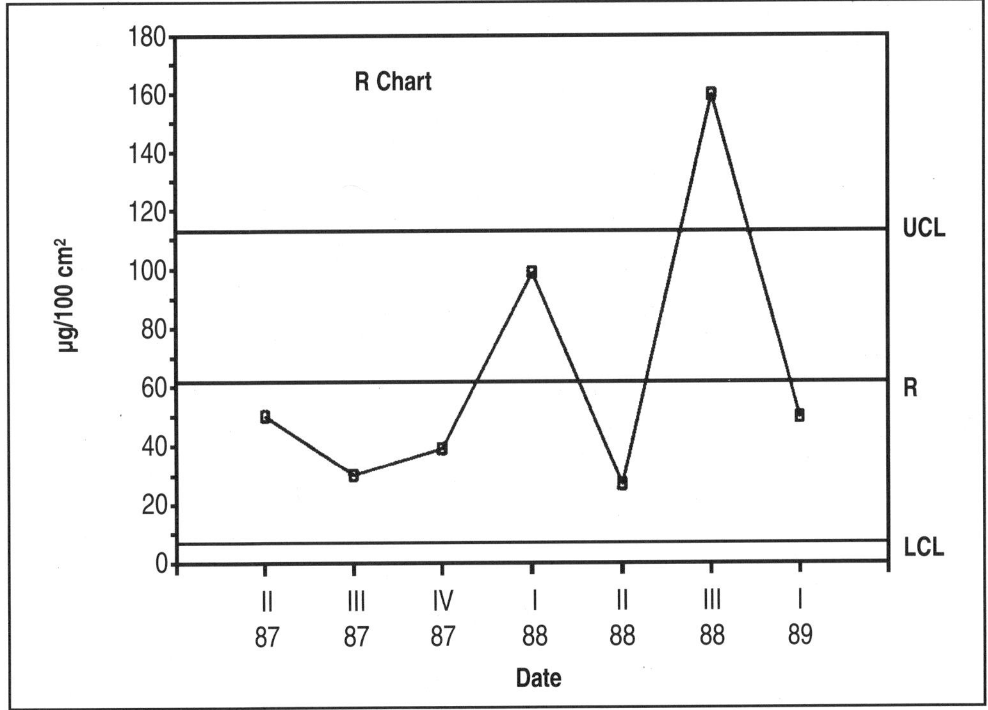

Figure X.2 — Range chart developed as an example of control chart analysis of a given set of wipe-testing data.

Table X.2 — Example Wipe Test Data for Control Chart Analysis

	Agent on wipe (µg)						
Quarter	*II*	*III*	*IV*	*I*	*II*	*IV*	*I*
Year	*'87*	*'87*	*'87*	*'88*	*'88*	*'88*	*'89*
Lunchroom	21	7	3.4	8	12.7	30.2	27.5
Engineer's office	49	9	38	50.5	4.4	112	33.5
Women's locker room	0.8	0.21	0.71	2.8	21.5	9.3	8.28
Lab	50	6.6	20	4.4	27.6	119	55.4
Lab office	29	5	23	3.0	12.7	56	19.9
Control room	44	23	18	98.9	8.2	77.1	37.3
Men's locker room	7.7	6.3	13.4	15.2	20.6	163	18.1
$\bar{X}$	28.8	8.2	16.6	26.1	15.4	80.9	28.6
R	49.2	22.8	37.3	95.9	23.2	153.7	47.1

$\bar{\bar{X}}$ = 29.2 µg

$\bar{R}$ = 61.3 µg

R Chart: Centerline = 61.3 µg
UCL = 1.924 (61.3) = 117.9 µg
LCL = 0.076 (61.3) = 4.7 µg

A review of these mean and range control charts indicates that the sample collected during the fourth quarter of 1988 was probably an outlier. Housekeeping was found to be poor around that period, elevating all wipe testing points. Changes were recommended in housekeeping practices as a control measure. This date's sample should not be used in recalculating the control chart values, and the remaining six campaigns should serve as the baseline for the future wipe test results.

Conclusion

An overview of control chart analysis was provided in this appendix. Experience and judgment is essential for control charting to be applied and interpreted properly.

References

1. **Hawkins, N.C., and B.D. Landenberger:** Statistical Control Charts: A Technique for Analyzing Industrial Hygiene Data. *Appl. Occup. Environ. Hyg. 6(8)*:689–795 (1991).

Appendix XI

Bibliography

EXPOSURE ASSESSMENT STRATEGIES

American Conference of Governmental Industrial Hygienists: *Topics in Biological Monitoring*. Cincinnati, Ohio: American Conference of Governmental Industrial Hygienists, 1996.

Blome, H.: Editorial: Workplace Assessment. *Ann. Occup. Hyg. 38(1)*:1-2 (1994).

Bonorden, J.: "Exposure Assessment Strategies Implementation: Hurdling the Barriers." Roundtable presentation at American Industrial Hygiene Conference & Exposition, Washington, D.C., May 22, 1996.

Booher, L.E.: "Exposure Assessment — Hurdling the Barriers." Paper presented at the American Industrial Hygiene Conference & Exposition, Washington, D.C., May 1996.

Burmaster, D.E., and K. von Stackelberg: Using Monte Carlo Simulations in Public Health Risk Assessment: Estimating and Presenting Full Distributions of Risk. *J. Expos. Anal. Environ. Epidem. 1*:491-512.

Burmaster, D.E., and R.H. Harris: The Magnitude of Compounding Conservatisms in Superfund Risk Assessments. *Risk Analysis 13(2)*:131 (1993).

Claycamp, H.G.: Commentary — Industrial Health Risk Assessment: Industrial Hygiene for Technology Transition. *Am. Ind. Hyg. Assoc. J. 57(5)*:423-427 (1996).

Damiano, J.: Quantitative Exposure Assessment Strategies and Data in the Aluminum Company of America. *Appl. Occup. Environ. Hyg. 10(4)*:289-298 (1995).

Hawkins, N.C., and J.S. Evans: Subjective Estimation of Toluene Exposures: A Calibration Study. *Appl. Ind. Hyg. 4*:61-68 (1989).

Hawkins, N.C., M.A. Jayjock, and J. Lynch: A Rationale Framework for Establishing the Quality of Human Exposure Assessment. *Am. Ind. Hyg. Assoc. J. 53(1):*34-41 (1992).

Hawkins, N.C., S.K. Norwood, and J.C. Rock: *A Strategy for Occupational Exposure Assessment.* Akron, Ohio: American Industrial Hygiene Association, 1991.

Heederik, D., and F. Hurley: Workshop Summary — Occupational Exposure Assessments: Investigating Why Exposure Measurements Vary. *Appl. Occup. Environ. Hyg. 9(1):*71-73 (1994).

Jayjock, M.A.: Assessment of Inhalation Exposure Potential from Vapors in the Workplace. *Am. Ind. Hyg. Assoc. J. 49(8):*380-385 (1988).

Jayjock, M.A.: Uncertainty Analysis in the Estimation of Exposure. *Am. Ind. Hyg. Assoc. J. 58(5):*380-382 (1997).

Norwood, S.K., M.G. Ott, C.N. Park, and G.C. van Beck: "Optimizing Sampling Strategies by Combining Traditional and Statistical Approaches." Paper presented at the American Industrial Hygiene Conference, Philadelphia, Pa., May 1983.

Rappaport, S.M.: Assessments of Long-Term Exposures to Toxic Substances in Air. *Ann. Occup. Hyg. 35(1):*61-121 (1991).

Rappaport, S.M., R.C. Spear, and J.W. Yager: Industrial Hygiene Data: Compliance, Dosage and Clinical Relevance. *West. J. Med. 137:*572-576 (1982).

Roach, S.A.: A Commentary on the December 1986 Workshop on Strategies for Measuring Exposure. *Am. Ind. Hyg. Assoc. J. 48(12):*A-322–A-332 (1987).

Roach, S.: *Health Risks from Hazardous Substances at Work — Assessment, Evaluation, and Control.* New York: Pergamon Press, 1992.

Roach. S.A.: A More Rational Basis for Air Sampling Programs. *Am. Ind. Hyg. Assoc. J. 27(1):*1-12 (1966).

Roach, S.A.: A Most Rational Basis for Air Sampling Programmes. *Ann. Occup. Hyg. 20:*65-84 (1977).

Rock, J.C.: Can Professional Judgment be Quantified? *Am. Ind. Hyg. Assoc. J. 47(6):*A-370 (1986).

Tait, K.: The Workplace Exposure Assessment Expert System (WORKSPERT). *Am. Ind. Hyg. Assoc. J. 53(2):*84-98 (1992).

Tait, K.: The Workplace Exposure Assessment Workbook. *Appl. Occup. Environ. Hyg. 8(1):*55-68 (1993).

Thompson, K.M., D.E. Burmaster, and E.A.C. Crouch: Monte Carlo Techniques for Quantitative Uncertainty

Analysis in Public Health Risk Assessments. *Risk Analysis 12:*53-63 (1992).

Wass, T.L.: "An Approach to the Process Characterization — Exposure Risk Assessment and Prioritization." Paper presented at the American Industrial Hygiene Conference & Exposition, Kansas City, Mo., May 1995.

GROUPING OF WORKERS

Cole, C.J.: Letter to the Editor. *Am. Ind. Hyg. Assoc. J. 55(9):*874-875 (1994).

Corn, M., and N.A. Esmen: Workplace Exposure Zones for Classification of Employee Exposures to Physical and Chemical Agents. *Am. Ind. Hyg. Assoc. J. 40(1):*47-54 (1979).

Gómez, M.R.: Letter to the Editor. *Am. Ind. Hyg. Assoc. J. 55(9):*875 (1994).

Kromhout, H., E. Symanski, and S.M. Rappaport: A Comprehensive Evaluation of Within- and Between-Worker Components of Occupational Exposure to Chemical Agents. *Ann. Occup. Hyg. 37:*253-270 (1993).

Rappaport, S.M.: Letter to the Editor. *Am. Ind. Hyg. Assoc. J. 55(9):*875-877 (1994).

Rappaport, S. M., H. Kromhout, and E. Symanski: Variation of Exposure Between Workers in Homogeneous Exposure Groups. *Am. Ind. Hyg. Assoc. J. 54(11):*654-662 (1993).

Rappaport, S.M., R.H. Lyles, and L.L. Kupper: An Exposure Assessment Strategy Accounting for Within- and Between-Worker Sources of Variability. *Ann. Occup. Hyg. 39:*469-495 (1995).

Scheffers, T.M.L.: Letter to the Editor. *Am. Ind. Hyg. Assoc. J. 55(9):*873-874 (1994).

SAMPLING STRATEGIES

Ayer, H.E.: Occupational Air Sampling Strategies. In *Air Sampling Instruments for Evaluation of Atmospheric Contaminants*, 7th Ed. (S.V. Hering, editor). Cincinnati, Ohio: American Conference of Governmental Industrial Hygienists, 1989.

British Occupational Hygiene Society: *Sampling Strategies for Airborne Contaminants in the Workplace* (Technical Guide No. 11) by I.G. Guest, J.W. Chessie, R.J. Gardner, and C.D. Money. Leeds, United Kingdom: H & H Scientific Consultants Ltd., 1993.

Buringh, E., and R. Lanting: Exposure Variability in the Workplace: Its Implications for the Assessment of Compliance. *Am. Ind. Hyg. Assoc. J. 52(1):*6-13 (1991).

Busch, K.A., and N.A. Leidel: Statistical Models for Occupational Exposure Measurements and Decision Making. In *Advances in Air Sampling*. Chelsea, Mich.: Lewis Publishers, 1988.

Corn, M.: Sampling Strategies for Prospective Surveillance: Overview and Future Directions. In *Advances in Air Sampling*. Chelsea, Mich.: Lewis Publishers, 1988.

Corn, M.: Strategies in Air Sampling. *Scand. J. Work, Environ. Health 11:*173-180 (1985).

Damiano, J.: A Guideline for Managing the Industrial Hygiene Sampling Function. *Am. Ind. Hyg. Assoc. J. 50(7):*366-371 (1989).

Gilbert, R.O.: *Statistical Methods for Environmental Pollution Monitoring.* New York: Van Nostrand Reinhold, 1987.

Leidel, N.A., K.A. Busch, and J.R. Lynch: *Occupational Exposure Sampling Strategy Manual* (DHEW [NIOSH] Pub. No. 77–173). Cincinnati, Ohio: National Institute for Occupational Safety and Health, 1977. [National Technical Information Service (NTIS) Pub. No. PB274792.]

Leidel, N.A., and K.A. Busch: Statistical Design and Data Analysis Requirements. In *Patty's Industrial Hygiene and Toxicology,* 3rd Ed., Vol. 3A (R.L. Harris, L.J. Cralley, and L.V. Cralley, editors). New York: John Wiley & Sons, 1994.

Lyles, R.H., and L.L. Kupper: On Strategies for Comparing Occupational Exposure Data to Limits. *Am. Ind. Hyg. Assoc. J. 57(1):*6-15 (1996).

Lynch, J.R.: Measurement of Worker Exposure. In *Patty's Industrial Hygiene and Toxicology,* 3rd Ed., Vol. 3A (R.L. Harris, L.J. Cralley, and L.V. Cralley, editors). New York: John Wiley & Sons, 1994.

Nicas, M., and R.C. Spear: A Task-Based Statistical Model of a Worker's Exposure Distribution: Part I — Description of the Model. *Am. Ind. Hyg. Assoc. J. 54(5):*211-220 (1993).

Nicas, M., and R.C. Spear: A Task-Based Statistical Model of a Worker's Exposure Distribution: Part II — Application to Sampling Strategy. *Am. Ind. Hyg. Assoc. J. 54(5):*221-227 (1993).

Rappaport, S.M.: Biological Considerations for Designing Sampling Strategies. In *Advances in Air Sampling*. Chelsea, Mich.: Lewis Publishers, 1988.

Rappaport, S.M., R.H. Lyles, and L.L. Kupper: An Exposure Assessment Strategy Accounting for Within- and Between-Worker Sources of Variability. *Ann. Occup. Hyg. 39:*469-495 (1995).

Rappaport, S.M, S. Selvin, and S.A. Roach: A Strategy for Assessing Exposures with Reference to Multiple Limits. *Appl. Ind. Hyg. 3:*310-315 (1988).

Rappaport, S.M., S. Selvin, R.C. Spear, and C. Keil: Air Sampling in the Assessment of Continuous Exposures to Acutely-Toxic Chemicals: Part I – Strategy. *Am. Ind. Hyg. Assoc. J. 42(11):*831-838 (1981).

Roach, S.A.: Alternate Ways of Monitoring Occupational Exposure. In *Exposure Assessment for Epidemiology and Hazard Control* (S.M. Rappaport and T.J. Smith, editors). Chelsea, Mich.: Lewis Publishers, 1990.

Rock, J.C.: Occupational Air Sampling Strategies. In *Air Sampling Instruments for Evaluation of Atmospheric Contaminants,* 8th Ed. (B.S. Cohen and S.V. Hering, editors). Cincinnati, Ohio: American Conference of Governmental Industrial Hygienists, 1995.

Soule, R.D.: Industrial Hygiene Sampling and Analysis. In *Patty's Industrial Hygiene and Toxicology,* 3rd Ed., Vol. 1 (G.D. Clayton and F.E. Clayton, editors). New York: John Wiley & Sons, 1978.

Still, K.R., and B. Wells: Quantitative Industrial Hygiene Programs: Workplace Monitoring. *Appl. Ind. Hyg. 4:*F-14–F-17 (1989).

Symanski, E., and S.M. Rappaport: An Investigation of the Dependence of Exposure Variability on the Interval Between Measurements. *Ann. Occup. Hyg. 38:*361-372 (1994).

Tuggle, R.M.: "A General Look at Action Levels." [Extended Abstract 75.] Paper presented at the American Industrial Hygiene Conference, St. Louis, Mo., May 1989.

Tuggle, R.M.: The NIOSH Decision Scheme. *Am. Ind. Hyg. Assoc. J. 42(7):*493-498 (1981).

Waters, M., S. Selvin, and S.M. Rappaport: "A Strategy Focussed Upon Exposures Received by Groups of Workers." [Extended Abstract 74.] Paper presented at The Workplace Exposure Assessment Strategies Session at the American Industrial Hygiene Conference, St. Louis, Mo., May 1989.

GOVERNMENT STANDARDS

American Industrial Hygiene Association: White Paper — A Generic Exposure Assessment Standard. *Am. Ind. Hyg. Assoc. J. 55(11):*1009-1012 (1994).

Australia National Occupational Health and Safety Commission: *Control of Workplace Hazardous Substances.*

Canberra, Australia: Australian Government Publishing Service, 1993.

Brief, R.S., and A.R. Jones: A Statistical Technique for Determining Compliance with Dual Hygienic Standards. *Am. Ind. Hyg. Assoc. J. 37(8):*474-478 (1976).

Comité Européen de Normalisation: *Workplace Atmospheres — General Requirements for the Performance of Procedures for Workplace Environment* (EN 482). Brussels, Belgium: Comité Européen de Normalisation, 1994.

Comité Européen de Normalisation: *Workplace Atmospheres — Guidance for the Assessment of Exposure by Inhalation to Chemical Agents for Comparison with Limit Values and Measurement Strategy* (EN 689). Brussels, Belgium: Comité Européen de Normalisation, 1995.

European Commission: "Vinyl Chloride Directive." 1978.

"Federal Mine Safety and Health Act of 1977 (FMSHAct)." Public Law 91–173 (1977).

"Formaldehyde — Appendix B," Title 29 *Code of Federal Regulations* Part 1910.1048. 1994.

"Generic Standard for Exposure Monitoring — Advance Notice of Proposed Rulemaking," *Federal Register 53:*37591-37598 (September 27, 1988).

National Institute for Occupational Safety and Health: *Criteria for a Recommended Standard — Occupational Exposure to Respirable Coal Mine Dust* (DHHS [NIOSH] Pub. No. 95–106). Cincinnati, Ohio: National Institute for Occupational Safety and Health, 1995.

"Occupational Exposure to Benzene; Final Rule." *Federal Register 52(176):*34460-34578 (1987).

"Occupational Exposure to Lead; Final Standard," *Federal Register 43(220):*52952-53014 (1978).

"The Occupational Safety and Health Act." Public Law 91–596. 91st Congress, S. 2193 (29 December 1970).

Occupational Safety and Health Administration: *OSHA Technical Manual.* Washington, D.C.: U.S. Government Printing Office, 1995.

Organization Resources Counselors, Inc.: *A Proposed Generic Workplace Exposure Assessment Standard.* Washington, D.C.: Organization Resources Counselors, Inc., 1992.

Rappaport, S.M.: The Rules of the Game: An Analysis of OSHA's Enforcement Strategy. *Am. J. Ind. Med. 6:*291-303 (1984).

Rock, J.C.: A Comparison Between OSHA-Compliance Criteria and Action-Level Decision Criteria. *Am. Ind. Hyg. Assoc. J. 43(5):*297-313 (1982).

Tait, K.: A Commentary on the AIHA Position Statement and White Paper on a Generic Exposure Assessment Standard. *Am. Ind. Hyg. Assoc. J. 55(11):*1014-1018 (1994).

United Kingdom Health and Safety Executive: *The Control of Substances Hazardous to Health (COSHH) Regulations and Approved Codes of Practice.* London: Her Majesty's Stationery Office Publications Centre, 1988.

United Kingdom Health and Safety Executive: *VCM and You.* London: Her Majesty's Stationary Office Publications Centre, 1988.

OCCUPATIONAL EXPOSURE LIMITS

American Conference of Governmental Industrial Hygienists: *Documentation of the Threshold Limit Values and Biological Exposure Indices.* Cincinnati, Ohio: American Conference of Governmental Industrial Hygienists. [Published annually.]

American Conference of Governmental Industrial Hygienists: *Threshold Limit Values (TLVs™) for Chemical Substances and Physical Agents and Biological Exposure Indices (BEIs™).* Cincinnati, Ohio: American Conference of Governmental Industrial Hygienists. [Published annually.]

American Industrial Hygiene Association: *Workplace Environmental Exposure Level (WEEL) Guides.* Fairfax, Va.: American Industrial Hygiene Association. [Published annually.]

Atherley, G.: A Critical Review of Time-Weighted Average as an Index of Exposure and Dose, and Its Key Elements. *Am. Ind. Hyg. Assoc. J. 46(9):*481-487 (1985).

Brief, R.S., and R.A. Scala: Occupational Exposure Limits for Novel Work Schedules. *Am. Ind. Hyg. Assoc. J. 36(6):*467-469 (1975).

Brief, R.S., and R.A. Scala: Occupational Health Aspects of Unusual Work Schedules: A Review of Exxon's Experiences. *Am. Ind. Hyg. Assoc. J. 47(4):*199-202 (1986).

Fairhurst, S.: The Uncertainty Factor in Setting of Occupational Exposure Standards. *Ann. Occup. Hyg. 39(3):*375-385 (1995).

Klaassen, C.D. (ed.): *Casarett and Doull's Toxicology — The Basic Science of Poisons,* 5th Ed. New York: McGraw-Hill, 1996.

Koizumi, A., T. Sekiguchi, M. Konno, and M. Ikeda: Evaluation of the Time Weighted Average of Air Contaminants with Special References to Concentration

Fluctuation and Biological Half Time. *Am. Ind. Hyg. Assoc. J. 41(10):*693-699 (1980).

Naumann, B.D., E.V. Sargent, B.S. Starkman, W.J. Fraser, G.T. Becker, and G.D. Kirk: Performance-Based Exposure Control Limits for Pharmaceutical Active Ingredients. *Am. Ind. Hyg. Assoc. J. 57(1):*33-42 (1996).

Paustenbach, D.J.: Occupational Exposure Limits, Pharmacokinetics, and Unusual Work Schedules. In *Patty's Industrial Hygiene and Toxicology,* 3rd Ed., Vol. 3A (R.L. Harris, L.J. Cralley, and L.V. Cralley, editors). New York: John Wiley & Sons, 1994.

Rappaport, S.M.: Smoothing of Exposure Variability at the Receptor: Implications for Health Standards. *Ann. Occup. Hyg. 29:*201-214 (1985).

Rappaport, S.M., R.C. Spear, and S. Selvin: The Influence of Exposure Variability on Dose Response Relationships. In *Inhaled Particles.* Oxford, United Kingdom: Pergammon Press, 1988. pp. 529-537.

Rekus, J.F.: The Real Meaning of Threshold Limit Values. *Occup. Haz.:*45-47 (June 1996).

Roach, S.A., and S.M. Rappaport: But They Are Not Thresholds: A Critical Analysis of the Documentation of Threshold Limit Values. *Am. J. Ind. Med. 17:*727-753 (1990).

Stokinger, H.E.: Intended Use and Application of the TLVs. In *Transactions of the Thirty-third Annual Meeting of the American Conference of Governmental Industrial Hygienists 33:*113-116 (1971).

Stokinger, H.E.: Threshold Limit Values. *Dang. Prop. Ind. Mater. Rep.:*8-13 (May/June 1981).

U.S. Environmental Protection Agency: *Guidelines for Reproductive Toxicity Risk Assessment* (EPA 630/4–96/00). Washington, D.C.: U.S. Environmental Protection Agency/Office of Research and Development, 1996.

STATISTICAL ANALYSIS

Aitchison, J., and J.A.C. Brown: *The Lognormal Distribution with Special Reference to its Uses in Economics.* Cambridge, United Kingdom: Cambridge University Press, 1957.

Armstrong, B.G.: Confidence Intervals for Arithmetic Means of Lognormally Distributed Exposures. *Am. Ind. Hyg. Assoc. J. 53(8):*481-485 (1992).

Attfield, M.D., and P. Hewett: Exact Expressions for the Bias and Variance of Estimators of the Mean of a Lognormal Distribution. *Am. Ind. Hyg. Assoc. J. 53(7):*432-435 (1992).

Brief, R.S., and A.R. Jones: A Statistical Technique for Determining Compliance with Dual Hygienic Standards. *Am. Ind. Hyg. Assoc. J. 37(8):*474-478 (1976).

Buringh, E., and R. Lanting: Exposure Variability in the Workplace: Its Implications for the Assessment of Compliance. *Am. Ind. Hyg. Assoc. J. 52(1):*6-13 (1991).

Cohen, A.C.: Tables for Maximum Likelihood Estimates: Singly Truncated and Singly Censored Samples. *Technometrics 3:*535-541 (1961).

Dewell, P.: *British Occupational Hygiene Society Technical Handbook No. 1: Some Applications of Statistics in Occupational Hygiene.* Leeds, United Kingdom: Science Reviews Ltd./H & H Scientific Consultants, 1989.

Dowdy, S., and S. Wearden: *Statistics for Research.* New York: John Wiley & Sons, 1983.

DuPont Company: *LOGAN — Workplace Exposure Evaluation Sytem User's Manual.* Newark, Del.: E.I. du Pont de Nemours & Co., 1990.

Esmen, N.A., and Y.Y. Hammad: Log-normality of Environmental Sampling Data. *J. Environ. Sci. Health A12(1&2):*29-41 (1977).

Esmen, N.A.: Mathematical Basis for an Efficient Sampling Strategy. In *Aerosols in the Mining and Industrial Work Environment*, Vol. I (V.A. Marple and B.Y.U. Liu, editors). 1983.

Esmen, N.A.: A Distribution-Free Double-Sampling Method for Exposure Assessment. *Appl. Occup. Environ. Hyg. 7:*613-621 (1992).

Evans, J.S., and N.C. Hawkins: The Distribution of Student's t-Statistic for Small Samples from Lognormal Exposure Distributions. *Am. Ind. Hyg. Assoc. J. 49(10):*512-515 (1988).

Filliben, J.J.: The Probability Plot Correlation Coefficient Test for Normality. *Technometrics 17:*111-117 (1975). [See **Looney, S.W., and T.R. Gulledge:** Use of the Correlation Coefficient with Normal Probability Plots. *Am. Statist. 39:*75-79 (1985) for an improved procedure.]

Francis, M., S. Selvin, R. Spear, and S. Rappaport: The Effect of Autocorrelation on the Estimation of Workers' Daily Exposures. *Am. Ind. Hyg. Assoc. J. 50(1):*37-43 (1989).

George, D.K., M.R. Flynn, and R.L. Harris: Autocorrelation of Interday Exposures at an Automobile Assembly Plant. *Am. Ind. Hyg. Assoc. J. 56(12):*1187-1194 (1995).

Gómez, M.R., and G. Rawls: Conference on Occupational Exposure Databases: A Report and Look at the Future. *Appl. Occup. Envir. Hyg. 10:*238-243 (1995).

Hawkins, N.C., and B.D. Landenberger: Statistical Control Charts: A Technique for Analyzing Industrial Hygiene Data. *Appl. Occup. Envir. Hyg. 6(8):*689-695 (1991).

Hewett, P.: Sample Size Formulae for Estimating the True Arithmetic or Geometric Mean of Lognormal Exposure Distributions. *Am. Ind. Hyg. Assoc. J. 56(3):*219-225 (1995).

Hewett, P., and G.H. Ganser: Simple Procedures for Calculating Confidence Intervals Around the Sample Mean and Exceedance Fraction Derived from Lognormally Distributed Data. *Appl. Occup. Environ. Hyg. 12(2):*132-142 (1997).

Hornung, R.W., and L.D. Reed: Estimation of Average Concentration in the Presence of Nondetectable Values. *Appl. Occup. Environ. Hyg. 5(1):*46-51 (1990).

Kumagai, S., and I. Matsunaga: Changes in the Distribution of Short-Term Exposure Concentrations with Different Averaging Times. *Am. Ind. Hyg. Assoc. J. 56(1):*24-31 (1995).

Kumagai, S., I. Matsunaga, and Y. Kusakai: Autocorrelation of Short-Term and Daily Average Exposure Levels in Workplaces. *Am. Ind. Hyg. Assoc. J. 54(7):*341-350 (1993).

Land, C.E.: Tables of Confidence Limits for Linear Functions of the Normal Mean and Variance. In *Selected Tables in Mathematical Statistics*, Vol. III (H. Harter and D. Owen, editors). 1975. pp. 385-419.

Leidel, N.A., and K.A. Busch: Statistical Design and Data Analysis Requirements. In *Patty's Industrial Hygiene and Toxicology,* 3rd Ed., Vol. 3A (R.L. Harris, L.J. Cralley, and L.V. Cralley, editors). New York: John Wiley & Sons, 1994.

Lippmann, M.: Exposure Data Needs in Risk Assessment and Risk Management: Database Information Needs. *Appl. Occup. Environ. Hyg. 10:*244-250 (1995).

Lyles, R.H., and L.L. Kupper: On Strategies for Comparing Occupational Exposure Data to Limits. *Am. Ind. Hyg. Assoc. J. 57(1):*6-15 (1996).

Lyles, R.H., L.L. Kupper, and S.M. Rappaport: A Lognormal Distribution-Based Exposure Assessment Method for Unbalanced Data. *Ann. Occup. Hyg. 41(1):*63-76 (1997).

Neter, J., W. Wasserman, and M.H. Kutner: *Applied Linear Statistical Models,* 3rd Ed. Homewood, Ill.: Richard D. Irwin, Inc., 1990.

Nicas, M., B.P. Simmons, and R.C. Spear: Environmental Versus Analytical Variability in Exposure Measurements. *Am. Ind. Hyg. Assoc. J. 52(12):*553-557 (1991).

Odeh, R.E., and D.B. Owen: Table 7. In *Statistics: Textbooks and Monographs Series,* Vol. 32 — Tables for Normal Tolerance Limits, Sampling Plans, and Screening. 1980.

Oldham, P.D., and S.A. Roach: A Sampling Procedure for Measuring Industrial Dust Exposure. *Br. J. Ind. Med. 9:*112-119 (1952).

Olsen, E.: Analysis of Exposure Using a Logbook Method. *Appl. Occup. Environ. Hyg. 9(10):*712-722 (1994).

Ott, W.R.: *Environmental Statistics and Data Analysis.* Boca Raton, Fla.: CRC Press, 1995.

Perkins, J.L., G.N. Cutter, and M.S. Cleveland: Estimating the Mean, Variance and Confidence Limits from Censored (<Limit of Detection) Lognormally-Distributed Exposure Data. *Am. Ind. Hyg. Assoc. J. 51(8):*416-419 (1990).

Rappaport, S.M.: Interpreting Levels of Exposures to Chemical Agents. In *Patty's Industrial Hygiene and Toxicology,* 3rd Ed, Vol. 3A (R.L. Harris, L.J. Cralley, and L.V. Cralley, editors). New York: John Wiley & Sons, 1994.

Rappaport, S.M. , H. Kromhout, and E. Symanski: Variation of Exposure Between Workers in Homogeneous Exposure Groups. *Am. Ind. Hyg. Assoc. J. 54(11):*654-662 (1993).

Rappaport, S.M., and S. Selvin: A Method for Evaluating the Mean Exposure from a Lognormal Distribution. *Am. Ind. Hyg. Assoc. J. 48(4):*374-379 (1987).

Rappaport, S.M, S. Selvin, and S.A. Roach: A Strategy for Assessing Exposures with Reference to Multiple Limits. *Appl. Ind. Hyg. 3:*310-315 (1988).

Royston, P.: A Pocket-Calculator Algorithm for the Shapiro-Francia Test for Non-normality: An Application to Medicine. *Statistics in Medicine 12:*181-184 (1993).

Scheffers, T.M.L.: "HYGINIST — A Computer Program for the Lognormal Evaluation of Air Exposure Data." Maastricht, The Netherlands: Scheffers IHPC, 1994. [Software.]

Selvin, S., and S.M. Rappaport: A Note on the Estimation of the Mean Value from a Lognormal Distribution. *Am. Ind. Hyg. Assoc. J. 50(12):*627-630 (1989).

Selvin, S., S. Rappaport, R. Spear, J. Schulman, and M. Francis: A Note on the Assessment of Exposure Using One-Sided Tolerance Limits. *Am. Ind. Hyg. Assoc. J. 48(2):*89-93 (1987).

Shapiro, S.S., and M.B. Wilk: An Analysis of Variance Test for Normality. *Biometrika 52:*591-611 (1965).

Spear, R.C., S. Selvin, and M. Francis: The Influence of Averaging Time on the Distribution of Exposures. *Am. Ind. Hyg. Assoc. J. 47(6):*365-368 (1986).

Tuggle, R.M.: Assessment of Occupational Exposure Using One-Sided Tolerance Limits. *Am. Ind. Hyg. Assoc. J. 43(5):*338-346 (1982).

Waters, M.A., S. Selvin, and S.M. Rappaport: A Measure of Goodness-of-Fit for the Lognormal Model Applied to Occupational Exposures. *Am. Ind. Hyg. Assoc. J. 52(11):*493-502 (1991).

Waters, M.A., S. Selvin, and S.M. Rappaport: "A Strategy Focussed Upon Exposures Received by Groups of Workers." [Extended Abstract 74.] Paper presented at the American Industrial Hygiene Conference, St. Louis, Mo., May 1989.

DERMAL EXPOSURE ASSESSMENT

Anonymous: "Worker Dermal Exposure to Trichloroketone — Laboratory Final Report." [Data submitted to U.S. Environmental Protection Agency for the Premanufacture Notification Program.] Washington, D.C.: U.S. Environmental Protection Agency/Office of Pollution Prevention and Toxics, 1996.

Burke, A. (ed.): Under Your Skin. *Ind. Saf. Hyg. News:*21-22 (July 1996).

Chester, G.: Evaluation of Agricultural Worker Exposure to, and Absorption of, Pesticides. *Ann. Occup. Hyg. 37(5):*509-523 (1993).

DeCock, J., D. Heedrik, H. Kromhout, and J.S.M. Boleij: Strategy for Assigning a 'Skin Notation': A Comment. *Ann. Occup. Hyg. 40:*611-614. (1996).

Fenske, R.A., and J.J. van Hemmen: Occupational Skin Exposure to Chemical Substances: Setting Limits. *Ann. Occup. Hyg. 38(4):*333-336 (1994).

Fenske, R.A.: Dermal Exposure Assessment Techniques. *Ann. Occup. Hyg. 37(6):*687-706 (1993).

Fenske, R.A., and C. Lu.: Determination of Handwash Removal Efficiency: Incomplete Removal of the Pesticide Chlorpyrifos from Skin by Standard Handwash. *Am. Ind. Hyg. Assoc. J. 55(5):*425-432 (1994).

Fiserova-Bergerova, V., J.T. Pierce, and P.O. Droz: Dermal Absorption Potential of Industrial Chemicals: Criteria for Skin Notation. *Am. J. Ind. Medicine 17:*617-635 (1990).

Kissel, J.C., K.Y. Richter, and R.A. Fenske: Field Measurement of Dermal Soil Loading Attributable to Various Activities: Implications for Exposure Assessment. *Risk Analysis 16(1):*115-125 (1996).

Klingner, T.D., and T. McCorkle: The Application and Significance of Wipe Samples. *Am. Ind. Hyg. Assoc. J. 55(3):*251-254 (1994).

Lansink, C.J.M., M.S.C. Beelen, J. Marquart, and J.J. van Hemmen: *Skin Exposure to Calcium Carbonate in the Paint Industry. Preliminary Modeling of Skin Exposure Levels to Powders Based on Field Data* (TNO Report V 96.064). Rijswijk, The Netherlands: TNO Nutrition and Food Research Institute, 1996.

Kiec-Swierczynska, M.: Preliminary Assessment of the Effect of Disinfectants on Skin Changes in Health Service Workers. *Med. Pr. 46:*149-154 (1995).

McArthur, B.: Dermal Measurement and Wipe Sampling Methods: A Review. *Appl. Occup. Environ. Hyg. 7(9):*599-606 (1992).

Ness, S.A.: *Surface and Dermal Monitoring for Toxic Exposures.* New York: Van Nostrand Reinhold, 1994.

Packham, C.L.: *Skin Care at Work — A Manual for the Prevention of Occupational Skin Disease,* 2nd Rev. Ed. Evesham, United Kingdom: Skin Care Services, 1994.

Perkins, J.L.: Chemical Protective Clothing: I. Selection and Use. *Appl. Ind. Hyg. 6:*222-230 (1987).

U.S. Environmental Protection Agency: *Dermal Exposure Assessment: Principles and Applications (*EPA/600/8–9–91). Washington, D.C.: U.S. Environmental Protection Agency/Office of Research and Development, 1992.

U.S. Environmental Protection Agency: *Development of Statistical Distributions or Ranges of Standard Factors Used in Exposure Assessments* (EPA 600/8–85/010). Washington, D.C.: U.S. Environmental Protection Agency/Office of Health and Environmental Assessments, 1985.

U.S. Environmental Protection Agency: *Exposure and Release Estimations for Filter Press and Tray Dryer Operations Based on Pilot Plant Data* (EPA 600/R–92/039). Washington, D.C.: U.S. Environmental Protection Agency/Risk Reduction Engineering Laboratory, 1992.

U.S. Environmental Protection Agency: *Exposure Assessment for Retention of Chemical Liquids on Hands* by Versar, Inc. (Contract No. 68–01–6271). Washington, D.C.: U.S. Environmental Protection Agency/Exposure Evaluation Division, 1992.

U.S. Environmental Protection Agency: *Exposure Factors Handbook* (EPA 600/8–89–043). Washington, D.C.: U.S. Environmental Protection Agency/Office of Health and Environmental Assessments, Exposure Assessment Group, 1989.

U.S. Environmental Protection Agency: *Occupational Dermal Exposure Assessment — A Review of Methodologies and Field Data. Final Report* (Contract No. 68–D2–0157, WA No. 2–50). Washington, D.C.: U.S. Environmental Protection Agency/Office of Pollution Prevention and Toxics, 1996.

U.S. Environmental Protection Agency: Pesticide Assessment Guidelines, Subdivision U, Application Exposure Monitoring. Washington, D.C.: U.S. Environmental Protection Agency/Office of Pesticide Programs, 1987.

U.S. Environmental Protection Agency: *Preparation of Engineering Assessment, Vol 1: CEB Engineering Manual.* Washington, D.C.: U.S. Environmental Protection Agency/Office of Toxic Substances, Chemical Engineering Branch, 1991.

VanRooij, J.G.M., J.G.C. de Roos, M.M. Bodelier-Bade, and F.J. Jongeneelen: Absorption of Polycyclic Aromatic Hydrocarbons through the Human Skin: Differences Between Anatomical Sites and Individuals. *J. Toxicol. Environ. Health 38:*355-368 (1993).

HEALTH HAZARD CONTROLS

American National Standards Institute: *American National Standard for the Safe Use of Lasers* (ANSI Z136.1–1993). New York: American National Standards Institute, 1993.

American Conference of Governmental Industrial Hygienists: *Industrial Ventilation: A Manual of Recommended Practice,* 22nd Ed. Cincinnati, Ohio: American Conference of Governmental Industrial Hygienists, 1995.

Birkner, L.R., and L.S. Salzman: Assessing Exposure Control Strategy Cost-Effectiveness. *Am. Ind. Hyg. Assoc. J. 47(1):*50-54 (1986).

Colormetric Laboratories, Inc.: "Implementation of a Dermal Exposure Protection Program." Des Plaines, Ill.: Colormetric Laboratories, Inc., 1995. [Brochure.] [CLI, 1261A Rand Road, Des Plaines, IL 60016.]

Lipton, S., and J. Lynch: *Handbook of Health Hazard Control in the Chemical Process Industry.* New York: John Wiley & Sons, 1994.

DATABASES

Beaumont, P.L., and H.L. Dalrymple: A Standard for the Presentation of Occupational Exposure Data. *Ann. Occup. Hyg. 36(1):*79-98 (1992).

Begin, D., M. Gerin, G. Adib, et al.: Development of an Occupational Exposure Data Bank on the Territory of a Department of Community Health in Montreal. *Appl. Occup. Environ. Hyg. 10(4):*355-360 (1995).

Botkin, A., and H. Conway: The Relevance of Exposure Data to Regulatory Impact Analyses: Overcoming Availability Problems. *Appl. Occup. Environ. Hyg. 10(4):*383-390 (1995).

Burns, D.K., and P.L. Beaumont: The HSE National Exposure Database — (NEDB). *Ann. Occup. Hyg. 33:*1-14 (1989).

Fehrenbacher, M.C.: EPA's Use of Occupational Exposure Databases for Screening Level Assessments Under TSCA. *Appl. Occup. Environ. Hyg. 10(4):*374-378 (1995).

Gómez, M.R.: Recommendations for Methods to Code Industry and Job Task in Routinely Collected Exposure Data. *Am. Ind. Hyg. Assoc. J. 55(8):*743-747 (1994).

Gómez, M.R., and G. Rawls: Conference on Occupational Exposure Databases: A Report and Look at the Future. *Appl. Occup. Envir. Hyg. 10:*238-243 (1995).

Holzner, C.L., R.B. Hirsh, and J.B. Perper: Managing Workplace Exposure Information. *Am. Ind. Hyg. Assoc. J. 54(1):*15-21 (1993).

Joint ACGIH–AIHA Task Group on Occupational Exposure Databases: Data Elements for Occupational Exposure Databases: Guidelines and Recommendations for Airborne Hazards and Noise. *Appl. Occup. Envir. Hyg. 11:*1294-1311 (1996).

Lippmann, M.: Exposure Assessment Strategies for Crystalline Silica Health Effects. *Appl. Occup. Environ. Hyg. 10:*981-990 (1995).

Nelson, T.J., and S.W. Dixon: "Management of Air Sampling Results." Paper presented at the American Industrial Hygiene Conference, Philadelphia, Pa., May 25, 1983.

Ott, M.G., S.K. Norwood, and R.R. Cook: The Collection and Management of Occupational Exposure Data. *Am. Statist. 39:*432-436 (1985).

Rajan, B., R. Alesbury, B. Carton, M. Gérin, H. Litske, H. Marquart, E. Olsen, T. Scheffers, R. Stamm, and T. Woldbaek: European Proposal for Core Information for the Storage and Exchange of Workplace Exposure Measurements on Chemical Agents. *Appl. Occup. Environ. Hyg. 12(1):*31-39 (1997).

Susie, P., and S. Schneider: Database Needs for a Task-Based Exposure Assessment Model for Construction. *Appl. Occup. Environ. Hyg. 10(4):*394-399 (1995).

Vincents, P., B. Carton, P. Fjeldstad, et al.: A Preliminary Comparison of Exposure Measurements Stored in European Databases on Occupational Air Pollutants and Definition of Core Information *Appl. Occup. Environ. Hyg. 10(4):*351-354 (1995).

EPIDEMIOLOGY

Harris, R.L.: *Guideline for Collection of Industrial Hygiene Exposure Assessment Data for Epidemiologic Use.* Washington, D.C.: Chemical Manufacturers Association, 1993.

Herrick, R.F., and P.A. Stewart: International Workshop on Retrospective Exposure Assessment for Epidemiological Studies. *Appl. Occup. Environ. Hyg. 6:*417-418 (1991).

National Institute for Occupational Safety and Health: *National Occupational Research Agenda.* Cincinnati, Ohio: National Institute for Occupational Safety and Health, 1996.

Rappaport, S.M.: Selection of the Measures of Exposure for Epidemiological Studies. *Appl. Occup. Environ. Hyg. 6(6):*448-457 (1991).

Rappaport, S.M., and T.J. Smith: *Exposure Assessment for Epidemiology and Hazard Control.* Chelsea, Michigan: Lewis Publishers, 1991.

Smith. T.J.: Exposure Assessment for Occupational Epidemiology. *Am. J. Ind. Med. 12(3):*249- 268 (1987).

Smith, T.J., S.K. Hammond, M. Hallock and S.R. Woskie: Exposure Assessment for Epidemiology: Characterization of Exposure. *Appl. Occup. Environ. Hyg. 6(6):*441-447 (1991).

Stewart, P.A., and M. Dosemeci: A Bibliography for Occupational Exposure Assessment for Epidemiologic Studies. *Am. Ind. Hyg. Assoc. J. 55(12):*1178-1187 (1994).

Stewart, P.A., A. Blair, M. Dosemeci, and M. Gómez: Collection of Exposure Data for Retrospective Occupational Epidemiologic Studies. *Appl. Occup. Environ. Hyg. 6(4):*280-289 (1991).

MODELING

Chemical Manufacturers Association: *PAVE – Program to Assess Volatile Emissions, Version 2.0.* Washington, D.C.: Chemical Manufacturers Association, 1992. [Software.]

Drivas, P.J., P.G. Simmonds, and F.H. Shair: Experimental Characterization of Ventilation Systems in Buildings. *Environ. Sci. Technol. 6:*609-614 (1972).

Fehrenbacher, M.C., and A.A. Hummel: Evaluation of the Mass Balance Model Used by the Environmental Protection Agency for Estimating Inhalation Exposure to New Chemical Substances. *Am. Ind. Hyg. Assoc. J. 57(6):*526-536 (1996).

Hummel, A.A., K.O. Braun, and M.C. Fehrenbacher: Evaporation of a Liquid in a Flowing Airstream. *Am. Ind. Hyg. Assoc. J. 57(6):*519-525 (1996).

Jayjock, M.A.: Back Pressure Modeling of Indoor Air Concentrations from Volatilizing Sources. *Am. Ind. Hyg. Assoc. J. 55(3):*230-235 (1994).

Jayjock, M.A., and N.C. Hawkins: A Proposal for Improving the Role of Exposure Modeling in Risk Assessment. *Am. Ind. Hyg. Assoc. J. 54(12):*733-741 (1993).

Lipton, S., and J. Lynch: *Handbook of Health Hazard Control in the Chemical Process Industry.* New York: John Wiley & Sons, 1994.

Liss, P.S., and P.G. Slater: Flux of Gases Across the Air-Sea Interface. *Nature 247:*181-184 (1974).

Lyman, W.J., W.F. Reehll, and D.H. Rosenblat: *Handbook of Chemical Property Estimation Methods.* New York: McGraw-Hill, 1982.

Meylan, W.M., and P.H. Howard: Bond Contribution Method for Estimating Henry's Law Constants. *Environ. Toxicol. Chem. 10:*1283-1293 (1991).

National Research Council: *National Research Council Committee on Advances in Assessing Human Exposure to Airborne Pollutants: Human Exposure Assessment for Airborne Pollutants — Advances and Opportunities.* Washington, D.C.: National Research Council/National Academy of Sciences, Board on Environmental Studies and Toxicology/Commission on Geoscience, Environment, and Resources, 1991.

Nicas, M., and R.C. Spear: Application of Mathematical Modeling for Ethylene Oxide Exposure Assessment. *Appl. Occup. Environ. Hyg. 7(11):*744-748 (1992).

Nicas, M.: Estimating Exposure Intensity in an Imperfectly Mixed Room. *Am. Ind. Hyg. Assoc. J. 57(6):*542-550 (1996).

Roach, S.A.: On the Role of Turbulent Diffusion in Ventilation. *Ann. Occup. Hyg. 24:*105-132 (1981).

Scheff, P.A., R.L. Friedman, J.E. Franke, L.M. Conroy, and R.A. Wadden: Source Activity Modeling of Freon Emissions from Open-Top Vapor Degreasers. *Appl. Occup. Environ. Hyg. 7:*127-134 (1992).

Schroy, J.M., and J.M. Wu: Emission from Spills. In *Proceedings on Control of Specific Toxic Pollutants.*

Gainesville, Fla.: Air Pollution Control Association/Florida Section, 1979.

Sparks, L.E.: Modeling Indoor Concentrations and Exposure. *Ann. N.Y. Acad. Sci. 641:*102-111 (1992).

Thibodeaux, L.J.: Exchange Rates Between Air and Water. In *Chemodynamics.* New York: Wiley-Interscience, 1979.

U.S. Environmental Protection Agency: *Evaporation Rate of Volatile Liquids* (PACE Laboratories Inc. Project 890501.315 [EPA/744–R–92–001]) by K.O. Braun and K.J. Caplan. Washington, D.C.: U.S. Environmental Protection Agency/Office of Pollution Prevention and Toxics, 1989. [National Technical Information Service (NTIS) Pub. No. PB92–232305.]

U.S. Environmental Protection Agency: *A Manual for the Preparation of Engineering Assessment.* Washington, D.C.: U.S. Environmental Protection Agency/Office of Toxic Substances, Chemical Engineering Branch, Economics and Technology Division, 1984.

U.S. Environmental Protection Agency: *Preparation of Engineering Assessment, Vol 1: CEB Engineering Manual.* Washington, D.C.: U.S. Environmental Protection Agency/Office of Toxic Substances, Chemical Engineering Branch, 1991.

Wadden, R.A., J.L. Hawkins, P.A. Scheff, and J.E. Franke: Characterization of Emission Factors Related to Source Activity for Trichloroethylene Degreasing and Chrome Plating Processes. *Am. Ind. Hyg. Assoc. J. 52(9):*349-356 (1991).

Wadden, R.A., and P.A. Scheff: *Indoor Air Pollution, Characterization, Prediction, and Control.* New York: John Wiley & Sons, 1983.

Wadden, R.A., P.A. Scheff, and J.E. Franke: Emission Factors of Trichloroethylene Vapor Degreasers. *Am. Ind. Hyg. Assoc. J. 50:(9)*496-500 (1989).

Zellers, E.T., and R. Sulewski: Modeling the Temperature Dependence of N-Methylpyrrolidone Permeation through Butyl- and Natural-Rubber Gloves. *Am. Ind. Hyg. Assoc. J. 54(9):*465-479 (1993).

HEALTH EFFECTS RATING SCHEMES

Centers for Disease Control and Prevention: *Classification of Etiologic Agents on the Basis of Hazard.* Atlanta, Ga.: Centers for Disease Control and Prevention/Office of Biosafety, 1976.

The Council of the European Communities: "Council Directives on the Minimum Safety and Health Requirements Regarding the Protection of Workers from Risks Related to Exposure to Biological, Chemical and Physical Agents" (Directive 80/1107/EEC [O.J. L 327]). *Off. J. European Communities,* 27 November 1980.
— 67/548/EEC (27 June 1967)
— 88/379/EEC, Council Directive (7 June 1988)
— 88/379/EEC (7 June 1988)
— 91/155/EEC (5 May 1991)
— 91/115/EEC, Annex V 3.1.1 (1 March 1991)
— 91/115/EEC, Supplemental Council Directive (5 March 1991)
— 92/32/EEC (1993)

Henry, B.J., and K.L. Schaper: PPG's Safety and Health Index System: A 10-Year Update of an In-Plant Hazardous Materials Identification System and Its Relationship to Finished Product Labeling, Industrial Hygiene, and Medical Programs. *Am. Ind. Hyg. Assoc. J. 51(9):*475-484 (1990).

Ignatowski, A.J., J.D. Hamilton, and E.D. Weiler: Review of International Criteria and Mixture Rules for Health Hazard Classification. *Regul. Toxicol. Pharmacol. 22:*231-242 (1995).

National Fire Protection Association: *Standard System for the Identification of the Fire Hazards of Materials* (NFPA 704). Quincy, Mass.: National Fire Protection Association, 1994.

National Paint and Coatings Association: "Hazardous Materials Identification System (HMIS)." National Paint and Coatings Association, 1500 Rhode Island Avenue, N.W., Washington, DC 20005.

Sowinski, E.J., et al.: Criteria for Identifying and Classifying Carcinogens, Mutagens and Teratogens. *Regul. Toxicol. Pharmacol. 7:*1-20 (1987).

Appendix XII

Glossary

absorbed dose The amount of a substance penetrating a worker's exchange boundaries (e.g., lungs, skin, gastrointestinal tract) after contact (exposure).

acceptable exposure Occupational exposure to a chemical, physical, or biological agent judged to present a minimal risk for illness or disease.

accuracy The measure of the correctness of data, as given by the difference between the measured value and the true value. Ideal accuracy is zero difference between measured and true value. Contrast with *precision*, the difference between one measured value and the mean of measured values. See *precision*, *measurement error*.

acute Having a sudden onset, sharp rise, and short course; may apply either to exposures in the workplace or to a physiological response.

administrative controls The restriction or redeployment of workers to reduce the exposure time for individuals (e.g., spreading the exposure over a larger group of workers).

agent A chemical, radiological, thermal, physical, or biological entity that may cause deleterious effects in an exposed worker. Also known as an "environmental agent."

analytical methods Methods used in laboratory analysis of individual industrial hygiene samples. Usually these are chemical analysis techniques used to quantify an agent collected on sampling media (e.g., gas chromatography).

area monitoring The measurement of an environmental agent at a fixed location or position.

area sample An environmental sample at a fixed point or position in the workplace; reflects workplace contaminant concentrations that might not correlate with personal samples of individual worker exposure.

arithmetic mean A measure of central tendency, calculated as the sum of all values in a population divided by the number of values in the population.

asphyxiant A substance that in sufficient concentration renders a person unconscious by preventing sufficient oxygenation of the blood. This may be by chemical or physical blocking of blood oxygenation.

authoritative OEL An occupational exposure limit recommended by a nonregulatory credible organization such as the ACGIH, AIHA, or NIOSH.

autocorrelation Correlation between sequential exposure values for an SEG. Autocorrelation occurs when the magnitude of exposure to an environmental agent in one time period is related to the magnitude of exposure in the preceding and/or subsequent periods. Autocorrelation can lead to inaccurate estimates of the mean and underestimates of variability if the exposure measurements are clustered in a limited time period (e.g., campaign monitoring).

average See *arithmetic mean.*

baseline monitoring The measurement of exposure levels and their variability for workers in a similar exposure group (SEG). Baseline monitoring generally uses a random sampling strategy directed at determining the exposure profile of an SEG for a given time period.

baseline Data that describe the magnitude and variability of exposures for a given SEG for a given time period. There should be at least six samples in a minimum baseline. Descriptive baseline statistics include number of samples, mean, variance, range, and percent of exposures exceeding the OEL guideline. The baseline often serves as a comparison for subsequent monitoring data.

basic characterization The collection and organization of information needed to describe the workplace, work force, and environmental agents so that exposures can be comprehended.

between-worker variability The worker-to-worker variability in environmental agent exposures for an SEG.

bias A systematic error inherent in, or caused by, some feature of a measurement system.

breathing zone A zone of air in the vicinity of a worker from which air is breathed. Personal breathing zone measurements of air contaminant concentrations frequently are made by directly placing monitors in the breathing zone of workers.

carcinogen An agent that potentially causes induction of tumors (cancer) following exposure.

ceiling limit A peak exposure limit established to describe the concentration that should not be exceeded during any part of the working day. See *occupational exposure limit.*

central limit theorem The sampling distribution of the mean approaches a normal distribution as the sample size increases, regardless of the shape of the underlying population distribution.

certified industrial hygienist An individual who has received the CIH designation from the American Board of Industrial Hygiene (ABIH). To receive ABIH certification, an individual must meet rigorous standards of special education and lengthy experience prior to proving, by written examination, competency in either the comprehensive practice of industrial hygiene or one of the specialties or "aspects." Abbreviated *CIH.*

chronic Marked by long duration or frequent recurrence; not acute. May refer either to workplace exposures or to the resulting disease or injury state.

coefficient of variation The sample standard deviation divided by the sample mean (or population parameters). When comparing variation between distributions with different means, coefficients of variation should be used. Sometimes expressed as a percentage. Abbreviated *CV.*

compliance monitoring Technique for evaluating compliance with governmental standards. Typically, the maximally exposed worker is identified and monitored for exposure to environmental agents. If that personal exposure is below the standard, all worker exposures are also presumed to be in compliance with the regulatory OEL.

compliance strategy An occupational exposure assessment strategy directed at assessing compliance with OELs. It usually uses worst-case monitoring with a focus on exposures during the time of survey.

comprehensive strategy An occupational exposure assessment strategy directed at assessing all exposures for all workers on all days.

concentration The amount of a contaminant (mass or volume) relative to a given air volume.

confidence interval A range of values (i.e., interval) that has a specified probability of including the true value of the parameter(s) of an underlying distribution.

confidence limits The upper and lower boundaries of a confidence interval. Upper confidence limit is abbreviated *UCL;* lower confidence limit is abbreviated *LCL.*

continuous air monitors Direct-reading systems used to monitor air concentrations of agents continuously with some present averaging time (e.g., consecutive 5-minute time-weighted averages). These monitors are sometimes linked to alarm systems that are triggered if workplace concentrations begin to approach hazardous levels for workers. Often, they are used to evaluate concentrations of acute agents (e.g., carbon monoxide) continuously.

control chart A chart that shows sequential data or sequential statistics as a function of the time of collection. Usually, decision (control) limits are plotted on the chart to facilitate detection of out-of-control situations (e.g., nonstationary distributions).

control strategies Tools to reduce and control workplace agent concentrations and exposures. Examples include substitution of a less toxic agent; engineering controls such as ventilation; use of personal protective equipment; administrative controls; and change in work practices.

correlation A number or function with a value between -1 and +1 measuring the relation between variables that tend to vary together in a way not expected on the basis of chance alone. Specifically, it is the covariance divided by the product of standard deviations.

critical SEG An SEG for which there is significant risk of inadvertently grouping some workers who incur unacceptable exposures to an environmental agent with workers judged to have acceptable exposures to the same environmental agent.

descriptive statistics Simple metrics of a sample distribution's characteristics such as central tendency (e.g., mean, median) and dispersion (e.g., standard deviation, variance, range). Other examples are number of samples and actual fraction of samples above an OEL.

diagnostic monitoring Workplace monitoring to identify the sources of unacceptable exposures and to understand how the sources, tasks, and other variables (e.g., production rates) contribute to worker exposure.

dose The amount of a substance available for interaction with metabolic processes of a worker following exposure and absorption. The amount of a substance crossing the exchange boundaries of the skin, lungs, or digestive tract is called "absorbed dose."

dose rate Dose per unit time (e.g., mg/day) taken into a worker's body.

dose-response curve A representation, usually in a graphical presentation, of the relationship between dose and probability of occurrence of a health effect or effects. Often these curves are actually based on exposure rather than dose.

dosimeter Instrument used to measure dose; many so-called dosimeters actually measure exposure rather than dose.

duration Length of time. One of three important parameters used to describe the extent and potential consequences of exposures; the other two parameters are frequency and magnitude of exposure.

effective exposure That concentration actually available at the interface of a worker's body (e.g., inside the respirator).

engineering controls Physical changes in process equipment or the installation of auxiliary equipment directed at enclosing, blocking, reducing, attenuating, or capturing emissions to maintain the environmental agent at an acceptable exposure level.

environmental agent See *agent*.

epidemiology The study of the relationships between disease agents and the health-related states of populations.

exceedance fraction The proportion of an exposure profile that exceeds a criterion such as an OEL.

excursion limits Peak exposure criteria established by the American Conference of Governmental Industrial Hygienists (ACGIH). In the absence of a short-term exposure limit (STEL) or ceiling limit, ACGIH recommends that "excursions in worker exposure levels may exceed 3 times the TLV–TWA for no more than a total of 30 minutes during a workday, and under no circumstances should they exceed 5 times the TLV–TWA, provided that the TLV–TWA is not exceeded."

exposure A worker's contact with a chemical, physical, or biological agent. Occupational exposures can occur via several pathways, including inhalation, ingestion, skin contact, and whole body radiation.

exposure assessment The process of defining exposure profiles and judging the acceptability of workplace exposures to environmental agents.

exposure assessment strategy A plan to guide industrial hygiene actions and decisions in accomplishing the goal of accurately evaluating each worker's exposures.

exposure history Qualitative and/or quantitative data describing the chronology of exposures for a worker or SEG.

exposure pathway The course an environmental agent takes from its source to the worker (e.g., inhalation, skin contact, ingestion, whole body exposure).

exposure profile Magnitude and variability of exposures for an SEG. This includes some understanding of the central tendency of the exposures (such as the mean exposure) and some understanding of the breadth, or variability, of the exposures (such as the range of exposures) or frequency with which the exposures exceed the OEL.

exposure rate Exposure per unit time (e.g., ppm/hour) potentially at the boundary of a worker's body (e.g., lungs, skin).

exposure rating Exposure level relative to the OEL.

frequency One of three important parameters used to describe the extent and potential consequences of exposures. The other two parameters are duration and magnitude of exposure.

full shift The complete length of a day's working schedule for one worker (e.g., full-shift exposure monitoring).

geometric mean The nth root of the product of n values. The geometric mean is the median of lognormally distributed data. The geometric mean and arithmetic mean of most distributions are not equal and should not be used interchangeably. Arithmetic mean is the correct parameter for evaluating cumulative exposure.

geometric standard deviation The antilog of the standard deviation of the logtransformed data (measure of variability for a lognormal distribution).

goodness-of-fit test A formal statistical test that evaluates whether sample data are consistent with a population or hypothetical statistical distribution.

health hazard A circumstance, condition, or situation that might result in illness or disease.

health hazard control A procedural change, facility, program, or practice directed at reducing to acceptable levels workplace exposures to chemical, physical, or biological agents. Health hazard controls involve the elimination of the hazardous agent or the effective interruption of the exposure pathway.

health effects data Toxicological, epidemiological, and clinical data that demonstrate potential harmful health effects from exposure to environmental agents; often observed in animal studies of agent exposure, although epidemiological and clinical human data are sometimes available.

hearing zone The physical area approximately 10 cm or less from either ear. Personal monitoring for noise is performed in a worker's "hearing zone."

homogeneous In statistics, having identical probability distribution functions.

homogeneous exposure group A group of employees who experience agent exposures similar enough that monitoring the agent exposures of any worker in the group provides data useful for predicting exposures to the remaining workers. The categorization of workers into these groups often involves categorization by process, job description, and agents, although finer separation can be attained by further dividing on the basis of task analysis. Abbreviated *HEG*.

hypothesis test A statistical test, based on a random sample from a population, that assigns a confidence level on a parameter of the population. In industrial hygiene, a hypothesis test often will be performed to compare summary measures of exposure data with standards or OELs.

independent Two random variables are said to be independent if the outcome of a trial on one variable does not affect the outcome of a trial on the other.

industrial hygiene The science and art of anticipating, recognizing, evaluating, and controlling health hazards in the workplace.

inferential statistics Parameters used to make estimates about the exposure distribution and underlying population.

internal OEL An occupational exposure limit established by a private organization for environmental agents for which there are no regulatory or authoritative OELs, or when the regulatory or authoritative OEL is dated or otherwise considered inadequate.

irreversible health effect An occupational illness or disease that is not repairable (i.e., cannot be expected to heal). Examples are silicosis and permanent hearing loss.

irritant A substance that can cause a typically reversible inflammatory reaction in epithelial tissues.

job A position or occupation held by one or more persons in an organization. In the hierarchy of many workplaces, a process or department frequently contains one or more jobs. One or more tasks or work activities are often assigned to each job.

limit of detection The smallest concentration or amount of a substance that can be differentiated from background levels by a given measurement process. Abbreviated *LOD.*

lognormal distribution The distribution of a random variable with the property such that the logarithms of its values are normally distributed.

long-term average–OEL The concentration of an environmental agent averaged over some period longer than a single work shift. Generally set to prevent against cumulative adverse health effects. Abbreviated *LTA–OEL.*

magnitude of exposure Intensity (concentration, amount, level, etc.) of contact with an environmental agent. One of three important parameters used to describe the extent and potential consequences of exposures; the other two parameters are duration and frequency.

mean The arithmetic average of a set of data; not used as a substitute for geometric mean.

mean test A statistical test that evaluates whether the sample arithmetic mean exposure equals a specified population mean value.

measurement error The difference between the true value and the value obtained by a measuring device. In the absence of systematic bias, the distribution of measurement errors is often considered measurement precision.

median The exposure measurement that divides a set of measurements into two equal parts, with half less than and half greater than this value.

mode The value in a set of measurements that occurs most frequently; the maximum value of a continuous probability density function. The mode of a lognormal distribution is less than the median, which is less than the mean. The mean, median, and mode of a normal distribution are equal.

model A mathematical, physical, or subjective representation of real phenomena (e.g., dilution ventilation models).

monitor Measure worker exposure to an environmental agent.

monitoring protocols Plans for implementing monitoring campaigns.

nonparametric Statistical methods that do not assume a particular statistical distribution for the statistic of interest (e.g., distribution-free methods).

nonrandom sample A sample taken in a manner that means some members of the defined population are more likely to be chosen than others.

nonroutine operation A process, job, or task characterized by some of the following: short lead time, short duration, transient work force, nonrepetitiveness, variable work sites, and variable work practices. Nonroutine operations include research and development, environmental remediation, and hazardous waste cleanup. Maintenance and repair duties are more often routine than nonroutine.

nonstationary Any process for which population statistics vary over time, space, or other independent variable. Nonstationary processes are not suited to analysis by statistical tools that explicitly assume an unchanging population distribution.

normal distribution An important symmetric probability distribution characterized completely by two parameters: the mean and the standard deviation. It has its highest ordinate at the center and tails off to zero in both directions, forming a bell-shaped curve.

null hypothesis The hypothesis of a population parameter to be tested (e.g., the population mean exposure is less than or equal to the OEL). The alternative hypothesis covers the complement of the null (e.g., the population mean exposure is greater than the OEL).

occupational disease An adverse, generally chronic and irreversible health effect associated with overexposure to chemical, physical, or biological agents in the workplace. Examples of occupational diseases are silicosis, bladder cancer, and berylliosis.

occupational exposure limit Abbreviated *OEL*. A generic term used to represent a pair of numbers: 1) the agent concentration or intensity that is allowable (based on health effects data), and 2) the period over which one averages workplace concentrations to evaluate whether the measured concentrations are less than the allowable limit. Some substances may have several occupational exposure limits (e.g., an 8-hour time-weighted average [TWA] and a short-term exposure limit [STEL] of 15 minutes). See *authoritative OEL, internal OEL, regulatory OEL, working OEL.*

occupational illness An adverse, generally transient and reversible health effect associated with overexposure to chemical, physical, or biological agents in the workplace. Examples of occupational illnesses are asthma, metal fume fever, heat cramps, and dermatitis.

overexposure An exposure greater than the OEL. The exposure should be evaluated over the appropriate averaging time.

parameter A quantity that describes a statistical population (e.g., mean and standard deviation, geometric mean, geometric standard deviation).

parametric Statistical tests are said to be parametric if an underlying statistical distribution, described by appropriate parameters, is based solely on computations involving these parameters.

peak exposure The highest exposure or the largest group of exposures experienced by workers during some defined exposure duration (usually short time periods).

personal monitoring Measurements collected in the breathing zones of workers or, in the case of noise, near the ears.

population Every element or member of a distribution. Usually a small portion of the population is sampled to estimate characteristics of that population.

population distribution A description of the relative frequencies of the elements of a population.

population statistics The true parameters calculated by including the entire population (e.g., population mean and standard deviation). In workplace exposure assessment, these parameters usually must be estimated from a representative sample of the population and, therefore, are not known exactly.

potency Health effect level per unit dose of the agent; in the most simple case, this would be the slope of a linear dose-response function).

potential health effect(s) The capability or possibility of adversely affecting an individual's health.

precision A measure of the reproducibility of a measured value under a given set of conditions. Accuracy usually refers to the size of deviations from the true mean, whereas precision refers to the size of deviations from the mean of observations.

prioritization Placement of industrial hygiene follow-up tasks in rank order of importance (e.g., the rank ordering of SEGs from those needing monitoring immediately down to those groups requiring no monitoring).

probability of noncompliance The likelihood of exceeding a regulatory OEL determined through application of an inferential statistical methodology published by the National Institute for Occupational Health and Safety (NIOSH).

probability paper Graph paper on which a specific family of distributions is represented by spacing along a probability axis. For example, samples from a lognormal distribution appear as a straight line when plotted on log-probability paper, and samples from a normal distribution appear as a straight line when plotted on linear-probability paper.

probability plot Plot in which sample observations are plotted on the x-axis and the sample probability of occurrence are plotted on the y-axis. If the plot results in a straight line, the sample conforms to the family of distributions represented by the probability paper.

process A stand-alone manufacturing or service operation.

professional judgment The application and appropriate use of knowledge gained from formal education, experience, experimentation, inference, and analogy. That capacity of an experienced professional to draw correct inferences from incomplete quantitative data, frequently on the basis of observations, analogy, and intuition.

qualitative Based on integration of information and judgment, rather than quantitative data.

quality assurance The system of activities that provides the user of the exposure assessment the assurance that data used as a basis for a decision meet defined quality standards (e.g., submittal of spiked or blank samples, laboratory proficiency testing, sampling records).

random samples Samples selected from a statistical population such that each sample item has an equal probability of being selected.

range The difference between the largest and smallest values in a measurement data set.

regulatory OEL An occupational exposure limit established by a governmental law or regulation.

representativeness The degree to which a sample is, or samples are, characteristic of the whole medium, exposure, or dose for which the samples are being used to make inferences.

reversible health effect An occupational illness that can be treated so that complete healing takes place.

risk The probability of deleterious health effects; risk is a function of exposure level and potency (health effect per unit exposure [or dose]).

risk assessment The scientific evaluation (in either qualitative or quantitative terms) of the chance of injury, illness, or disease resulting from exposure to a particular form of matter or energy.

route of exposure The manner in which an environmental agent may enter or contact the body. The routes of exposure include inhalation, ingestion, skin contact, and whole or partial body irradiation.

sample The portion, part, or subset of the population drawn for observation or the measurement chosen for statistical analysis and study. Sample data often are used to make inferences about the true values of population parameters.

sample parameters Estimators of population parameters based on observation of a subgroup of the population (e.g., sample means and sample standard deviation).

sampling Selecting members of a statistical population for examination.

sampling frequency The interval between collection of successive samples.

short-term exposure limit The concentration to which workers can be exposed for a short period without suffering 1) irritation; 2) chronic or irreversible tissue damage; or 3) narcosis of sufficient degree to increase the likelihood of accidental injury, impair self-rescue, or materially reduce work efficiency — provided the daily TLV–TWA is not exceeded. It usually is defined as a 15-minute TWA exposure that should not be exceeded at any time during a workday even if the 8-hour TWA is within the TLV–TWA. An averaging period other than 15 minutes may be recommended when warranted by observed biological effects. Abbreviated *STEL.*

similar exposure group Group of workers having the same general exposure profile for the agent(s) being studied because of the similarity and frequency of the tasks they perform, the materials and processes with which they work, and the similarity of the way they perform the tasks. Abbreviated *SEG.*

similar exposure interval A period in which the distribution of exposures for a SEG would be expected to be stationary. Abbreviated *SEI.*

skew A property of a statistical distribution indicating lack of symmetry; a distribution is said to be skewed to the right or left if observations are concentrated to the left or right of the mean, respectively. A distribution is skewed right (positive skew) when the mean is greater than the median and is skewed to the left (negative skew) when the mean is less than the median.

standard deviation The positive square root of the variance of a distribution; the parameter measuring spread of values about the mean. It can be estimated from the slope of the straight line through data plotted on probability paper.

stationary A random process is said to be stationary if its distribution is independent of the time of observation.

stationary population An underlying population that does not change during the exposure assessment period.

statistic A characteristic of a sample, such as sample mean and sample standard deviation; used to characterize the underlying population.

statistical power One minus the probability that a given test causes acceptance of the null hypothesis; this is the same as the probability of rejecting the null hypothesis by a test when the alternative is true.

statistical significance The statistically based probability that the null hypothesis is true. If that probability is small (e.g., less than 5%) the null hypothesis is rejected.

strategy A plan to guide actions to accomplish a stated goal.

student's t-distribution A family of probability distributions distinguished by their degrees of freedom and used as the sampling distribution of arithmetic means when the population standard deviation is unknown. As sample size increases, the t-distribution approaches a normal distribution.

surveillance Ongoing scrutiny to detect changes in distribution or trends of disease or exposures in order to initiate more focused studies or control measures.

systematic bias The selection of samples in which nonrandom or confounding variables might lead to an inaccurate or distorted exposure profile.

tail That part of a distribution represented by extreme values with a low probability of occurrence. See *skew*.

task A work element or series of work elements.

teratogen An agent for which exposures might result in fetal health effects (e.g., birth defects).

threshold limit value Abbreviated *TLV*. Refers to OELs established by the American Conference of Governmental Industrial Hygienists (ACGIH), representing conditions under which it is believed nearly all workers may be repeatedly exposed day after day without adverse effect. Threshold limit values include time-weighted average (TWA) limits, short-term exposure limits (STELs), ceiling limits, and excursion limits.

time-weighted average–OEL A full-shift average OEL such as the ACGIH threshold limit value–time-weighted average (TLV–TWA). The TLV–TWA is defined as the time-weighted average concentration for a conventional 8-hour workday and a 40-hour workweek to which nearly all workers may be exposed repeatedly, day after day, without adverse health effect. Abbreviated *TWA–OEL.*

tolerance interval An interval that contains a stated fraction of the values of a population distribution with stated probability; refers to the probability that the random variable lies within the stated interval (e.g., 95% probability that no more than 5% of the daily exposures exceed the standard). Contrast with *confidence interval*, which refers to probability (confidence) that a parameter of the underlying distribution lies within the stated interval.

tolerance limit The upper or lower limits of a tolerance interval. A tolerance limit enables one to quantify confidence in a percentile estimate. Upper tolerance limit is abbreviated *UTL*; lower tolerance limit is abbreviated *LTL.*

toxic Causes deleterious health effects in living organisms.

toxicity The degree (health effects per unit exposure) to which a chemical or biological agent causes deleterious health effects in living organisms.

toxicokinetics The study of the time course of absorption, distribution, metabolism, and excretion of a foreign substance (e.g., drug or chemical) in an organism's body (i.e., effect of the organism on the chemical).

toxicology The study of the adverse health effects caused by chemicals in humans and animals.

unacceptable exposure A condition in which a significant risk (occupational illness, etc.) is associated with an SEG's exposure profile; the probability of adverse health effects is significant, or there is evidence of adverse health effects associated with exposure to an environmental agent.

uncertain exposure A condition in which acceptability of an exposure cannot be determined because of a lack of exposure, toxicity, or other information.

validation Verification of the correctness of the methods used for sampling and laboratory analysis of an agent under conditions of use; also, demonstration that a model accurately predicts real-world phenomena by comparing model prediction with actual data.

variance The mean of the square of the differences between the mean value of population and randomly selected values from the same population. Units are squares of the data units, such as cm^2 or m^2.

warning properties Properties of an agent that enable an educated worker to identify potential overexposures. For example, odor thresholds at or below the OEL can alert workers to the agent's presence; however, an odor threshold above the OEL means the worker will have no warning of potential overexposure.

wipe testing Collection of chemical, mineralogical, or radiological agents on wipe media (typically a wipe of filter paper on an area 100 cm^2); results are useful indices of contamination level, but they are not direct estimators of exposure.

within-worker variability The variability (e.g., day-to-day, minute-to-minute) of exposure to an environmental agent for an individual worker.

work history A historical representation of various processes, jobs, and tasks for the extent of an employee's career.

work practice controls Prescribed work methods and procedures directed at controlling a health hazard (e.g., wetting down a surface to reduce particulate release).

working OEL An informal occupational exposure limit created in the course of performing an exposure assessment. Working OELs are established in the absence of formal OELs, or they may be established in the presence of a formal OEL when there is significant uncertainty of the adequacy of the formal OEL.

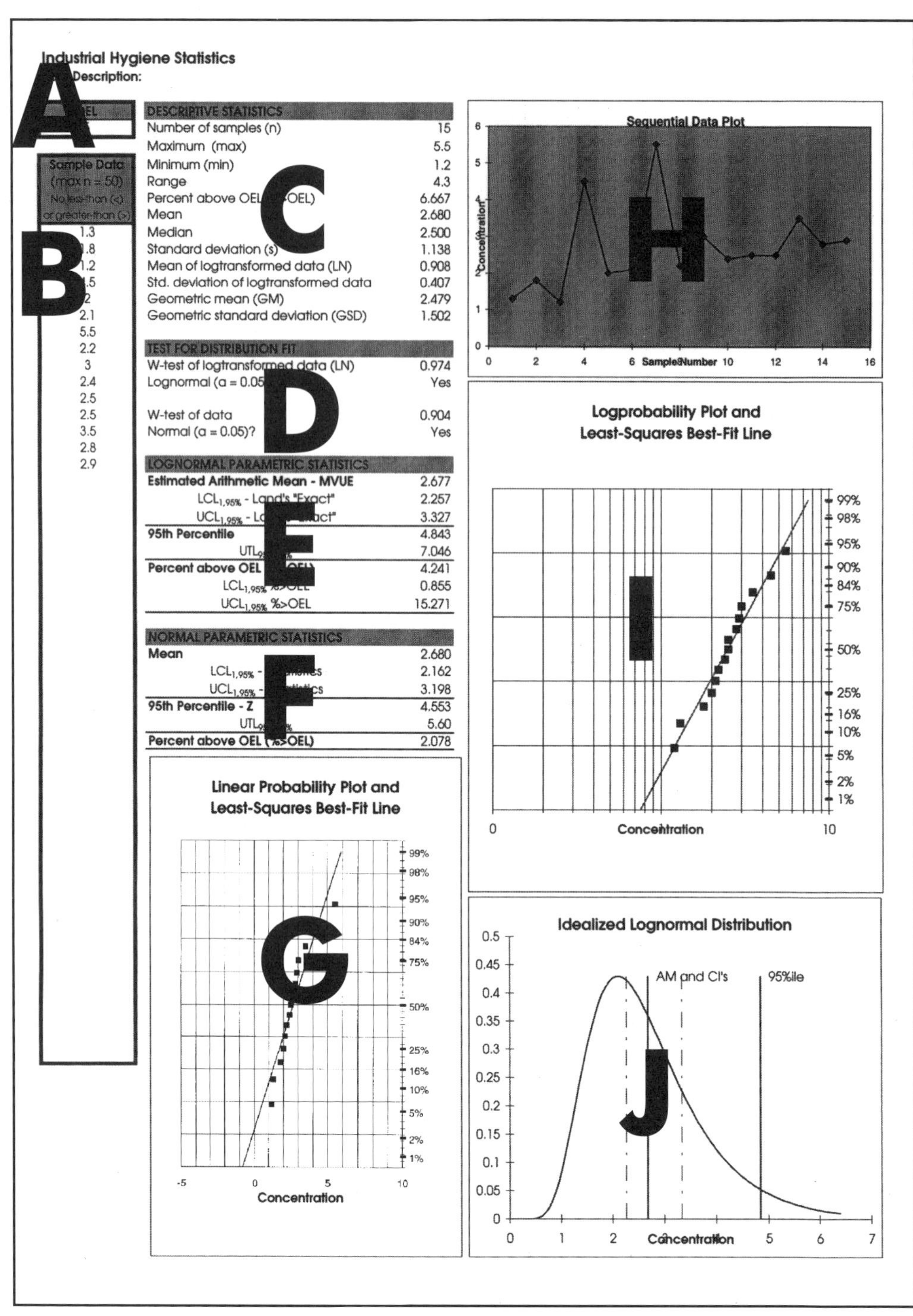

Figure XIII.1 — Industrial hygiene statistics spreadsheet: (A) Enter OEL; (B) enter monitoring results; (C) descriptive statistics calculated; (D) W-test; (E) lognormal parametric statistics calculated; (F) normal parametric statistics calculated; (G) linear probability plot; (H) sequential data plot; (I) logprobability plot; (J) idealized lognormal distribution plot.

Appendix XIII

Instructions: Industrial Hygiene Statistics Spreadsheet

So readers can begin using the statistical tools discussed in this text, we have included a simple spreadsheet program that will help in calculating key descriptive and inferential statistics (see Figure XIII.1). The OEL and monitoring data must be entered. The spreadsheet is limited to a maximum of 50 monitoring results, and it will not handle less-than, greater-than, or zero values. (It may be appropriate to handle less-than values by entering them as 70% or 50% of the detection limit, depending on your estimate of the GSD — see Chapter 7 for more detail.)

Use of the spreadsheet and examples of its output are included below.

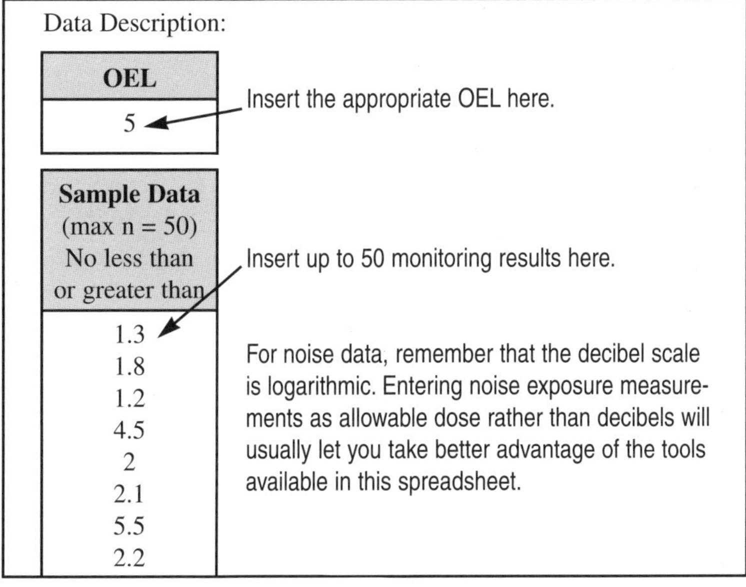
Data Description:
OEL
5
Insert the appropriate OEL here.
Sample Data
(max n = 50)
No less than
or greater than
Insert up to 50 monitoring results here.
1.3
1.8
1.2
4.5
2
2.1
5.5
2.2
For noise data, remember that the decibel scale is logarithmic. Entering noise exposure measurements as allowable dose rather than decibels will usually let you take better advantage of the tools available in this spreadsheet.

Figure XIII.2 — Industrial hygiene statistics (A,B).

Number of samples (n)	15	
Maximum (max)	5.5	
Minimum (min)	1.2	
Range	4.3	
Percent above OEL (%>OEL)	6.667	
Mean	2.680	Descriptive statistics are automatically calculated here (see Appendix IV).
Median	2.500	
Standard deviation (s)	1.138	
Mean of logtransformed data (LN)	0.908	
Std. deviation of logtransformed data (LN)	0.407	
Geometric mean (GM)	2.479	
Geometric standard deviation (GSD)	1.502	

Figure XIII.3 — Descriptive statistics (C).

W-test of logtransformed data (LN)	0.974	Lognormal and normal distribution fit tests are automatically calculated (see Appendix V).
Lognormal (a = 0.05)?	Yes	
W-test of data	0.904	
Normal (a = 0.05)?	Yes	

Figure XIII.4 — Test for distribution fit (D).

Estimated Arithmetic Mean – MVUE	2.677	The lognormal distribution arithmetic mean is estimated (MVUE method) and one-sided 95% confidence limits calculated using Land's method (see Appendix VI).
$LCL_{1,95\%}$ – Land's "Exact"	2.257	
$UCL_{1,95\%}$ – Land's "Exact"	3.327	
95th Percentile	4.843	The 95th percentile is estimated and the 95%,95% upper tolerance limit calculated (see Appendix VII).
$UTL_{95\%,95\%}$	7.046	
Percent above OEL (%>OEL)	4.241	
$LCL_{1,95\%}$ %>OEL	0.855	The percent exceedance and one-sided 95% confidence limits are calculated (see Appendix VII).
$UCL_{1,95\%}$ %>OEL	15.271	

Figure XIII.5 — Lognormal parametric statistics (E).

Mean	2.680	Parameter estimates are made assuming a normal distribution as well.
$LCL_{1,95\%}$ – t statistics	2.162	
$UCL_{1,95\%}$ – t statistics	3.198	
95th Percentile – Z	4.553	
$UTL_{95\%,95\%}$	5.60	
Percent above OEL (%>OEL)	2.078	

Figure XIII.6 — Normal parametric statistics (F).

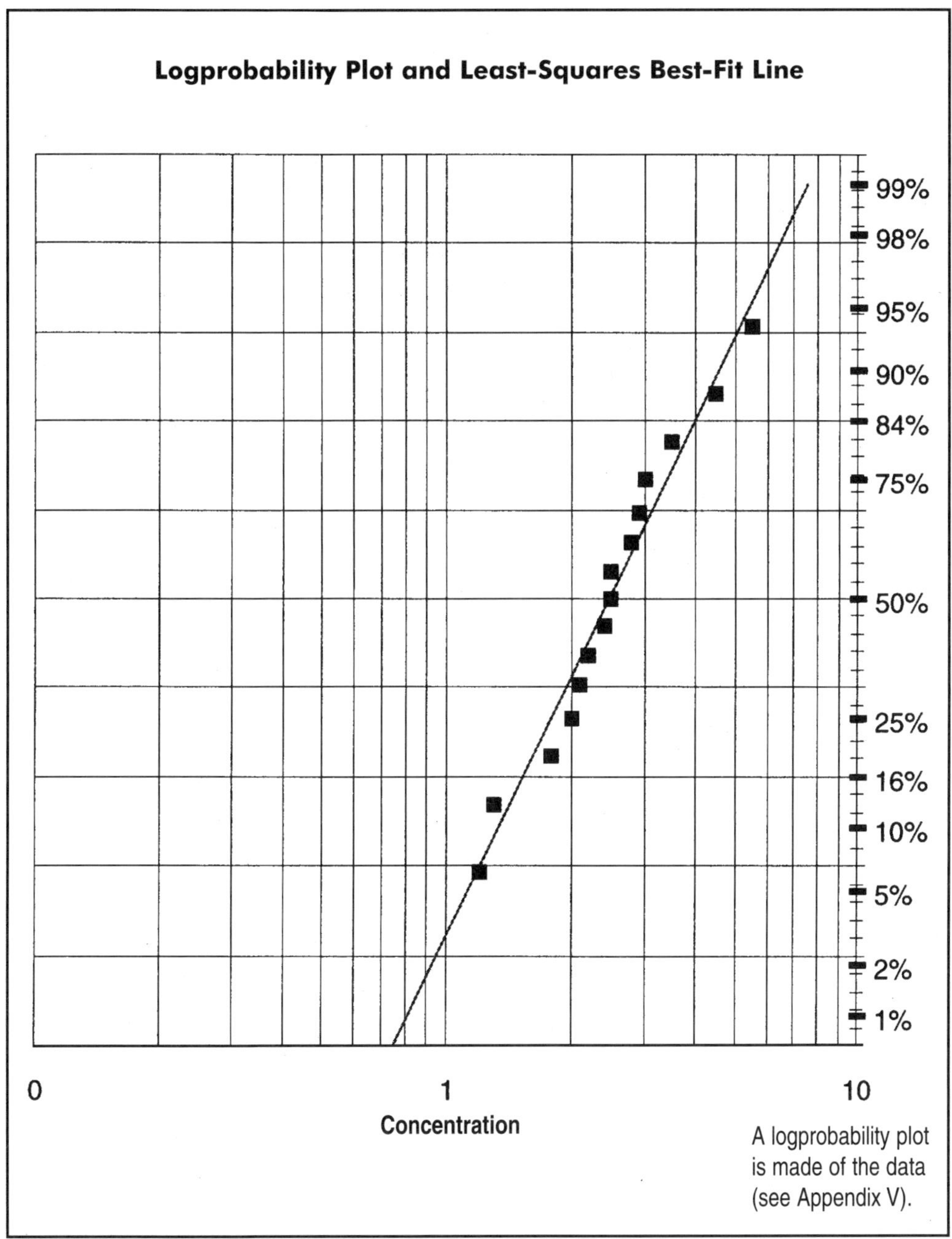

Figure XIII.7 — Logprobability plot and least-squares best-fit line (I).

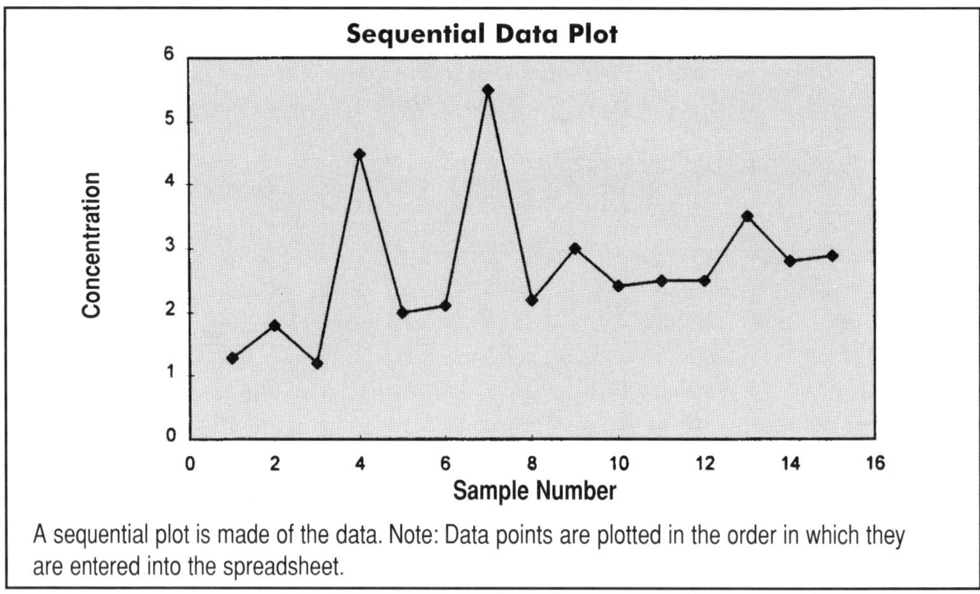

A sequential plot is made of the data. Note: Data points are plotted in the order in which they are entered into the spreadsheet.

Figure XIII.8 — Sequential data plot (H).

Idealized Lognormal Distribution

AM and CI's

95th percentile

0.45, 0.4, 0.35, 0.3, 0.25, 0.2, 0.15, 0.1, 0.05, 0

0, 1, 2, 3, 4, 5, 6, 7

Concentration

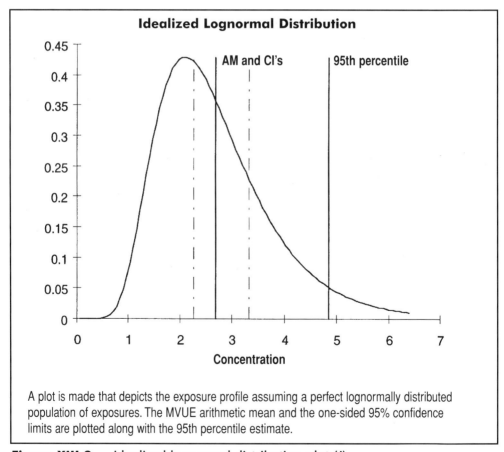

A plot is made that depicts the exposure profile assuming a perfect lognormally distributed population of exposures. The MVUE arithmetic mean and the one-sided 95% confidence limits are plotted along with the 95th percentile estimate.

Figure XIII.9 — Idealized lognormal distribution plot (J).

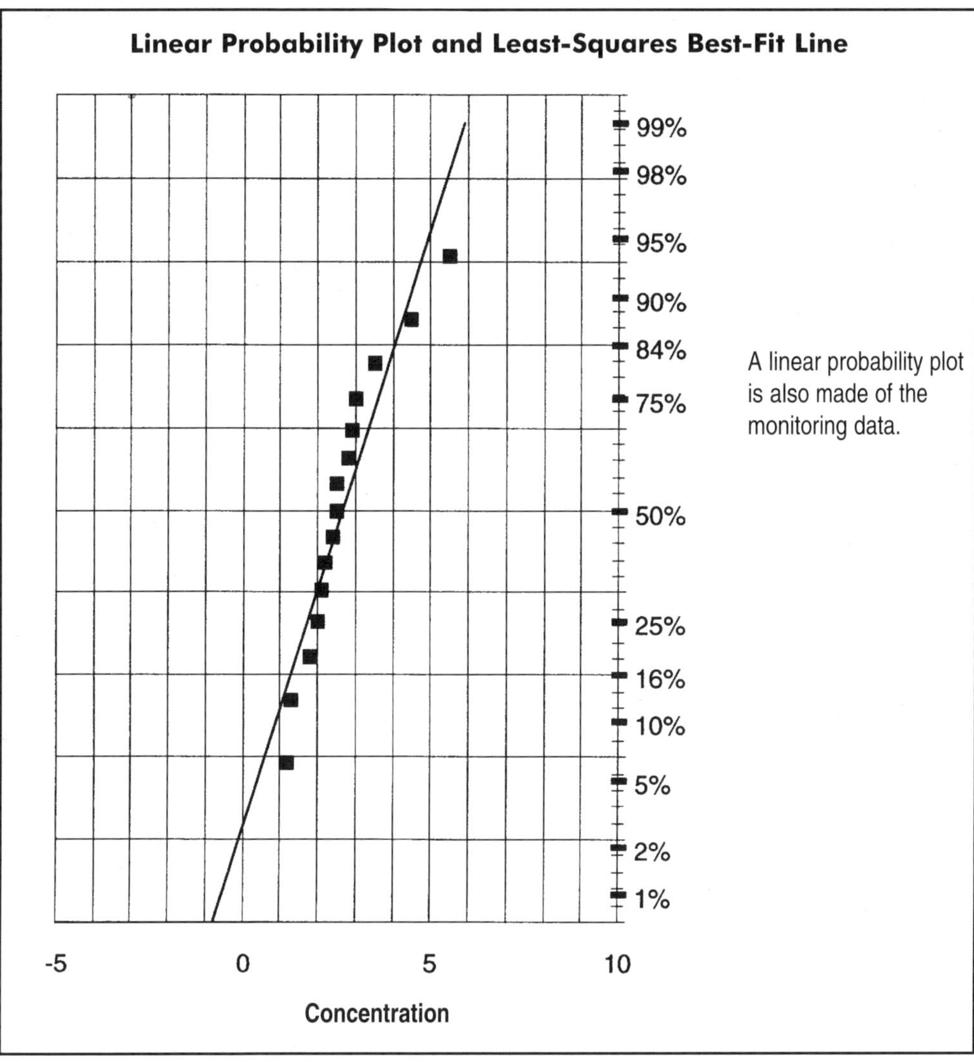

Figure XIII.10 — Linear probability plot and least-squares best-fit line (G).

Sources

1. **Gilbert, R.O.:** *Statistical Methods for Environmental Pollution Monitoring.* New York: Van Nostrand Reinhold, 1987.
2. **Hewett, P., and G.H. Ganser:** Simple Procedures for Calculating Confidence Intervals Around the Sample Mean and Exceedance Fraction Derived from Lognormally Distributed Data. *Appl. Occup. Environ. Hyg. 12(2)*:132-142 (1997).

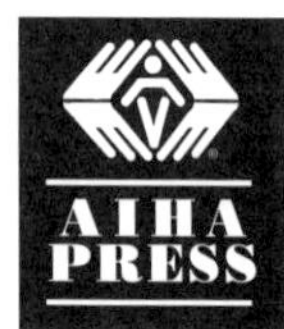

Design by James Myers

Composed at AIHA in QuarkXpress® with electronic output to film.

Typefaces
Body Text: 11/12, Times
Heads: 14/15, Futura Medium

Printed by Jarboe Printing Company
Cover: 80# White Litho coated one side and laminated; PMS# 3305 and black inks.
Text: 50# White Opaque, black ink.
Case bound and sewn with reinforced end sheets.

The inside pages are 50% chlorine compound-free, 50% recycled content, including 10% post-consumer waste.

The entire book has been printed with alcohol-free soybean inks.

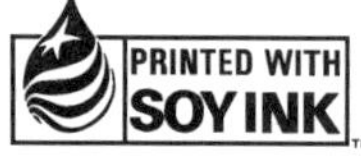